Statistics for Social and Behavioral Sciences

Statistics for Social and Behavioral Sciences (SSBS) includes monographs and advanced textbooks relating to education, psychology, sociology, political science, public policy, and law.

More information about this series at http://www.springer.com/series/3463

Kristian Kleinke • Jost Reinecke • Daniel Salfrán •
Martin Spiess

Applied Multiple Imputation

Advantages, Pitfalls, New Developments and Applications in R

Springer

Kristian Kleinke
Department of Education Studies
and Psychology
University of Siegen
Siegen, Germany

Jost Reinecke
Faculty of Sociology
University of Bielefeld
Bielefeld, Germany

Daniel Salfrán
Institute of Psychology
University of Hamburg
Hamburg, Germany

Martin Spiess
Institute of Psychology
University of Hamburg
Hamburg, Germany

ISSN 2199-7357 ISSN 2199-7365 (electronic)
Statistics for Social and Behavioral Sciences
ISBN 978-3-030-38163-9 ISBN 978-3-030-38164-6 (eBook)
https://doi.org/10.1007/978-3-030-38164-6

Mathematics Subject Classification (2010): 62-07, 62F10, 62F12, 62F15, 62F40, 62F35, 62J12

This Springer imprint is published by the registered company Springer Nature Switzerland AG.
The registered company address is: Gewerbestrasse 11, 6330 Cham, Switzerland

Preface

Empirical data are seldom completely observed. How to adequately analyse data sets affected by missing values is usually not the focus of courses at bachelor or master level, and thus applied researchers often resort to simple ad hoc solutions like complete case analysis or (unconditional) mean imputation, which in the former case is often inappropriate and is virtually always inappropriate in the latter case. PhD students and applied researchers often tell us that they have read about multiple imputation (MI) but that they have found it cumbersome to learn the application of MI in an autodidactic way. This book will provide helpful tutorials in this regard. But it is not only the question about *how* to apply MI techniques. It is also important to know *when* to apply MI—in which scenarios it is appropriate to use the method, and when it is not. To this end, applied researchers should be at least aware of the possible problems caused by missing values and have a basic understanding of the theory of multiple imputation, that is, what MI tries to correct and what the underlying assumptions are.

The intention behind writing this book was to meet both ends, i.e. to provide a detailed introduction to the basic concepts and statistical underpinnings, and to demonstrate the practical application of MI based on the underlying theory.

The statistical concepts behind the method of multiple imputation are explained in Chaps. 1–4. Each of the chapters consists of an in-depth description and discussion of the theory and the various concepts needed to understand *why* and *when* MI works (or not) and to enable users to decide whether a certain method or software may work for his or her particular application. Each concept is illustrated with examples. Readers who only want to get a brief overview over the theory may find a summary section at the end of each chapter.

Chapters 5 and 6 describe and explain the *how*. Should readers—at first—not be interested in the statistical background, they can start with the applied Chaps. 5 and 6 to learn how to apply the techniques to empirical data sets and come back to the theory part when needed (various cross-references will direct readers to the respective sections, where they can find further details and explanations). In our tutorials, we explicitly did not want to use nice and well-behaved examples that work and run through nicely without further ado. Instead we base our examples on a real-life problem and illustrate, what decisions and sometimes also trade-offs applied researchers have to make when analysing empirical data, where convenient model assumptions are often not entirely met.

While we walk readers through the steps of creating multiple imputations with the respective MI packages and functions in R, we discuss the advantages and disadvantages of these methods with regard to the particular problem at hand.

This book is intended for students at graduate and postgraduate level, and for applied empirical researchers in all fields of social and health sciences. To get the best out of this book, we assume that readers already have basic knowledge in statistics and some experience with statistical software. We use R throughout this book (https://www.R-project.org). The supplementary material of the book is available from github (https://github.com/kkleinke). Readers who are not yet familiar with R may find the following references helpful: An excellent online resource to get new users started is Phillips (2018). A very comprehensive book about R is Adler (2010). Furthermore, there are many textbooks on special topics available, e.g. introductory statistics with R (Dalgaard, 2008), statistical analysis with R (Everitt & Hothorn, 2006), linear models with R (Faraway, 2004, 2006), multilevel analysis in R (Gelman & Hill, 2007) and latent variable modeling (Beaujean, 2014).

We would like to thank Maximilian Wächter, one of our master students in sociology, who read Chap. 5 and gave valuable feedback on how to improve the tutorials given in this chapter. We are also grateful to Milena Tzvetkova for assistance in typesetting the LaTeX document.

Siegen, Germany — Kristian Kleinke
Bielefeld, Germany — Jost Reinecke
Hamburg, Germany — Daniel Salfrán
Hamburg, Germany — Martin Spiess
November 2019

References

Adler, J. (2010). *R in a nutshell*. Beijing: O'Reilly.

Beaujean, A. A. (2014). *Latent variable modeling using R: A step by step guide*. New York, NY: Routledge.

Dalgaard, P. (2008). *Introductory statistics with R* (2nd ed.). New York, NY: Springer.

Everitt, B., & Hothorn, T. (2006). *A handbook of statistical analysis using R*. Boca Raton, FL: Chapman & Hall.

Faraway, J. J. (2004). *Linear models with R*. Boca Raton, FL: Chapman & Hall.

Faraway, J. J. (2006). *Extending linear models with R*. Boca Raton, FL: Chapman & Hall.

Gelman, A., & Hill, J. (2007). *Data analysis using multilevel/hierarchical models*. Cambridge, UK: Cambridge University Press.

Phillips, N. D. (2018). *YaRrr! The Pirate's Guide to R*. https://bookdown.org/ndphillips/YaRrr/

Contents

Chapter 1
Introduction and Basic Concepts

1.1 Overview

The purpose of this chapter is to characterize and describe missing data situations, to introduce terminology used in this field, e.g., the terms item nonresponse, unit nonresponse and attrition, and review the most common statistical approaches to inference from samples to populations. Missing data patterns (univariate, monotone, arbitrary) are described as far as they are relevant for choosing an appropriate technique to compensate for missing data. Since the scope of the method of multiple imputation is rather general, those aspects of the most common statistical approaches relevant to understanding when and how multiple imputation works are reviewed. The different statistical approaches and the potential usefulness of methods to compensate for missing data are demonstrated through simple examples and illustrations.

1.2 Introduction

Most data sets are subject to nonresponse, for example, because units selected into a sample refuse to participate in a survey, decline to answer certain questions in a questionnaire or simply because the (technical) measuring instrument has a defective contact. In any of these cases, statistical inference has to deal with the fact that not all information has been observed. As will be seen later, one even deals with this problem, although implicitly and in a rather crude way, if the problem is simply ignored.

Dealing with the problem of missing values means that assumptions are to be made about the process leading to nonresponse and that model assumptions for valid inferences are necessary in addition to those required for inferences based on

K. Kleinke et al., *Applied Multiple Imputation*,
Statistics for Social and Behavioral Sciences,
https://doi.org/10.1007/978-3-030-38164-6_1

completely observed data sets. Hence the best strategy to avoid additional modeling and estimation steps including potentially inadequate assumptions about processes which are not of primary interest and whose violation may nevertheless invalidate statistical inferences is to avoid the occurrence of missing values. Unfortunately, this is often not possible, in which case a book like the present one may be of some help in dealing with nonresponse. Before different methods and in particular the method of multiple imputation will be discussed, however, some basic concepts have to be introduced.

1.3 Unit and Item Nonresponse

Missing values may be characterized as values of variables surveyed for an intended statistical analysis but being not observed for all of the selected statistical units. Slightly more general, missing values are unobserved data values of scientifically interesting variables that are assumed to exist and cannot be derived in a deterministic way from observed values. This characterization is still not a clear-cut definition of the phenomenon of missing values, but it includes the most common situations.

Examples of missing data are unanswered questions in a survey questionnaire, not recorded reactions in an experiment or if impossible or implausible values (outliers) are deleted. Depending on the context, 'don't know' or 'does not apply' answers may mask the refusal to provide the corresponding information (e.g., Rubin, Stern, & Vehovar, 1995). Further examples are values which are not observed because units are exposed only to parts or blocks of a larger questionnaire ('missing by design'), or if units selected into a sample refuse to participate. Not observing units under one or more conditions in the context of causal inference in non-experimental settings can also be interpreted as a missing data problem.

The distinction of (single) missing data values or 'item nonresponse' and 'unit nonresponse' where entire units are not observed does not mean that both concepts are mutually exclusive: unit nonresponse can be interpreted as an extreme form of item nonresponse and there are even ambiguous situations. For example, in a panel survey units may be observed in the first waves but drop out in one of the later waves. These units are partly observed: Information is available for the first waves of the panel but not for later waves (if the units do not return), a phenomenon also called panel attrition.

Since item and unit nonresponse describe just different realizations of the same concept, both versions of missing values can in principle be treated by the same techniques. Due to the availability of specific techniques and the complexity of these techniques depending on the situation, however, different techniques are usually adopted to treat item or unit nonresponse (see Chap. 3).

1.4 Patterns of Observed and Missing Values

The pattern of missing and observed values plays an important role with respect to the theoretical justification and the application of techniques to compensate for missing values. Therefore, in this section, we will consider the relevant patterns of observed and missing values.

As a starting point let us consider two variables, one being not completely observed. For example, we could be interested in the relationship between the number of children living in a household and hourly wage. Although all the statistical units, e.g., households, report the number of children, hourly wage is not observed for all households. This pattern of missing values would be called a univariate missing pattern. A simple extension would include more than one variable, which would still be called a univariate missing pattern if only one variable were not completely observed (see left graphic in Fig. 1.1).

A further generalization would be to consider more variables with missing values. One version of considerable interest is a monotone missing pattern, which can be defined as follows: Given a rectangular data set with rows indicating statistical units $i = 1, \ldots, n$ and columns denoting variables. Then a missing pattern is called monotone if the data set can be arranged by sorting rows and/or columns such that, going from left to right, if a missing value occurs in a row all the following values in that row are missing as well (see Fig. 1.1). This definition works, of course, in the other direction as well.

A prominent example of a monotone missing pattern is panel attrition, as long as attrition is an absorbing state, i.e., if once a unit dropped out it is not observed in

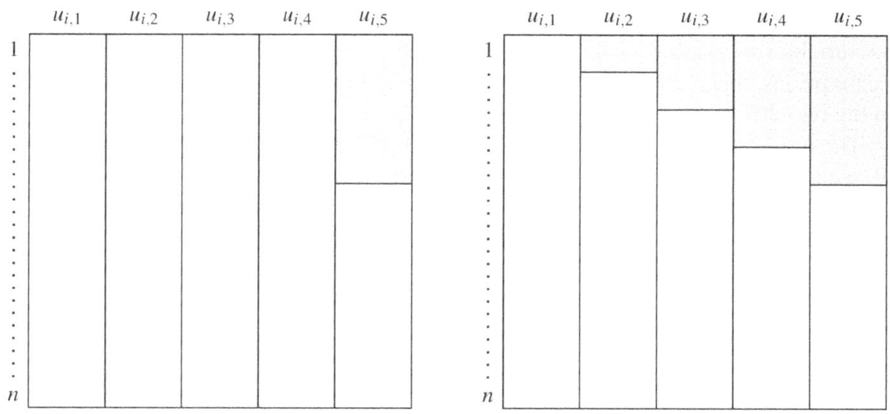

Fig. 1.1 Monotone missing patterns: $i = 1, \ldots, n$ units, variables $u_{i,1}, \ldots, u_{i,5}$. Left graphic: Missings in variable $u_{i,5}$ (univariate missing pattern). Right graphic: Missing values in more than one variable, monotone missing pattern. Observed part: white portions, missing part: grey portions

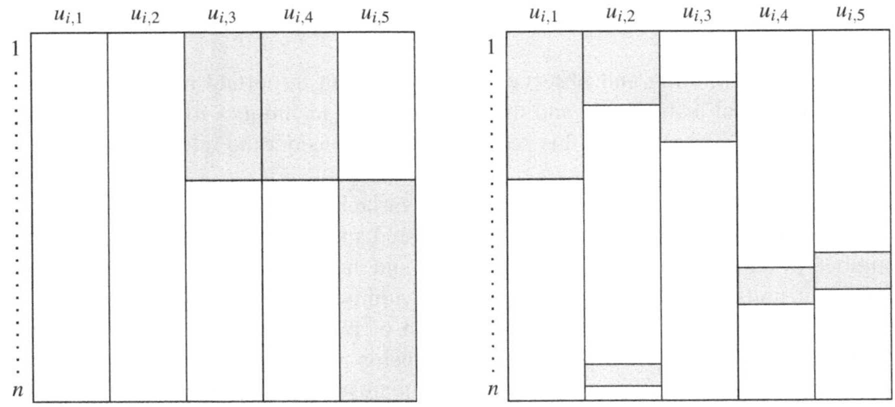

Fig. 1.2 Missing patterns: $i = 1, \dots, n$ units, variables $u_{i,1}, \dots, u_{i,5}$. Left graphic: Missings in more than one variable (block missing pattern). Right graphic: Missing values in more than one variable, arbitrary missing pattern. Observed part: white portions, missing part: grey portions

later waves of a panel study. Obviously, a univariate missing pattern is a monotone pattern.

The left graphic in Fig. 1.2 shows a block structure which may arise from multiple matrix sampling sometimes also referred to as split questionnaire design (see Gonzalez & Eltinge, 2007): Variables $u_{i,1}$ and $u_{i,2}$ are observed for all units, however, for the first n_1 units $u_{i,3}$ and $u_{i,4}$ are not observed but $u_{i,5}$ is observed and vice versa for the remaining $n - n_1$ units. Matrix sampling is usually adopted to reduce the burden of survey participants. The same data structure results from statistical file matching, where two (or more) different data sets are matched based on variables $u_{i,1}$ and $u_{i,2}$ observed for all units (e.g., Rubin, 1987). Under certain assumptions, this pattern simplifies the task of compensating the unobserved values in the two different response groups.

The most common pattern, however, is probably an arbitrary pattern, an example of which is given in the right graphic of Fig. 1.2. Arbitrary patterns cannot be reduced to the patterns discussed above. Consider the simple example with two variables: Number of children living in the household and hourly wage. The missing pattern would be arbitrary if for some households the number of children is missing but hourly wage is observed and if for other households the number of children is missing but hourly wage is observed.

1.5 Inferential Approaches and Concepts

In this section, we will shortly describe the most common statistical approaches and concepts as far as they are relevant for understanding how and when a method to compensate for missing data should be applied, particularly the method of multiple imputation proposed by Rubin (1987, 1996), and how the downstream statistical analysis could proceed. In this section we assume no missing values.

Statistical inference can follow a design-based or a model-based approach. Official statistics often adopts the design-based approach with known sampling probabilities to estimate totals, means or portions of certain characteristics in a finite population. On the other hand, the more common approach in applied scientific research is model-based where unknown parameters in a statistical model are estimated (we consider only situations with a finite number of parameters).

1.5.1 Design-Based Approach

In design-based statistics, the characteristic of interest, e.g., hourly wage, is not treated as a random variable, the values in the finite population are considered to be fixed. For example, the population statistic of interest could be the portion of poor families in a given country at a certain point in time.

In principle all the values of the characteristic of interest could be surveyed, and the population statistic of interest could directly be calculated. Due to restricted financial and time resources, this is often not possible and thus samples have to be selected. Drawing random samples guarantees that statistical inferences about a population can be justified. Within this framework, the only random variable is the selection indicator,

$$s_j = \begin{cases} 1 \text{ if unit } j \text{ is selected into the sample,} \\ 0 \text{ otherwise,} \end{cases}$$

where j denotes the jth population unit. Usually, sampling in this context is without replacement, which is the case considered here (otherwise we would have to take into account that the same units can be selected more than once). Hence, a sample is the set of units for which $s_j = 1$. The population statistic of interest can be estimated using a function of the fixed values selected into the sample and the random selection indicator. In this setting, the sampling design, which specifies for each possible sample its selection probability, is usually known. Thus, no unknown model parameters need to be estimated. However, this is the ideal case. If units or values are missing or if the observed values are not error-free with respect to the characteristic of interest, then statistical models are needed to assist the analysis (e.g., Särndal, Swensson, & Wretman, 1992).

Estimators, or more general, functions of variables and characteristics of interest, like test statistics or confidence intervals, of the design-based approach are evaluated based on their frequentist properties. This means, their properties are evaluated over an infinite, or in finite populations an excessive large, number of repetitions of the sampling process under hypothetically identical conditions. Concepts considered are the mean of an estimator and thus its bias, the standard error, variance, the actual fraction of falsely or correctly rejecting a null hypothesis or the actual coverage of the true value by confidence intervals. For a better readability, we will omit the phrase 'or an excessive large number' in the sequel. It should be noted, however, that this would be more precise in the case of finite populations as there are only a finite—although, given most population sizes excessive—number of possible samples induced by a given sampling design.

Alternatively, the properties of functions of variables can be evaluated based on the observed values in the sample only (non-frequentist evaluation). How this is done will be described below.

1.5.2 Model-Based Approaches

Whereas the design-based approach is usually adopted in official statistics, a model-based approach prevails in many areas of empirical research. For example, if inferences about relationships or dependencies between two or more variables are of interest, then statistical analyses are usually based on statistical models. As an example, one could be interested in the effect of the variable 'years of schooling' on the variable 'hourly wage'. In this case, a model for the relationship of the two variables could be assumed where—besides an unknown nuisance parameter—only the effect of the former variable onto the latter is unknown. In a next step the unknown model parameters would be estimated.

One way to learn about the parameter of interest would be to maximize the likelihood function with respect to the unknown parameter. The starting point to derive the likelihood function, or likelihood for short, is the density or probability function of the variables given the parameter of scientific interest and possibly a nuisance parameter (e.g., an error variance). The likelihood is this function but with roles of variables and parameters reversed: The variables are fixed at their observed values while the parameter may vary. A maximum likelihood estimator for the unknown (assumed to be fixed) true parameter is that function of the variables, which maximizes this likelihood function (assuming that this maximum exists and, for simplicity, that it is unique). The value of this function for a specific data set is the estimate for the unknown true value of the parameter. Often any function proportional to the likelihood where the multiplier does not depend on any of the parameters is also called a likelihood.

Under a direct- or pure-likelihood inference, which is the non-frequentist version of the likelihood approach, only the observed values of the variables are considered, other possible samples are ignored. By considering the likelihoods for varying values of the parameter relative to the likelihood at the maximum likelihood estimate, plausible values for the estimator may be found. From these comparisons likelihood regions and likelihood intervals, also denoted as support regions or support sets, are derived.

However, the likelihood approach may also be combined with a frequentist evaluation ('frequentist likelihood inference'). In that case, the maximum likelihood estimator is calculated as described above, but now also statements are made about the distribution of the estimator over repeated sampling or about statistics like bias, variance, standard error or coverage rates of confidence intervals over repeated sampling.

There are many other non-likelihood model-based methods in use assuming fixed parameters and evaluated from a frequentist point of view. Examples are (non-linear) least squares, generalized methods of moments or generalized estimating equations (e.g., Liang & Zeger, 1986; Newey & McFadden, 1994).

Another model-based way to learn about the parameters is via the Bayesian approach. In contrast to the model-based approaches described above, Bayesian analysis is not about fixed true parameters. Instead, knowledge about parameters is expressed in form of distributional models. The prior distribution reflects the knowledge (or ignorance) about the parameters before any data values are observed. This statement should not be taken literally, however, as prior knowledge about parameters is hardly precise enough to justify the specification of a distribution. Hence the prior distribution is usually an approximation to prior knowledge. Often the term 'belief' instead of 'knowledge' is used in this context (e.g., Welsh, 1996), but since the former is an important concept within a more general approach (e.g., Shafer, 1976) we will use the term 'knowledge' in the sequel.

Following Bayes' theorem, the prior distribution is multiplied by the likelihood described above divided by a function which does not depend on the parameters, leading—by Bayes' theorem—to the posterior distribution, which is the distribution of the parameters in light of the data. The process can be interpreted as a learning process in the sense that it models how observing informative data increases our knowledge about the parameters if appropriate models are chosen.

Within a subjective Bayesian school each researcher may adopt his or her own prior distribution, that should however be the result from a coherent procedure. For example, a betting game could be conducted to quantify the prior knowledge. Another school may be called 'rational' (e.g., Welsh, 1996, p. 60). Within this school, a prior distribution should reflect available information independent from the individual researcher. This approach works even if no knowledge is available and can thus be interpreted as formalizing the ignorance about a parameter. Often, however, the prior distribution is chosen based on a compromise between its mathematical tractability and its adequateness of expressing the available prior knowledge.

An interesting class of prior distributions are conjugate priors. A prior distribution is called a conjugate prior, if both the prior and the posterior distribution are in the same class of distributions. If a conjugate prior distribution is mathematically easy to handle, which is not always the case, then it is particularly attractive because the learning process over several cycles is straightforward. The class of noninformative prior distributions are attractive if prior ignorance about parameters is to be modeled. As an example consider the case of an one-dimensional parameter. Based on the idea that if nothing is known about a (continuous) parameter the value of the prior distribution should be the same for each possible parameter value, a flat density function could be chosen. This is an example of a noninformative improper prior if the parameter space is an infinite interval. It is improper because the integral of the density is infinite. Otherwise, if it would be equal to one, it would be a proper prior distribution. Choosing an improper prior distribution may still be attractive as it may lead to a proper posterior distribution and to valid inferences which are mainly based on information from the observed data set. The effect of such a vague prior is small as compared to the observed information in the data.

As an estimate for the unknown parameter of interest, usually the mean of the posterior distribution is adopted. Lower and upper quantiles of the posterior distribution are used to generate 'credible intervals' which can be interpreted as covering the true parameter with a certain, more or less subjective (posterior) probability. Note that only the observed values of the variables are used for inferences and evaluation, although Bayes estimators and credible intervals can also be evaluated from a frequentist perspective (e.g., Efron, 2015; Rubin, 1996).

1.6 Statistical Inference and Missing Data

Often research in empirical sciences focuses on certain aspects of populations. For researchers which are not interested in response behaviour, missing values are therefore just annoying as they may cause difficulties with standard software and can lead to invalid inferences if not properly accounted for. Thus, the main objective of any method to compensate for missing values should be to allow valid inferences even in the context of incompletely observed data sets. A secondary objective may be the possibility to apply easy-to-use (standard) analysis software.

In any case, if a data set is affected by missing values then, to allow valid inferences, additional assumptions or knowledge are necessary with respect to the mechanism that generated the missing values ('missing data mechanism'). An important decision in the analysis process is whether the missing data mechanism can safely be ignored for valid inferences. Unfortunately this decision is not easy: It mainly depends on the missing data mechanism itself, which is often neither part of the theoretical considerations nor justified by empirical evidence. Note that the missing data mechanism may even be different for different units or variables. To make things worse, even if a missing data mechanism can be ignored, this does not mean that the same analysis tools can be applied to the incompletely observed data set as would have been to analyse a fully observed data set. The missing data mechanism and its possible ignorability will be treated at length in Chap. 2.

In some situations the missing data mechanism may be known, e.g., due to the adopted research design like in matrix sampling. In most cases, however, very little is known about the missing data mechanism and inferences are either based on implicit or explicit assumptions about this mechanism. Therefore, another important issue in applications is the robustness of inferences of scientific interest with respect to a possibly incorrect model of the missing data mechanism. This, however, is not the only source for a possible invalidation of the statistical inference. When a method to compensate for missing data is adopted, then there are often additional models to estimate beyond those that are of interest and the compatibility of these models with the model of applied scientific interest becomes relevant with respect to robustness considerations.

If the missing data mechanism cannot be ignored, then a strategy to compensate for the missing values has to be chosen. This strategy depends on the missing data mechanism, the assumed model of applied scientific interest including all assumptions, the availability of resources (e.g., software, programming skills, time), but also on the adopted inferential concept.

1.7 The Method of Multiple Imputation

A widely accepted method to compensate for missing values is the method of multiple imputation proposed by Rubin (1987, 1996). Like other theory-based methods, the method of multiple imputation can in principle be adopted to compensate for missing values in most situations. However, in the way the method is currently implemented in available software packages, the probability of not observing values should, after conditioning on all other relevant variables, not depend on these unobserved values (see Chap. 2 for a detailed discussion). For a thorough treatment of the underlying classification of missing data mechanisms, see Rubin (1976) and Seaman, Galati, Jackson, and Carlin (2013).

The basic idea underlying multiple imputation is to generate several (M) plausible values ('imputations') for each missing value to generate M completed data sets. These M data sets are then analysed with standard software for completely observed data sets and the M results are combined according to some simple rules (Rubin, 1987). The point is to generate the imputations in a way that allows valid statistical inferences based on these combining rules.

Hence, the idea is that although a data set is affected by nonresponse, standard software can be used to analyse the data. Thus, once a data set is multiply imputed the analysis is straightforward. In fact, the method of multiple imputation was developed assuming an institute that sets up a database and has access to sufficient resources, knowledge and possibly to data sources not publicly available but beneficial to sensibly generate imputations. The data analyst and the data-set provider (the institute) were assumed to be different entities (Reiter & Raghunathan, 2007; Rubin, 1996). Thanks to many functions available in standard software and fast computers, however, even generating multiple imputations became very fast and easy, so that multiple imputations are often generated by the data analyst (Reiter & Raghunathan, 2007).

The simplicity with which imputations can be generated even using standard software, the availability of options to generate imputations in many different situations, the simple application of the combining rules and the speed of modern computers may be one of the reasons for the fast spread of the method. However, it should not be forgotten that it is a statistical method that relies on assumptions, some of which are difficult to check. If one or more of the assumptions are not met, then inferences may be invalid.

1.8 Illustration of Concepts and Techniques

Suppose that, as described in Sect. 1.4, a data set is available with variables 'hourly wage in Euro' (WAGE) and 'number of children living in the household' (NCHILD) for $n = 15$ units.

The (simulated) data are given in Table 1.1. Unfortunately, both variables are affected by missing values which are denoted by a dot. The data set is already sorted in a way to easily detect the pattern of observed and missing values.

1.8.1 Unit and Item Nonresponse, (Non)response Pattern

Looking at the pattern of observed and missing values in Table 1.1, it can be seen that for the unit with identification number 1 we did neither observe the number of children living in the household nor wage. If there is no other information available for this unit, as in our example, then this is an instance of unit nonresponse.

Table 1.1 also reveals that the pattern of missing and observed values is not monotone. This is due to observation with ID 6 for which the number of children is not observed. Hence, the missing data pattern is arbitrary. If this value would have been observed, then the pattern would have been monotone.

1.8.2 Design-Based Approach

Up to now only the data set can be described and no inference about a population or a model is possible. However, suppose that the above given values resulted from selecting a probability sample by random sampling without replacement from a population with $N = 1000$ units where for a given draw, each unit that has not yet been selected has the same probability of being selected into the sample. Suppose we are interested in the average hourly wage in this population.

Table 1.1 Simulated hourly wage (WAGE) in Euro and number of children living in the household (NCHILD) values for $n = 15$ individuals (ID denotes the unit identification number)

ID	NCHILD	WAGE	ID	NCHILD	WAGE	ID	NCHILD	WAGE
1	.	.	6	.	16.13	11	4	13.42
2	1	.	7	3	15.36	12	3	14.39
3	1	.	8	4	13.08	13	4	14.46
4	3	.	9	2	15.55	14	4	15.11
5	1	.	10	3	16.37	15	3	16.10

Missing values are denoted as '.'

Note that there is no model to estimate and the sampling design is known: Given the number of population units, the sampling plan and the sample size, the probability of observing each unit can be calculated. Given a population of size N, sample size n and if sampling is without replacement, where each unit has the same probability of being selected from the set of eligible units, the probability that unit j, $j = 1, \ldots, N$, is selected from the population into a sample is $\pi_j = \Pr(s_j = 1) = n/N$ for all j, where s_j is the selection indicator introduced in Sect. 1.5. Note that j indexes the units in the population. To address units in a sample we will use another index, as the values of index j in the sample can be arbitrary values from $\{1, \ldots, N\}$. Let i be this index. Hence by definition, we will simply use y_i, $i = 1, \ldots, n$, to address the values selected into a sample.

To estimate the statistic of interest, we could adopt the approach proposed by Horvitz and Thompson (1952) and estimate the average hourly wage in the finite population by

$$\widehat{\text{aver}}_{\text{inc}} = \frac{1}{N}\sum_{j=1}^{N}\frac{s_j}{\pi_j}y_j = \frac{1}{N}\sum_{i=1}^{n}\frac{y_i}{\pi_j} = \frac{1}{N}\sum_{i=1}^{n}\frac{y_i}{n/N} = \frac{1}{n}\sum_{i=1}^{n}y_i\,, \tag{1.1}$$

where y_j are the wage values in the population and y_i are the elements of the subset of these values selected into the sample. However, at this point the properties of this estimator are still unknown. Hence we do not know, if our inferences are valid based on this estimator.

Design based statisticians consider the values of the interesting characteristics, y_j for all N, as fixed values. Thus, s_j is the only random variable. For the frequentist evaluation adopted in the design-based approach, we hypothetically repeat the random selection procedure an infinite number of times according to the same sampling design and, in a first step, consider the expectation of the estimator,

$$E(\widehat{\text{aver}}_{\text{inc}} \mid y_1, \ldots, y_N) = E\left(\frac{1}{N}\sum_{j=1}^{N}\frac{s_j}{\pi_j}y_j\right) = \frac{1}{N}\sum_{j=1}^{N}\frac{E(s_j)}{\pi_j}y_j = \frac{1}{N}\sum_{j=1}^{N}y_j\,,$$

which is equal to the corresponding mean in the population. Hence, this estimator is unbiased and the values of $\widehat{\text{aver}}_{\text{inc}}$ realized in successive samples vary randomly around the population mean.

In a second step, the variance of this estimator over the hypothetically infinite number of repetitions can be derived, which in terms of general selection probabilities is

$$\text{var}(\widehat{\text{aver}}_{\text{inc}}) = \frac{1}{N^2}\left(\sum_{j=1}^{N}\frac{1-\pi_j}{\pi_j}y_j^2 + \sum_{j=1}^{N}\sum_{\substack{k=1 \\ j\neq k}}^{N}\frac{\pi_{j,k}-\pi_j\pi_k}{\pi_j\pi_k}y_jy_k\right),$$

where $\pi_{j,k} = \Pr(s_j = 1, s_k = 1)$. Given the sampling design in the example, $\pi_{j,k} = n(n-1)/[N(N-1)]$ and the variance simplifies to

$$\text{var}(\widehat{\text{aver}}_{\text{inc}}) = \frac{N-n}{nN(N-1)} \sum_{j=1}^{N} \left(y_j - \frac{1}{N} \sum_{j=1}^{N} y_j \right)^2$$

which can be estimated by

$$\widehat{\text{var}}(\widehat{\text{aver}}_{\text{inc}}) = \frac{N-n}{nN(n-1)} \sum_{i=1}^{n} \left(y_i - \frac{1}{n} \sum_{i=1}^{n} y_i \right)^2$$

(see Horvitz & Thompson, 1952). To generate confidence intervals we can approximate the distribution of the (hypothetically infinitely many) estimates by the t-distribution or, in large samples, by the normal distribution (Särndal et al., 1992). Alternatively, a bootstrap technique could be adopted to generate confidence intervals without specifying a certain distribution (e.g., Efron & Tibshirani, 1993). In fact, the technique is based on repeated sampling of units with replacement into bootstrap samples from the units observed in the sample and does not require the assumption of a specific distribution. For each bootstrap sample the statistic of interest is calculated resulting in a distribution of values over the bootstrap samples. For the present example this statistic is the mean based on the actual values observed in the bootstrap sample minus the mean from the original sample and this difference divided by the estimated standard deviation based on the bootstrap sample ('bootstrap-t method'). The quantiles from this empirical distribution are then taken to calculate the bootstrap-t confidence interval (see Efron & Tibshirani, 1993).

The above data set is not completely observed: Five out of the selected wage values are missing. Therefore, the question is how to deal with the missing values. The simplest way would be to use the ten observed values. Adopting this strategy, the estimated mean for this data set is $\widehat{\text{aver}}_{\text{inc}} = 15$ with estimated variance $\widehat{\text{var}}(\widehat{\text{aver}}_{\text{inc}}) = 0.13$. Assuming a t-distribution with $df = 9$ degrees of freedom gives the symmetric 0.95-confidence interval [14.19, 15.81]. To avoid any distributional assumption, we calculated confidence intervals using the bootstrap-t method with 999 bootstrap samples (see, e.g., Cameron & Trivedi, 2005; Lange, 2010), resulting in a 0.95-confidence interval of [13.81, 15.87], which is a little bit wider. Hence, if our distributional assumption holds approximately and the sampling design was realized as described above, both confidence intervals should cover the population mean with probability of approximately (at least) 0.95. Note that both confidence intervals are realizations of random intervals and the bootstrap interval does not require the strong distributional assumption.

However, if we ignore the fact that missing data occurred, we actually assume that the observed part of the sample was generated according to the same mechanism according to which the sample was originally sampled. But if, for example, individuals with missing hourly wage tended not to provide this information because

Table 1.2 Simulation results

	Mean	Empirical variance	Theoretical variance	Mean variance estimates	Coverage t-distr.	Coverage bootstrap
Population	16.259					
Complete sample	16.257	0.160	0.159	0.160	0.946	0.948
Incomplete sample	15.645	0.254	0.240[a]	0.200	0.764	0.832

Based on complete data sets (complete sample) and incompletely observed data sets (incomplete sample): Means of estimates $\widehat{\text{aver}}_{\text{inc}}$, variance of estimates over simulations (empirical variance), theoretical variance of the estimator $\widehat{\text{aver}}_{\text{inc}}$, average of variance estimates and coverage rates of 0.95-confidence intervals assuming a t-distribution (t-distr.) and adopting the bootstrap-t method (bootstrap). Number of simulations is 100,000. Mean hourly wage in the population ($N = 1000$) is given in the first row of the table

[a]Note that the theoretical variance is calculated ignoring the missing data mechanism

their wage is low, then the assumption that the above described sampling design was realized for the observed part of the sample as well is wrong. As a consequence, the estimator $\widehat{\text{aver}}_{\text{inc}}$ may be biased and the confidence interval may not cover the true value with probability of approximately (at least) 0.95. Based on the estimation results for this single data set only, we can however not decide whether the results allow valid inferences or not.

On the other hand, with the help of simulations we can get an idea, whether the frequentist properties claimed for the estimator $\widehat{\text{aver}}_{\text{inc}}$ hold or not. Of course it is not possible to repeat the process of sample selection, generating missing values, calculating $\widehat{\text{aver}}_{\text{inc}}$ and the confidence interval for an infinite number of times. However, by choosing a large number of simulations, one can get an impression about the frequentist properties of the estimator.

To illustrate this, we generated 100,000 samples of size $n = 15$ each according to the sampling design described above from the population of $N = 1000$ units from which the above data set was selected, created 33% missing values in the wage values, analysed the data sets before and after the missing values were generated and recorded the results.[1] Since the data are simulated, we know the true mean of hourly wage in the population and the theoretical variance (see Table 1.2).

For the complete sample, before values are set to missing, the results in Table 1.2 illustrate the advantageous properties of $\widehat{\text{aver}}_{\text{inc}}$ and its variance estimator. It seems to be unbiased and the coverage of the population mean is close to 0.95 for both ways the confidence intervals are calculated. Thus, inferences based on the complete sample can considered to be valid.

Considering the results based on the observed part of the data set, we first note that these samples are smaller than the complete data sets, so the variance of $\widehat{\text{aver}}_{\text{inc}}$ is larger than for the complete data set. For the incompletely observed data sets, we

[1]All the simulated data used in this book are generated using the pseudo-random number generators provided by the software package R and all simulations are done with R (R Core Team, 2018).

find the average of the estimates to be below the true values and the coverage rates of both methods to calculate confidence intervals to be much too low, which may be due to—besides the biased estimator—an underestimation of the true variance of the estimator (see Table 1.2). Note also, that the empirical variance of the estimator is larger than the theoretical variance, which may be due to the fact that the latter is derived assuming that the above sampling design is realized for the observed part of the sample, i.e., the missing data mechanism is ignored. Depending on how the missing values are generated, however, this may be wrong, resulting in a differing variance of $\widehat{\text{aver}}_{\text{inc}}$. Note also that the mean estimated variance assuming ignorability of the missing data mechanism is smaller than the empirical variance. As a consequence of these results, we would systematically underestimate the mean hourly wage and confidence intervals would be systematically too short.

1.8.3 Model-Based Approaches

In this section, we will consider the likelihood and the Bayesian approach to make inferences about the mean of hourly wage. In contrast to the design-based approach, the characteristics WAGE and NCHILD are now considered to be random variables and the values in the sample are the realized values. The set of observed values is a subset of the realized values.

Within the framework of model-based approaches, a statistical model is assumed that approximately and at least partly describes how the realized values are generated ('data generating process'). In our example, we will assume that the variables y_i, $i = 1, \ldots, n$, can be interpreted as continuous variables, that they are mutually independent and all follow the same normal distribution. The normal distribution is uniquely determined by two parameters, the location parameter (mean, μ) and the scale parameter (variance, σ^2), and is denoted as $N(\mu, \sigma^2)$. Assuming that the normal model approximates the population of interest sufficiently well, our goal is to make inferences about μ. Note that we are now interested in a theoretical model parameter and not in a statistic that could be observed if we only had enough resources. Since hourly wage is the only variable we consider and therefore ambiguities are not possible, we denote the parameter of interest by μ and avoid the reference to the variable WAGE.

1.8.3.1 Likelihood Inference

In the first example we adopt a non-frequentist likelihood approach and assume for simplicity the variance of the variable WAGE to be known. For a clear presentation, we collect all variables y_i, $i = 1, \ldots, n$ in a vector $\mathbf{y} = (y_1, \ldots, y_n)^T$.

The density function of y_i, $i = 1, \ldots, n$, is

$$\begin{aligned} f(\mathbf{y} \mid \mu, \sigma^2) &= \prod_{i=1}^{n} \frac{1}{\sqrt{2\pi\sigma^2}} \exp\left\{-\frac{(y_i - \mu)^2}{2\sigma^2}\right\} \\ &= \prod_{i=1}^{n} \frac{1}{\sigma}\phi\left(\frac{y_i - \mu}{\sigma}\right) , \end{aligned} \tag{1.2}$$

where $\phi(z) = (2\pi)^{-1/2}\exp(-z^2/2)$ is the density function of the standard normal distribution and π is the irrational number π starting with 3.1415.

In general, the likelihood function is proportional to the density function, the multiplicity not depending on the parameters to be estimated, but with reversed roles of $\mathbf{y}$ and the unknown parameters: Variables y_i are now fixed at their observed values and parameters may vary. This is indicated by denoting the likelihood function by $L(\mu, \sigma^2; \mathbf{y})$, or $L(\mu, \sigma^2)$ for short. Since σ^2 is assumed to be known, only μ needs to be estimated. This leads to the likelihood function for μ,

$$L(\mu) = L(\mu; \mathbf{y}) = \prod_{i=1}^{n} \frac{1}{\sigma}\phi\left(\frac{y_i - \mu}{\sigma}\right) \propto \prod_{i=1}^{n} \exp\left\{-\frac{(y_i - \mu)^2}{2\sigma^2}\right\} . \tag{1.3}$$

The maximum likelihood estimator (MLE) is the function of $\mathbf{y}$ that maximizes this likelihood function. In many cases, this means that the first derivative of the log-likelihood function with respect to the unknown parameter is set equal to zero and solved for the unknown parameter. We will denote the estimator of μ by $\hat{\mu}$. However, it is often easier to maximize the (natural) logarithm of the likelihood function (log-likelihood function), which in the above example is,

$$l(\mu) = l(\mu; \mathbf{y}) \propto \sum_{i=1}^{n} -\frac{(y_i - \mu)^2}{2\sigma^2}$$

and leads to the same MLE as maximizing the likelihood function.

If the first derivative of $l(\mu)$ with respect to μ is set equal to zero and solved for the unknown parameter we arrive at the MLE for μ,

$$\hat{\mu} = \bar{y} = \frac{1}{n}\sum_{i=1}^{n} y_i , \tag{1.4}$$

which is the same function of $\mathbf{y}$ as (1.1) and, for a given data set, leads to the same point estimate. However, if we would assume another data generating process, e.g., a skew normal distribution, then we may arrive at a different estimating function.

In a direct-likelihood approach, inferences are based on relative likelihoods (likelihood ratios). A specific version is the normalized likelihood, which is the likelihood function for some μ divided by the value of the likelihood function at the point estimate. Thus, inferences are justified solely based on the observed data and, of course, based on model assumptions.

For the example with σ^2 known, we have in general terms

$$L(\mu)/L(\hat{\mu}) = \frac{\prod_{i=1}^{n} \frac{1}{\sigma}\phi\left(\frac{y_i-\mu}{\sigma}\right)}{\prod_{i=1}^{n} \frac{1}{\sigma}\phi\left(\frac{y_i-\hat{\mu}}{\sigma}\right)} = \prod_{i=1}^{n} \exp\left\{-\frac{1}{2\sigma^2}\left[(y_i-\mu)^2-(y_i-\hat{\mu})^2\right]\right\}$$

$$= \exp\left\{-\frac{1}{2}\frac{(\bar{y}-\mu)^2}{\sigma^2/n}\right\} ,$$

which is equal to the density function of $\bar{y}$ up to the factor $(2\pi\sigma^2/n)^{-1/2}$, given the model assumption is correct.

For inferences about a general parameter vector $\boldsymbol{\theta}$, likelihood sets or regions can be calculated. A likelihood set consists of all parameter values $\boldsymbol{\theta}$, for which $L(\boldsymbol{\theta})/L(\hat{\boldsymbol{\theta}})$, where $\hat{\boldsymbol{\theta}}$ is the MLE of $\boldsymbol{\theta}$, is equal to or larger than a certain value p, i.e., $L(\boldsymbol{\theta})/L(\hat{\boldsymbol{\theta}}) \geq p$ (e.g., Welsh, 1996, pp. 97–98). Such a region is called a p% likelihood set. In the above example with one continuous parameter, the region $L(\mu)/L(\hat{\mu}) \geq p$ simplifies to an interval,

$$\left[\bar{y} - \sqrt{-\frac{2\sigma^2 \ln p}{n}},\ \bar{y} + \sqrt{-\frac{2\sigma^2 \ln p}{n}}\right] .$$

Choosing, $p = 0.147$, which is supposed to lead to a likelihood interval being close to a 0.95-confidence interval (see Kalbfleisch, 1985, p. 18), $\hat{\mu} = 15$ and given the known variance $\sigma^2 = 2.34$, results in the likelihood interval [14.05, 15.95], slightly wider than the t-confidence interval in Sect. 1.8.2 but close to the bootstrap-t interval. Other values for p could be chosen as well.

Note that evaluation of the estimate and thus inferences about the fixed but unknown model parameter μ are based on the observed data set (and modeling assumptions) only, i.e., there are no (hypothetical) replications. Further, in the example, we ignore the missing data mechanism and treat all observed values as realizations from a normal distribution. The results are very similar to those from the design-based approach, which were obviously invalid as shown by the frequentist evaluation provided in Table 1.2.

In many applications, however, estimation functions based on a likelihood function are evaluated following the frequentist strategy. Let us now assume that besides μ also the variance is unknown. The MLE of μ is again (1.4) and the MLE for σ^2 is

$$\hat{\sigma}^2 = \frac{1}{n}\sum_{i=1}^{n}(y_i-\mu)^2 .$$

Table 1.3 Simulation results

	Mean	Empirical variance	Theoretical variance	Mean variance estimates	Coverage t-distr.	Coverage bootstrap
Population	16.300					
Complete sample	16.303	0.158	0.156	0.156	0.946	0.949
Incomplete sample	15.721	0.247	0.234[a]	0.196	0.801	0.870

Based on complete data sets (complete sample) and incompletely observed data sets (incomplete sample): Means of estimates $\hat{\mu}$, variance of estimates over simulations (empirical variance), theoretical variance of the estimator $\hat{\mu}$, average of variance estimates and coverage rates of 0.95-confidence intervals assuming a t-distribution (t-distr.) and adopting the bootstrap-t method (bootstrap). Number of simulations is 100,000. True value of μ is given in the first row of the table
[a]Note that the theoretical variance is calculated ignoring the missing data mechanism

Unfortunately, this estimator is biased in small samples as it underestimates the true variance by a factor $1 - 1/n$, the bias vanishing in large samples. Thus we can correct for this bias by multiplying this estimator with $n/(n-1)$.

Adopting a frequentist evaluation strategy, the variance of $\hat{\mu}$ is $\text{var}(\hat{\mu}) = \sigma^2/n$ and can be estimated by $\widehat{\text{var}}(\hat{\mu}) = \hat{\sigma}^2/n$. A symmetric, two-sided confidence interval is then given by

$$[\hat{\mu} - t_{n-1,1-\alpha/2}\hat{\sigma}/\sqrt{n},\ \hat{\mu} + t_{n-1,1-\alpha/2}\hat{\sigma}/\sqrt{n}]\ ,$$

where $t_{n-1,1-\alpha/2}$ is the $1 - \alpha/2$-quantile of the t-distribution with $df = n - 1$ degrees of freedom. For the example we find $\hat{\mu} = 15$, $\hat{\sigma}^2 = 1.295$ and, with $t_{n-1,1-\alpha/2} = 2.262$, finally the 0.95%-confidence interval [14.19, 15.81]. Note that these (rounded) results are equal to the results we found for the design-based estimator. This should not be surprising as the estimators for the mean of hourly wage are identical and the estimators of the variance of the estimators are equal up to the factor $(N - n)/N$, which is close to one if N is large and n, is small.

Creating again 100,000 data sets of size $n = 15$, but now from the underlying model instead of the finite population, generating 33% missing values according to the same missing data mechanism as in Sect. 1.8.2, the frequentist properties of the MLEs can be illustrated. Table 1.3 presents the results of estimating the unknown parameters, calculating the means, the variances of the estimators $\hat{\mu}$, the means over estimated variances and the coverage rates of t-confidence and bootstrap-t confidence intervals with $\alpha = 0.05$ over the simulations. The column 'theoretical variance' gives the true variances of $\hat{\mu}$ based on the true value of σ^2, but, for the incomplete sample, ignores the missing data mechanism.

As in the design-based case, the results for the incomplete data sets ignoring the missing data mechanism are invalid. The mean of the estimates for μ are too low, the variance estimator obviously underestimates the theoretical variance and even more so the empirical variance. As a consequence of the bias of the estimators for μ and its variance, the coverage rates of both ways to calculate confidence intervals are too low, although the bootstrap-t interval is closer to the nominal 0.95-level than the

t-confidence interval. The frequentist properties of the MLE estimators for μ and σ^2 based on the data set without missing values seem to be acceptable throughout.

Model-based inference is not necessarily based on a likelihood function. Non-likelihood approaches are available and are used in applications often based on frequentist evaluation criteria. Examples are generalized estimating equations (GEE, Liang & Zeger, 1986) or generalized methods of moments (GMM, Avery, Hansen, & Hotz, 1983).

1.8.3.2 Bayesian Inference

Instead of assuming a fixed unknown parameter value for μ, prior knowledge (or ignorance) about this parameter is explicitly taken into account by specifying a prior distribution for this parameter, denoted as $p(\mu)$.

In the example, we could choose the prior distribution, based on knowledge from already existing research complemented by assumptions, to be the $N(\nu, \tau^2)$ distribution, where $\nu = 16.3$ and $\tau^2 = 0.234$.

By Bayes' theorem the posterior distribution can be written as

$$p(\mu \mid \mathbf{y}) = \frac{f(\mathbf{y} \mid \mu)p(\mu)}{\int_{-\infty}^{\infty} f(\mathbf{y} \mid \mu)p(\mu)\,d\mu} = \frac{f(\mathbf{y} \mid \mu)p(\mu)}{f(\mathbf{y})} \propto f(\mathbf{y} \mid \mu)p(\mu)\,, \tag{1.5}$$

where $f(\mathbf{y} \mid \mu)$ is the density function of $\mathbf{y}$ conditional on μ and $f(\mathbf{y})$ is the, with respect to μ, marginal density of $\mathbf{y}$. Thus $f(\mathbf{y})$ does not depend on μ and does not affect inferences with respect to μ. As in the case of likelihood inference, the variables $\mathbf{y}$ are fixed at their observed values. However, μ is considered to be a random variable in (1.5). Since μ varies, $f(\mathbf{y} \mid \mu)$ is also called the likelihood.

With the above assumptions, the prior distribution for μ is

$$p(\mu) = \frac{1}{\sqrt{2\pi\tau^2}} \exp\left\{-\frac{(\mu-\nu)^2}{2\tau^2}\right\}$$

and the likelihood is given by (1.3). Hence the posterior distribution for μ simplifies and is proportional to

$$\begin{aligned} f(\mathbf{y} \mid \mu)p(\mu) &= \left[\prod_{i=1}^{n} \frac{1}{\sqrt{2\pi\sigma^2}} \exp\left\{-\frac{(y_i-\mu)^2}{2\sigma^2}\right\}\right] \frac{1}{\sqrt{2\pi\tau^2}} \exp\left\{-\frac{(\mu-\nu)^2}{2\tau^2}\right\} \\ &\propto \exp\left\{-\left(\frac{n(\bar{y}-\mu)^2}{2\sigma^2} + \frac{(\mu-\nu)^2}{2\tau^2}\right)\right\} = \exp\left\{-\frac{(\mu-\tilde{\nu})^2}{2\tilde{\tau}^2}\right\}, \end{aligned}$$

where $\tilde{\nu} = \tilde{\tau}^2(n\bar{y}/\sigma^2 + \nu/\tau^2)$ and $\tilde{\tau}^2 = (n/\sigma^2 + 1/\tau^2)^{-1}$ (for details, see Cameron & Trivedi, 2005, p. 422f.). The posterior distribution of μ in the light of data $\mathbf{y}$ is thus proportional to the density of a normal distribution for μ with mean $\tilde{\nu}$ and variance $\tilde{\tau}^2$. The normal prior chosen in this example is thus a conjugate prior.

Both, the posterior mean $\tilde{\nu}$ and variance $\tilde{\tau}^2$ are weighted sums of the prior information and the observed or known information. If n increases, the weight of the observed or known information increases relative to the weight given to the prior information with respect to the posterior mean but also with respect to the posterior variance. For fixed n and σ^2, $\tilde{\tau}^2$ increases with the prior variance τ^2 but is always smaller than the variance of $\bar{y}$, $\text{var}(\bar{y}) = \sigma^2/n$. Thus the posterior precision, defined by $1/\tilde{\tau}^2$, increases with the prior precision $1/\tau^2$ and is always higher than the sample precision n/σ^2. Hence, choosing a flat prior (large τ^2) decreases the weight given to the prior information with respect to both, the posterior mean and variance.

In the example using the observed part of the sample we would take the mean of the posterior distribution as an estimate for the mean of WAGE. With the results and given values from above, we get

$$\tilde{\tau}^2 = (10/2.34 + 1/0.234)^{-1} = 0.117 \,,$$
$$\tilde{\nu} = 0.117(10 \times 15/2.34 + 16.3/0.234) = 15.65$$

and

$$\mu \mid \mathbf{y} \sim N(15.65, 0.117) \,.$$

Further, a '0.95%-credible interval' may be calculated by taking the 0.025 and the 0.975 quantiles of the posterior distribution as lower and upper bounds. Given the assumption of a random parameter, a prior distribution and the observed values $y_i, i = 1, \ldots, n$, a 0.95%-credible interval provides the often desired statement that the probability of the actual parameter value for μ, in our example, lies within this interval is at least 0.95. For the example, we get [14.98, 16.32] as a 0.95%-credible interval.

Thanks to using the parameter values from which the data were generated, the estimate for mean hourly wage is in between the estimates of the other approaches and the posterior variance is smaller than the estimated variances based on the other approaches. Hence, the upper bound of the credible interval is close to the mean from which the data were simulated and is covered by this interval.

If no information about μ were available, we could model our ignorance by a noninformative prior that assigns the same value to each possible value of μ, $p(\mu) \propto c$, $-\infty < \mu < \infty$, which is an improper prior distribution because $\int_{-\infty}^{\infty} p(\mu)\, d\mu = \infty$. It turns out, however, that adopting this improper prior distribution leads to a proper posterior distribution which is proportional to

$$
\begin{aligned}
p(\mathbf{y} \mid \mu)p(\mu) \propto \exp\left\{-\frac{\sum_{i=1}^{n}(y_i-\mu)^2}{2\sigma^2}\right\} &= \exp\left\{-\frac{1}{2\sigma^2}\sum_{i=1}^{n}(y_i-\mu)^2\right\} \\
&= \exp\left\{-\frac{1}{2\sigma^2}\sum_{i=1}^{n}(y_i-\bar{y}+\bar{y}-\mu)^2\right\} \\
&= \exp\left\{-\frac{1}{2\sigma^2}\left[\sum_{i=1}^{n}(y_i-\bar{y})^2+n(\bar{y}-\mu)^2\right]\right\} \propto \exp\left\{-\frac{n(\mu-\bar{y})^2}{2\sigma^2}\right\},
\end{aligned}
$$

because $p(\boldsymbol{\mu}) = c$ and $(\sum_{i=1}^{n}(y_i - \bar{y})^2)/(2\sigma^2)$ are absorbed into the constant.

The posterior distribution $p(\mu \mid \mathbf{y})$ is now the $N(\bar{y}, \sigma^2/n)$-distribution. In the example we get as the posterior mean and variance $\bar{y} = 15$ and $\sigma^2/n = 0.234$. Note that both values are very close to $\tilde{\nu}$ and $\tilde{\tau}^2$ if $\tau^2 \to \infty$. Thus the noninformative prior can be viewed as a rough approximation to the normal prior in this example. The 0.95%-credible interval is now equal to [14.05, 15.95].

1.9 Outline

The remaining chapters are about the method and techniques of multiple imputation to compensate for missing values developed by Rubin (1987, 1996). Although many techniques to generate single or multiple imputations are available, this book concentrates on the generation of multiple imputations such that inferences are valid using the combining rules derived in Rubin (1987). Other techniques to generate imputations that allow valid inferences will not be treated as they usually require more complicated versions of combining rules, but see, for example, Robins and Wang (2000).

Chapters 5 and 6 describe how to generate multiple imputations in various situations with packages available from within R (R Core Team, 2018). R is a dynamic open source system including many user written packages to analyse data but also to generate imputations. Thus, R includes several packages and functions to generate imputations. The downside of the open strategy is that it is well possible that some functions may not allow the generation of imputations such that analyses of the applied scientific interest allow valid inferences. It should be noted, however, that this is also not guaranteed if commercial software based on a closed concept is used.

However, it turns out that being able to apply currently available software to generate (multiple) imputations is not enough to justify valid inferences. Instead, it is important to understand the main concepts of multiple-imputation theory, where some aspects are often ignored. To successfully apply the method of multiple imputation, it is also essential to know about possible restrictions, fallacies and pitfalls.

Hence, not only the handling of available software will be described, which is not straightforward in general, but also the main concepts of the theory of multiple imputation will be presented with the help of examples. Unfortunately even simple examples get complicated as soon as missing values occur. Therefore, several examples will be based on simulations illustrating the frequentist properties of estimators, confidence intervals and test statistics.

In the following chapters we will see that the relative ease with which multiple imputations can be generated may be deceptive: Not all of the available imputation functions realize a proper imputation method and even those who do, may fail to do so in certain situations (see Chap. 4). In applications it is therefore important to know about the underlying assumptions and possible fallacies of the method and technique applied. Therefore, Chaps. 2–4 not only introduce the theoretical concepts underlying the method of multiple imputation, but also consider several aspects of the method of multiple imputation to be aware of when generating multiple imputations. This includes open questions, some misconceptions but also possible pitfalls. Finally, some technical details, basics and intermediate results can be found in the appendix.

References

Avery, R. B., Hansen, L. P., & Hotz, V. J. (1983). Multiperiod probit models and orthogonality condition estimation. *International Economic Review, 24*(1), 21–35.

Cameron, A. C., & Trivedi, P. K. (2005). *Microeconometrics: Methods and applications*. Cambridge, UK: University Press.

Efron, B. (2015). Frequentist accuracy of Bayesian estimates. *Journal of the Royal Statistical Society: Series B, 77*(3), 617–646.

Efron, B. & Tibshirani, R. J. (1993). *An introduction to the bootstrap*. New York, NY: Chapman & Hall.

Gonzalez, J. M., & Eltinge, J. L. (2007). Multiple matrix sampling: A review. In *Proceedings of the Section on Survey Research Methods* (pp. 3069–3075). Alexandria, VA: American Statistical Association.

Horvitz, D. G., & Thompson, D. J. (1952). A generalization of sampling without replacement from a finite universe. *Journal of the American Statistical Association, 47*(260), 663–685.

Kalbfleisch, J. G. (1985). *Probability and statistical inference, Vol. 2: Statistical inference* (2nd ed.). New York, NY: Springer.

Lange, K. (2010). *Numerical analysis for statisticians* (2nd ed.). New York, NY: Springer.

Liang, K.-Y., & Zeger, S. L. (1986). Longitudinal data analysis using generalized linear models. *Biometrika, 73*(1), 13–22.

Newey, W. K., & McFadden, D. L. (1994). Large sample estimation and hypothesis testing. In R. F. Engle & D. L. McFadden (Eds.), *Handbook of econometrics* (Vol. IV, pp. 2111–2245). Amsterdam: Elsevier.

R Core Team. (2018). *R: A language and environment for statistical computing*. Vienna: R Foundation for Statistical Computing. https://www.R-project.org.

Reiter, J. P., & Raghunathan, T. E. (2007). The multiple adaptations of multiple imputation. *Journal of the American Statistical Association, 102*(480), 1462–1471.

Robins, J. M., & Wang, N. (2000). Inference for imputation estimators. *Biometrika, 87*(1), 113–124.
Rubin, D. B. (1976). Inference and missing data. *Biometrika, 63*(3), 581–590.
Rubin, D. B. (1987). *Multiple imputation for nonresponse in surveys*. New York, NY: Wiley.
Rubin, D. B. (1996). Multiple imputation after 18+ years. *Journal of the American Statistical Association, 91*(434), 473–489.
Rubin, D. B., Stern, H. S., & Vehovar, V. (1995). Handling "don't know" survey responses: The case of the Slovenian plebiscite. *Journal of the American Statistical Association, 90*(431), 822–828.
Särndal, C.-E., Swensson, B., & Wretman, J. (1992). *Model assisted survey sampling*. New York, NY: Springer.
Seaman, S., Galati, J., Jackson, D., & Carlin, J. (2013). What is meant by "missing at random"? *Statistical Science, 28*(2), 257–268.
Shafer, G. (1976). *A mathematical theory of evidence*. Princeton, NJ: Princeton University Press.
Welsh, A. H. (1996). *Aspects of statistical inference*. New York, NY: Wiley.

Chapter 2
Missing Data Mechanism and Ignorability

2.1 Overview

In this chapter the concept of a missing data mechanism and the classification of missing data as being missing completely at random (MCAR), missing at random (MAR) or missing not at random (MNAR) is introduced. Consequences of different possible missing data mechanisms are considered and illustrated with simple examples. In addition, conditions are given for analysing data sets without the need to explicitly model the missing data mechanism ("ignorability"). We also review diagnostic tools for incomplete data sets, both descriptive and based on a statistical test.

2.2 Introduction

As we saw in the last chapter, missing values may not only decrease sample size, but may lead to invalid inferences. A decision about how to deal with a missing data situation needs therefore to be well justified. This in turn requires knowledge about the implications of the missing data mechanism, which will be introduced in Sect. 2.3.

A rough but often sufficient classification of missing data mechanisms is given in Sects. 2.3.1–2.3.3. Section 2.4 discusses conditions under which the missing data mechanism can be ignored and what this actually means. Unfortunately, for valid statistical inferences, it does not in general mean that the analysis techniques for completely observed data sets can safely be applied to the incompletely observed data set. Following the presentation of these predominantly classical results (see Rubin, 1976, 1987), Sect. 2.5 is devoted to a more detailed discussion of the missing

K. Kleinke et al., *Applied Multiple Imputation*, Statistics for Social and Behavioral Sciences, https://doi.org/10.1007/978-3-030-38164-6_2

data mechanism. Finally, in Sect. 2.6 we will consider some diagnostic tools. But first some notation needs to be introduced.

2.2.1 Some Notation

Units selected into a sample will be indexed by $i = 1, \ldots, n$, variables collected for each unit by $l = 1, \ldots, q$. Hence, $u_{i,l}$ denotes the lth variable of the ith unit. For simplicity, we will assume that for each unit the same number of variables is surveyed. This can easily be generalized, however, to a varying number of observed variables over units. If needed, for example, if panel data or more general clustered data sets are considered, additional indices may be used.

Variables $u_{i,1}, \ldots, u_{i,q}$ will often be collected into a $(q \times 1)$ (column) vector $\mathbf{u}_i = (u_{i,1}, \ldots, u_{i,q})^T$. The vectors $\mathbf{u}_i$, $i = 1, \ldots, n$ can be stacked over each other to form an $(nq \times 1)$ vector, $\mathbf{u} = (\mathbf{u}_1^T, \ldots, \mathbf{u}_n^T)^T$ (cf. Appendix A.1). Every statistic of scientific interest, like parameter estimators, test statistics or confidence intervals are functions of $\mathbf{u}$. For the sake of simplicity, we will not distinguish notationally between a variable and its realized value as this should be apparent from the context.

Similar to the selection indicator in Chap. 1, the response indicator r takes on the value one, if the corresponding variable value is observed, and zero otherwise. Therefore, if the response indicator does not explicitly indicate just unit nonresponse or address only a specific subset of the variables, there are q response indicators for each unit, $r_{i,1}, \ldots, r_{i,q}$. Thus we have

$$r_{i,l} = \begin{cases} 1 \text{ if } & u_{i,l} \text{ is observed,} \\ 0 \text{ otherwise .} \end{cases}$$

The response indicators can be collected into vectors, $\mathbf{r}_i$, which in turn can be stacked over each other resulting in an $(nq \times 1)$-vector $\mathbf{r} = (\mathbf{r}_1, \ldots, \mathbf{r}_n)^T$. So, $\mathbf{u}_i$ and $\mathbf{r}_i$ will usually have the same dimension.

If a data set is affected by nonresponse, then not all of the realized values in $\mathbf{u}$ are observed. The convention in R (R Core Team, 2018) is to assign these events the value *NA* for 'not available'. However, we will follow this convention only in R-output, otherwise we will use a dot, '.', for each missing value. Thus, if a data set is not completely observed $\mathbf{u}$ is a vector with valid variable values and '.' entries, whereas $\mathbf{r}$, a vector of ones and zeros, is always completely observed. For simplicity and to avoid any confusion, we will define the vector $\mathbf{u}_{(1)}$ which consists of all the variables in $\mathbf{u}$ whose values are observed in a given sample, and $\mathbf{u}_{(0)}$ consisting of all the variables whose values are not observed (cf. Rubin, 1976). Expressed differently, $\mathbf{u}_{(1)}$ is the vector of variables selected into the observed subsample, i.e., for which $r_{i,l} = 1$, and $\mathbf{u}_{(0)}$ is the vector of variables not selected into the observed subsample, i.e., for which $r_{i,l} = 0$.

2.3 The Missing Data Mechanism

For inferential statistics one has to model the data generating process. This allows well-founded statements about the underlying state or process if the model approximates the true data generating process sufficiently well. Since the event of observing or not observing variable values can be interpreted as the result of a data generating process for binary variables, modeling this process is no exception. The missing data mechanism can be any process that generates binary response variables r, which take on the value one if the value of a corresponding variable u is observed and zero otherwise. Thus, it is similar to the selection indicator described in Sect. 1.5.1. In fact, the process from the realized sample to the observed subsample can be interpreted as an additional sampling step. The underlying process may be known, however, like in matrix sampling (Gonzalez & Eltinge, 2007) or unknown, which is the case in most data collection situations. Apart from very specific applications, the missing data mechanism is considered to be a random process.

Thus the hypothesized missing data mechanism may be conceptualized as a probability function,

$$g(\mathbf{r} \mid \mathbf{u}, \boldsymbol{\gamma}) , \tag{2.1}$$

where $\boldsymbol{\gamma}$ is an unknown parameter that takes on values in an appropriate parameter space governing the missing data mechanism and (2.1) models the probability of observing $\mathbf{r}$ conditional on the observed values in $\mathbf{u}$ for each value of $\boldsymbol{\gamma}$.

Further considerations of (2.1) may proceed either for fixed or for varying $\mathbf{r}$, $\mathbf{u}_{(1)}$ and $\mathbf{u}_{(0)}$ (see Seaman et al., 2013). Fixing $\mathbf{r}$ at the observed pattern of missing and observed values was used by Rubin (1976) to derive the weakest conditions under which the missing data mechanism can be ignored. Under fixed $\mathbf{r}$, (2.1) models the probability of observing the realized pattern in $\mathbf{r}$ conditional on the realized values in $\mathbf{u}$ and for some $\boldsymbol{\gamma}$. Fixing $\mathbf{r}$ at the observed values is close to common practice under a frequentist evaluation of inferences where the size of an observed sample is considered to be fixed. In contrast, a stronger version considers varying $\mathbf{r}$, in which case (2.1) is a statement about the conditional distribution of the variable $\mathbf{r}$ given the realized values of $\mathbf{u}$ and not about realized values of $\mathbf{r}$ only. Hence, (2.1) models the probability of any possible pattern in $\mathbf{r}$ conditional on the realized values in $\mathbf{u}$. Even stronger, (2.1) may be a model not only for all possible $\mathbf{r}$, but also for all possible $\mathbf{u}$ at each value of $\boldsymbol{\gamma}$.

Regardless of whether (2.1) is assumed to model the relationship of the variable $\mathbf{r}$ or the observed values in $\mathbf{r}$ conditional on $\mathbf{u}$, it is often assumed that the realized values of different units have been generated by the same processes independently from each other. With this assumption (2.1) becomes

$$g(\mathbf{r} \mid \mathbf{u}, \boldsymbol{\gamma}) = \prod_{i=1}^{n} g(\mathbf{r}_i \mid \mathbf{u}_i, \boldsymbol{\gamma}) . \tag{2.2}$$

Considering (2.2) to hold for all possible values of $\mathbf{u}_i$ at the observed values of $\mathbf{r}_i$, i.e., for the observed part of the sample, is probably closest to standard assumptions made in statistical analyses. In fact, many statistical models assume $\mathbf{u}_i$ to be independent and even identically distributed (iid), which is stronger than the assumptions needed in this section. For example, consider the variable $u_{i,1}$, mean hourly wage of the ith individual (WAGE) collected from $i = 1, \ldots, n$ sampled individuals. In many model-based analyses one would assume that the variables $u_{i,1}$ are independent and follow the same distribution for all i.

In the next three subsections we will consider a widely used categorization of missing data mechanisms that goes back to Rubin (1976) and is relevant with respect to the way how missing values are handled.

2.3.1 Missing Completely at Random (MCAR)

The missing values are missing completely at random (MCAR) if for the realized pattern in $\mathbf{r}$ for each value of $\boldsymbol{\gamma}$ the function $g(\mathbf{r} \mid \mathbf{u}, \boldsymbol{\gamma})$ takes on the same value, which is the probability of the observed pattern, for all possible values of $\mathbf{u}$. This leads to

Definition 2.1 Missing data are missing completely at random (MCAR) if for fixed $\mathbf{r}$ and for each $\boldsymbol{\gamma}$

$$g(\mathbf{r} \mid \mathbf{u}, \boldsymbol{\gamma}) = g(\mathbf{r} \mid \boldsymbol{\gamma}) \quad \text{for all possible } \mathbf{u} \,. \tag{2.3}$$

This definition goes back to Rubin (1976), although the term 'missing completely at random' is not used in that paper (but see the first edition of Little & Rubin, 2002, published in 1987).

Note that Definition 2.1 is a statement about the observed and treated-as-fixed pattern of observed and missing values in $\mathbf{r}$. Due to some confusion in the literature Seaman et al. (2013) called missing values generated according to the above mechanism 'realized MCAR' to emphasize that $\mathbf{r}$ is fixed at the observed pattern. If $\mathbf{r}$ is not fixed and the above definition holds for all possible values of $\mathbf{r}$, then the missing values are denoted as being 'everywhere MCAR' by Seaman et al. (2013). In that latter case, the variables $\mathbf{r}$ and $\mathbf{u}$ are independent. This implies realized MCAR. But realized MCAR does not imply everywhere MCAR, so everywhere MCAR is a stronger assumption than realized MCAR.

For both situations, i.e., treating $\mathbf{r}$ as fixed or random, we may adopt the more restrictive iid assumption so that (2.1) simplifies to

$$g(\mathbf{r} \mid \mathbf{u}, \boldsymbol{\gamma}) = \prod_{i=1}^{n} g(\mathbf{r}_i \mid \boldsymbol{\gamma}) \tag{2.4}$$

for each $\boldsymbol{\gamma}$ and all $\mathbf{u}$.

Example 2.1 (Data Missing Completely at Random (MCAR)) As a simple example consider the two variables WAGE and NCHILD. Assume that WAGE is not completely observed but NCHILD is. Then the missing WAGE values are MCAR if the probability of observing or not observing a wage value is the same for all possible values of the variable NCHILD and all the observed WAGE variables. □

To illustrate the effect of this missing data mechanism for fixed **r**, we generated independently $n = 10{,}000$ pairs of data values $(x_i, y_i)^T$ from a bivariate normal distribution with means equal to zero, variances equal to one and a correlation of 0.6. In a second step, approximately 30% of the x-values were deleted completely at random by generating r_i from a Bernoulli distribution with $\Pr(r_i = 1) = 0.7$ independently for all i. If $r_i = 0$, then the corresponding value of x_i was deleted.

Figure 2.1 illustrates the effect of missing data being MCAR on various aspects of the bivariate distribution of $(x_i, y_i)^T$. Results for the realized data set, i.e., the complete-data set before any values are deleted, are depicted in solid lines, those based on the completely observed $(x_i, y_i)^T$ pairs in dashed lines.

However, the dashed lines are barely visible because they are almost completely covered by the solid lines. In fact, although the completely observed data set is smaller than the realized one, it is a non-selective random subsample from the realized sample. If the missing data are MCAR, then differences in the distributions are not systematic and standard analysis techniques will allow valid inferences as long as the assumed statistical models are approximately correct.

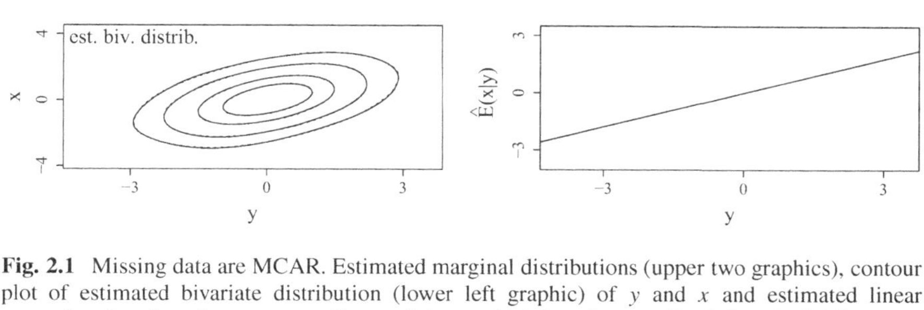

Fig. 2.1 Missing data are MCAR. Estimated marginal distributions (upper two graphics), contour plot of estimated bivariate distribution (lower left graphic) of y and x and estimated linear regression function from x on y (lower right graphic) based on realized data (solid line) and completely observed part of the sample (dashed line)

2.3.2 Missing at Random (MAR)

The missing values are missing at random (MAR) if for the realized pattern in $\mathbf{r}$ for each value of $\boldsymbol{\gamma}$ the function $g(\mathbf{r} \mid \mathbf{u}_{(1)}, \mathbf{u}_{(0)}, \boldsymbol{\gamma})$ takes on the same value for all possible values of $\mathbf{u}_{(0)}$. This leads to

Definition 2.2 Missing data are missing at random (MAR) if for fixed $\mathbf{r}$ and for each $\boldsymbol{\gamma}$

$$g(\mathbf{r} \mid \mathbf{u}_{(1)}, \mathbf{u}_{(0)}, \boldsymbol{\gamma}) = g(\mathbf{r} \mid \mathbf{u}_{(1)}, \boldsymbol{\gamma}) \quad \text{for all possible } \mathbf{u}_{(0)} \tag{2.5}$$

(see Rubin, 1976). That is, the probability of the observed pattern of missing and observed values in $\mathbf{r}$ is the same for any of the possible values of $\mathbf{u}_{(0)}$ conditional on the observed values in $\mathbf{u}_{(1)}$ for each value of $\boldsymbol{\gamma}$. Like in the MCAR case this definition is a statement about the observed and treated-as-fixed pattern of observed and missing values.

Redefining (2.5) to hold for all patterns of $\mathbf{r}$ and all values of $\mathbf{u}_{(1)}$ and $\boldsymbol{\gamma}$, we arrive at what is called 'everywhere MAR' by Seaman et al. (2013). Note that when the pattern of $\mathbf{r}$ changes then so does the subset of observed variables in $\mathbf{u}$, but also the dimensions of $\mathbf{u}_{(1)}$ and $\mathbf{u}_{(0)}$ may change. Everywhere MAR means that the missing data are MAR for each possible pattern of $\mathbf{r}$ and each possible value of $\mathbf{u}_{(1)}$, so $\mathbf{r}$ and $\mathbf{u}_{(0)}$ are independent conditional on $\mathbf{u}_{(1)}$. Again, everywhere MAR implies realized MAR but not vice versa.

Example 2.2 (Data Missing at Random (MAR)) In the example with the two variables WAGE and NCHILD assume that the two variables are negatively correlated. If individuals with a smaller number of children living in the same household tend to not answer the wage question, then the missing WAGE values are MAR. Note that although higher wages are less likely to be observed in the sample, within each class defined by the number of children, the probability for a missing wage value does not change over the possible values of WAGE. Thus the missing WAGE values are MCAR conditional on the number of children living in the same household. □

To illustrate the effect of the mechanism that leads to missing data being MAR for fixed $\mathbf{r}$, we again generated $n = 10{,}000$ pairs of data values $(x_i, y_i)^T$ independently from the same distribution as described in Sect. 2.3.1. In the second step, approximately 30% of the x-values were deleted at random by first generating values for a variable r_i^* as a linear function of y_i plus an independently generated noise variable from the standard normal distribution. The binary indicator variable r_i was set to zero if r_i^* exceeded a prespecified threshold. If $r_i = 0$, then the corresponding values of x_i was deleted.

Figure 2.2 illustrates the effect of missing data being MAR on the various aspects of the bivariate distribution of $(x_i, y_i)^T$. Both, the estimated marginal distribution of those y_i-values for which the corresponding x_i-values are observed (upper left graphic, dashed line) and the estimated marginal distribution of observed x_i-values (upper right graphic, dashed line) differ from the corresponding estimated marginal

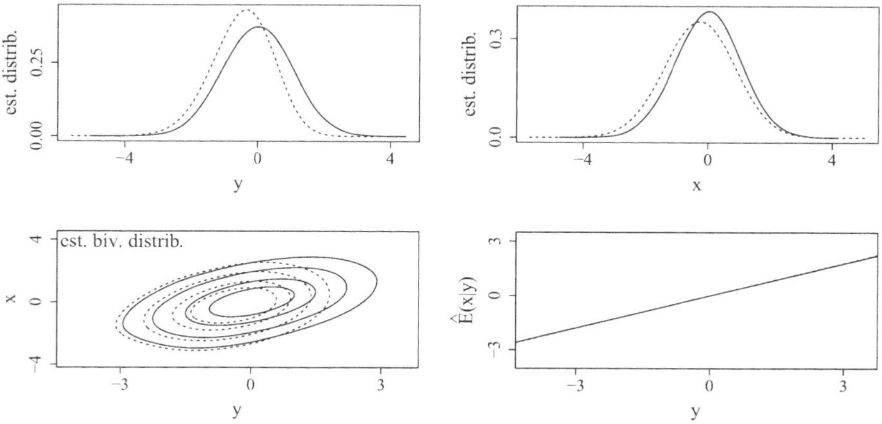

Fig. 2.2 Missing data are MAR. Estimated marginal distributions (upper two graphics), contour plot of estimated bivariate distribution (lower left graphic) of y and x and estimated linear regression function from x on y (lower right graphic) based on realized data (solid line) and completely observed part of the sample (dashed line)

distributions of the fully observed variables y_i (upper left graphic, solid line) and x_i (upper right graphic, solid line). Similarly, the estimated bivariate distribution based on the complete-data set and the completely observed part of the data set differ markedly as can be seen from the contour plots in the lower left graphic of Fig. 2.2.

Hence, estimators like the mean, the variance or the correlation if based on the completely observed pairs $(x_i, y_i)^T$ will be biased. On the other hand, the regression relationship of x_i on y_i in the completely observed part of the data set is not systematically different from the corresponding relationship in the realized sample. This is due to the fact that if the missing data are MAR, then conditional on $\mathbf{u}_{(1)}$, which is $(y_1, \ldots, y_n, \mathbf{x}_{(1)}^T)^T$ in the example, the probability of not observing $\mathbf{u}_{(0)}$, here $\mathbf{x}_{(0)}$, is the same for all possible $\mathbf{u}_{(0)}$-values. Thus the missing x_i values are MCAR conditional on the observed y_i and x_i values, but unconditionally MAR.

The observation that the regression relationship between x_i and y_i values seems to be not affected by the missing data being MAR will be important when methods to compensate for missing values are considered. In fact, the unbiasedness of this relationship can be used to compensate for nonresponse (for a more extensive discussion, see Chap. 4).

2.3.3 *Missing Not at Random (MNAR)*

Definition 2.3 Missing values are missing not at random (MNAR) if missing values are neither MCAR nor MAR.

In that case, the probability of the observed pattern in **r** depends on at least one variable whose value is not observed. Instead of 'missing not at random' sometimes the expression 'not missing at random' (NMAR) is used.

Example 2.3 (Data Missing Not at Random (MNAR)) Consider again the two variables WAGE and NCHILD. If individuals with high wage tend to not answer the wage question even within the group of households with the same number of children, then the missing values would be MNAR. □

To also illustrate the effect of this mechanism that leads to missing data being MNAR for fixed **r**, we generated $n = 10{,}000$ pairs of data values $(x_i, y_i)^T$ independently from the same distribution as described in Sects. 2.3.1 and 2.3.2. Again, in the second step, approximately 30% of the x-values were deleted randomly by first generating values for a variable r_i^* as a linear function now of x_i plus an independently generated noise variable from the standard normal distribution. The binary indicator variable r_i was set to zero if r_i^* exceeded a prespecified threshold. If $r_i = 0$, then the corresponding value of x_i was deleted.

In all four graphics of Fig. 2.3 the difference between the results based on the complete-data set before any values are deleted and the completely observed part of the data set after values in the x_i's are deleted are obvious. Now not only the estimated marginal and bivariate distributions seem to be distorted but also the regression relationship. That is, under missing data being MNAR, all the aspects

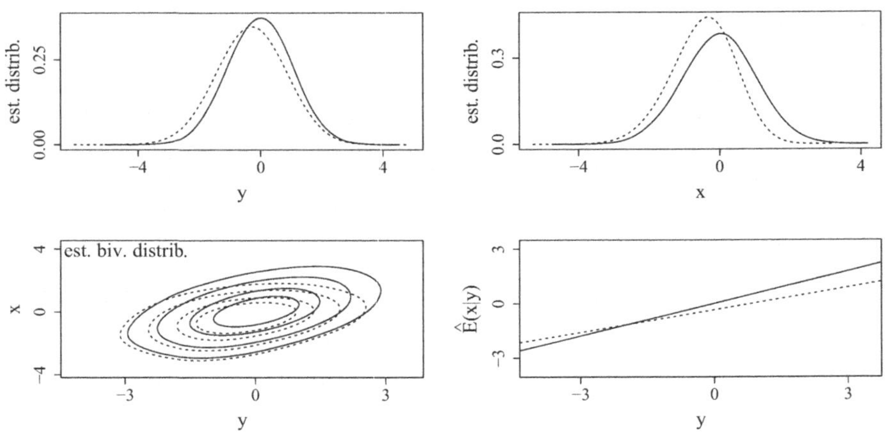

Fig. 2.3 Missing data are MNAR. Estimated marginal distributions (upper two graphics), contour plot of estimated bivariate distribution (lower left graphic) of y and x and estimated linear regression function from x on y (lower right graphic) based on realized data (solid line) and completely observed part of the sample (dashed line)

of the bivariate distribution in the completely observed part of the data set differ as compared to the complete-data case. Unlike in the MAR case, relationships between observed variables that could be used to (approximately) recover the state if there were no missing values are systematically distorted. To compensate for missing data being MNAR, in fact, strong external knowledge about the missing data mechanism is needed.

2.4 Ignorability of the Missing Data Mechanism

Given the categorization in the last section, the interesting question is: When can the missing data mechanism safely be ignored? The first step to answer this question is to look at the procedure that simply ignores the missing data mechanism. This usually means that $\mathbf{r}$ is fixed at its observed pattern and the observed values in $\mathbf{u}_{(1)}$ are assumed to be realizations from the marginal distribution

$$\int f(\mathbf{u} \mid \boldsymbol{\theta})\, d\mathbf{u}_{(0)} \tag{2.6}$$

(cf. Rubin, 1976), where $f(\mathbf{u} \mid \boldsymbol{\theta})$ is the assumed distribution of $\mathbf{u}$ depending on some parameter $\boldsymbol{\theta}$ from an appropriate parameter space, and we follow the inaccurate but simplifying notation in the corresponding literature and do not distinguish between continuous and discrete variables. To simplify the presentation we also write $\int f(\mathbf{u} \mid \boldsymbol{\theta})\, d\mathbf{u}$ instead of $\int \cdots \int f(u_1, \ldots, u_n \mid \boldsymbol{\theta})\, du_1 \cdots du_n$ for multiple integrals throughout the book.

If there are discrete variables in $\mathbf{u}_{(0)}$, then integration is replaced by taking the sum for these particular variables. Note that both, $\mathbf{u}_{(1)}$ and $\mathbf{u}_{(0)}$ are actually functions of $\mathbf{u}$ and $\mathbf{r}$.

Example 2.4 (Ignoring the Missing Data Mechanism) Assume a random sample of size $n = 5$ is selected from a population with $N = 10{,}000$ units ($j = 1, \ldots, N$) and for each of the $i = 1, \ldots, n$ sampled units the reaction time in some concentration task (RT) and mean hourly wage (WAGE) is recorded. The selection probability is identical for each eligible unit at each draw, and since the sample is small relative to the size of the population, we approximate sample selection without replacement by selection with replacement. The selection probability is thus approximately $\Pr(s = 1) = 1/N$ for each j at each draw, and selection of one unit is treated as being independent from the selection of any other unit.

The variables $u_{j,1}$ (RT) and $u_{j,2}$ (WAGE) are assumed to be realizations of bivariate normally distributed variables with correlation $\rho \neq 0$ and, since selection of the units is independent from $u_{j,1}$ and $u_{j,2}$, the sampling mechanism can be ignored. Therefore, we assume that $\mathbf{u}_i = (u_{i,1},\ u_{i,2})^T$ is iid normally distributed for all i.

If we are interested in the means and variances of RT and WAGE and the correlation ρ, then we could start with the likelihood function for the unknown parameters μ_1, μ_2, σ_1^2, σ_2^2 and ρ, collected in $\boldsymbol{\theta}$,

$$L(\boldsymbol{\theta}) = \prod_{i=1}^{5} f(u_{i,1}, u_{i,2} \mid \boldsymbol{\theta}) \ , \tag{2.7}$$

where $f(u_{i,1}, u_{i,2}|\boldsymbol{\theta})$ denotes the bivariate normal density function (see Appendix A.2.4). We would then estimate all the necessary parameters by maximizing the log-likelihood function.

Suppose that at the time that the data are to be analysed, one of the values of WAGE, say the value in the fifth draw, $u_{5,2}$, is unreadable. Ignoring the missing data mechanism means assuming $\mathbf{u}_i$, $i = 1, \ldots, 4$ and $u_{5,1}$, collected in $\mathbf{u}_{(1)}$ were generated from the same distribution from which the sample without any missing value would have been generated and the missing data mechanism needs not to be taken into account. The marginal distribution of $\mathbf{u}_{(1)}$ ignoring the missing data mechanism can be written as

$$\int f(\mathbf{u} \mid \boldsymbol{\theta})\, d\mathbf{u}_{(0)} = \int \left[\prod_{i=1}^{4} f(u_{i,1}, u_{i,2} \mid \boldsymbol{\theta})\right] f(u_{5,2} \mid u_{5,1}, \boldsymbol{\theta}_{2|1}) f(u_{5,1} \mid \boldsymbol{\theta}_1)\, du_{5,2} \ ,$$

where $\boldsymbol{\theta}_{2|1}$ is the vector of parameters of the regression from $u_{5,2}$ on $u_{5,1}$ and $\boldsymbol{\theta}_1 = (\mu_1\ \sigma_1^2)$. Thus the likelihood function would be

$$L(\boldsymbol{\theta}) = \left[\prod_{i=1}^{4} f(u_{i,1}, u_{i,2} \mid \boldsymbol{\theta})\right] f(u_{5,1} \mid \boldsymbol{\theta}_1) \ . \tag{2.8}$$

Note that this likelihood is different from the corresponding likelihood for the complete-data set with $n = 5$.

Thus, even when the missing data mechanism can be ignored this does not mean that the analysis of scientific interest is the same as if there were no missing values. In our example, estimation would be based on the same model as for the complete-data set, although with less observations, if the term $f(u_{5,1} \mid \boldsymbol{\theta}_1)$ would be ignored. This would still allow valid inferences if $u_{5,2}$ is MCAR. If instead $u_{5,2}$ is MAR, i.e., if the probability of observing $u_{5,2}$ depends on $u_{5,1}$, then the term $f(u_{5,1} \mid \boldsymbol{\theta}_1)$ should not be ignored if μ_1, σ_1^2 and ρ is intended to be estimated because ignoring $u_{5,1}$ would introduce a missing value which is MNAR. □

Example 2.4 shows that if the missing data mechanism can safely be ignored, this may lead to the same analysis as for the completely observed data set with just less observations. But this is not necessarily the case if the missing values are MAR, as is shown for the parameters governing both, the common distribution of WAGE and RT and the marginal distribution of RT. Analysing the observed part of the data set may then require more complex statistical models.

When discussing ignorability of the missing data mechanism, several aspects have to be taken into account. One is the distinctness of $\boldsymbol{\theta}$, the parameter of the model of scientific interest, and $\boldsymbol{\gamma}$, the parameter governing the missing data mechanism. Following Rubin (1976), the parameters $\boldsymbol{\theta}$ and $\boldsymbol{\gamma}$ are distinct, if they are not linked with each other. The assumed to be fixed parameters would not be distinct if, for example, the effect of RT on $\mathbf{r}$ increases with the strength of the effect of RT on WAGE (see also Sect. 2.4.2). If both parameters are interpreted as being not random, like in classical model-based statistics, distinctness means that each parameter is free to take on every possible value regardless of the values of the other parameter. If both parameters are considered to be random, like in Bayesian statistics, then distinctness is equivalent to assuming stochastic independence of $\boldsymbol{\theta}$ and $\boldsymbol{\gamma}$. Besides the distinctness of parameters, additional factors are the statistical approach, whether a frequentist evaluation strategy is adopted and whether inferences are made conditional on the pattern of observed and missing values or not.

2.4.1 Frequentist Approach

The frequentist approach considers a function of the observed variables, like an estimator for an unknown parameter or population value, a test statistic or a confidence interval and evaluates these statistics over a hypothesized infinite number of repetitions of exactly the same random experiment. Usually, the number of observations is fixed. Hence the relevant distribution is not (2.6), but the marginal distribution of the variables with observed values conditional on the observed pattern of missing and observed values,

$$\int \frac{f(\mathbf{u}_{(1)}, \mathbf{u}_{(0)} \mid \boldsymbol{\theta}) g(\mathbf{r} \mid \mathbf{u}_{(1)}, \mathbf{u}_{(0)}, \boldsymbol{\gamma})}{\int f(\mathbf{u} \mid \boldsymbol{\theta}) g(\mathbf{r} \mid \mathbf{u}, \boldsymbol{\gamma})\, d\mathbf{u}}\, d\mathbf{u}_{(0)} \tag{2.9}$$

(cf. Rubin, 1976), where $\boldsymbol{\theta}$ is the unknown parameter of interest, $g(\mathbf{r} \mid \mathbf{u}_{(1)}, \mathbf{u}_{(0)}, \boldsymbol{\gamma})$ is the (assumed) missing data mechanism evaluated at the observed value of $\mathbf{r}$ and $\int f(\mathbf{u} \mid \boldsymbol{\theta}) g(\mathbf{r} \mid \mathbf{u}, \boldsymbol{\gamma})\, d\mathbf{u} > 0$ is the marginal probability of the observed pattern of observed and missing values.

Rubin (1976) shows that for fixed $\mathbf{r}$, the distribution of a function of $\mathbf{u}_{(1)}$ using (2.6) is equal to the conditional distribution for the same statistic under (2.9) if the missing data are MCAR. The driving force behind this argument is that $\int f(\mathbf{u} \mid \boldsymbol{\theta}) g(\mathbf{r} \mid \mathbf{u}, \boldsymbol{\gamma})\, d\mathbf{u} = g(\mathbf{r} \mid \mathbf{u}_{(1)}, \mathbf{u}_{(0)}, \boldsymbol{\gamma})$ because, for each $\boldsymbol{\gamma}$, $g(\mathbf{r} \mid \mathbf{u}, \boldsymbol{\gamma})$ takes on the same value for all possible $\mathbf{u}_{(1)}$ and $\mathbf{u}_{(0)}$. Hence, if the missing values are MCAR and inferences are based on fixing $\mathbf{r}$ at the observed pattern in the realized data set, then the missing data mechanism can safely be ignored for frequentist inferences.

However, if missing values are MAR or MNAR at the observed pattern in $\mathbf{r}$, then (2.9) does not simplify to (2.6) because $\int f(\mathbf{u} \mid \boldsymbol{\theta}) g(\mathbf{r} \mid \mathbf{u}, \boldsymbol{\gamma})\, d\mathbf{u} \neq g(\mathbf{r} \mid \mathbf{u}_{(1)}, \mathbf{u}_{(0)}, \boldsymbol{\gamma})$. In that case, the distribution of any function of $\mathbf{u}_{(1)}$ conditional on $\mathbf{r}$ depends on $\mathbf{r}$. Hence, the missing data mechanism cannot in general be ignored for (conditional) frequentist inferences because the probability functions for the pattern of observed and missing values do not cancel out. With increasing sample size, however, the influence of $\mathbf{r}$ on the distribution of functions of $\mathbf{u}_{(1)}$ may decrease so that approximately valid frequentist inferences are possible if missing values are MAR.

If inferences are not conditional on the observed pattern in $\mathbf{r}$ but unconditional, then the relevant distribution for functions of $\mathbf{u}_{(1)}$ is

$$\int f(\mathbf{u} \mid \boldsymbol{\theta}) g(\mathbf{r} \mid \mathbf{u}_{(1)}, \mathbf{u}_{(0)}, \boldsymbol{\gamma})\, d\mathbf{u}_{(0)} . \tag{2.10}$$

Note that the unconditional view corresponds to the everywhere MCAR- or MAR-versions. Missing values are MNAR in this context, if they are not everywhere MCAR or MAR. If inferences are unconditional with respect to $\mathbf{r}$, then the missing data mechanism has to be taken into account in general unless $g(\mathbf{r} \mid \mathbf{u}_{(1)}, \mathbf{u}_{(0)}, \boldsymbol{\gamma}) = 1$ (see Rubin, 1976). Consider (2.10) and assume that missing values are MCAR, then

$$\int f(\mathbf{u} \mid \boldsymbol{\theta}) g(\mathbf{r} \mid \mathbf{u}_{(1)}, \mathbf{u}_{(0)}, \boldsymbol{\gamma})\, d\mathbf{u}_{(0)} = g(\mathbf{r} \mid \boldsymbol{\gamma}) \int f(\mathbf{u} \mid \boldsymbol{\theta})\, d\mathbf{u}_{(0)}$$

and therefore the distribution of every function of $\mathbf{u}_{(1)}$ would depend on $\mathbf{r}$. On the other hand, it turns out that the effect of ignoring the missing data mechanism depends on characteristics like sample size, the missing data mechanism and the function of $\mathbf{u}_{(1)}$ considered. Thus, analyses may still approximately be valid in large samples even when missing values are MCAR or MAR and inferences are unconditional, as will be seen in the next subsection. Strictly speaking for unconditional inferences, a minimum number of observed values are required. Thus, inferences are conditional on a minimum of observed values, the number of which depends on the parameters and models to be estimated.

Example 2.5 (Ignorability and Frequentist Inference (Example 2.4 Cont.)) Consider Example 2.4 and note that there is a missing value only in $u_{5,2}$ and the values of all other variables are observed. Hence the indicator variables r_i are only needed for the variable WAGE, so that $\mathbf{r} = (r_1, \ldots, r_5)^T$ indicates whether values of WAGE variables are observed or not. We now explicitly account for the missing data mechanism and write $g(\mathbf{r} \mid \mathbf{u}_1, \ldots, \mathbf{u}_5) = \prod_{i=1}^{5} g(r_i \mid \mathbf{u}_i)$ for the probability of the observed pattern $\mathbf{r}$ assuming independence conditional on the realized values in $\mathbf{u}_i$, $i = 1, \ldots, 5$.

Then, ignoring the parameters notationally, the density function of the variables $\mathbf{u}_i$ whose values are observed conditional on the pattern of observed and missing values in the $u_{i,1}$ variables, $\mathbf{r} = (1, 1, 1, 1, 0)^T$, is

$$f(\mathbf{u}_{(1)} \mid \mathbf{r}) = \frac{\left[\prod_{i=1}^{4} f(\mathbf{u}_i) g(r_i \mid \mathbf{u}_i)\right]\left[\int f(u_{5,2} \mid u_{5,1}) f(u_{5,1}) g(r_5 \mid u_{5,1}, u_{5,2})\, du_{5,2}\right]}{\prod_{i=1}^{5} \int f(\mathbf{u}_i) g(r_i \mid \mathbf{u}_i)\, d\mathbf{u}_i} .$$

Assuming that for fixed $\mathbf{r}$ and for all possible $\mathbf{u}_i$, $g(r_i \mid \mathbf{u}_i) = g(r_i)$ implies that the missing value is MCAR and thus that the probability functions for $\mathbf{r}$ cancel out, so that

$$f(\mathbf{u}_{(1)} \mid \mathbf{r}) = \left(\prod_{i=1}^{4} f(\mathbf{u}_i)\right) f(v_{5,1}) \, ,$$

which is equal to the marginal distribution of the variables whose values are observed ignoring the missing data mechanism which leads to likelihood function (2.8) (see Example 2.4).

On the other hand, assuming $g(r_i \mid u_{i,1}, u_{i,2}) = g(r_i \mid u_{i,1})$ for all possible values of $u_{i,2}$ and for fixed $\mathbf{r}$, the missing value is MAR,

$$\begin{aligned} f(\mathbf{u}_{(1)} \mid \mathbf{r}) &= \frac{\left[\prod_{i=1}^{4} f(\mathbf{u}_i) g(r_i \mid \mathbf{u}_i)\right]\left[\int f(u_{5,2} \mid u_{5,1}) f(u_{5,1}) g(r_5 \mid u_{5,1}, u_{5,2})\, du_{5,2}\right]}{\prod_{i=1}^{5} \int f(\mathbf{u}_i) g(r_i \mid \mathbf{u}_i)\, d\mathbf{u}_i} \\ &= \frac{\left[\prod_{i=1}^{4} f(\mathbf{u}_i) g(r_i \mid \mathbf{u}_i)\right]\left[f(u_{5,1}) g(r_5 \mid u_{5,1})\right]}{\prod_{i=1}^{5} \int f(\mathbf{u}_i) g(r_i \mid \mathbf{u}_i)\, d\mathbf{u}_i} \end{aligned}$$

and the probability functions for r_i do not cancel out. Hence any function of the variables whose values are observed depends on the missing data mechanism. In general, therefore, the missing data mechanism cannot be ignored in these cases. The same is true when the missing values are MNAR or when inferences are not conditional on $\mathbf{r}$ as can easily be verified. □

2.4.2 Likelihood Approach

If a direct-likelihood approach is adopted, functions of the variables, like estimators, and thus inferences are not evaluated over repeated sampling. Instead, the likelihood at the estimate for an unknown but assumed to be fixed parameter is considered based on the observed data set and compared to the likelihood at other values of the unknown parameter via likelihood ratios (see Rubin, 1987).

Ignoring the missing data mechanism, in this context, means that only the variables $\mathbf{u}_{(1)}$ whose values are observed are considered relevant for inferences. The corresponding marginal likelihood function would be

$$L(\boldsymbol{\theta}) = \int f(\mathbf{u} \mid \boldsymbol{\theta})\, d\mathbf{u}_{(0)}, \quad \boldsymbol{\theta} \in \boldsymbol{\Theta} \, , \tag{2.11}$$

where $\boldsymbol{\theta}$ is an unknown parameter and $\boldsymbol{\Theta}$ its parameters space. However, in the presence of missing data, there are additional random variables, $\mathbf{r}$, that need to be considered as well. Hence, the correct likelihood function would be

$$L(\boldsymbol{\theta}, \boldsymbol{\gamma}) = \int f(\mathbf{u} \mid \boldsymbol{\theta}) g(\mathbf{r} \mid \mathbf{u}, \boldsymbol{\gamma})\, d\mathbf{u}_{(0)} \quad \boldsymbol{\theta}, \boldsymbol{\gamma} \in \boldsymbol{\Omega}\ , \tag{2.12}$$

where $\boldsymbol{\Omega}$ is the joint parameter space of $\boldsymbol{\theta}$ and $\boldsymbol{\gamma}$.

If the missing values are MCAR, then (2.12) simplifies to

$$L(\boldsymbol{\theta}, \boldsymbol{\gamma}) = f(\mathbf{u}_{(1)} \mid \boldsymbol{\theta}) g(\mathbf{r} \mid \boldsymbol{\gamma}) \quad \boldsymbol{\theta}, \boldsymbol{\gamma} \in \boldsymbol{\Omega}$$

and if they are MAR to

$$L(\boldsymbol{\theta}, \boldsymbol{\gamma}) = f(\mathbf{u}_{(1)} \mid \boldsymbol{\theta}) g(\mathbf{r} \mid \mathbf{u}_{(1)}, \boldsymbol{\gamma}) \quad \boldsymbol{\theta}, \boldsymbol{\gamma} \in \boldsymbol{\Omega}\ .$$

Therefore, in both cases and if $g(\mathbf{r} \mid \boldsymbol{\gamma}) > 0$, the likelihood ratio used to evaluate the maximum likelihood estimate $\hat{\boldsymbol{\theta}}$ for $\boldsymbol{\theta}$ relative to some other value $\tilde{\boldsymbol{\theta}}$, $L(\hat{\boldsymbol{\theta}}, \boldsymbol{\gamma})/L(\tilde{\boldsymbol{\theta}}, \boldsymbol{\gamma})$ is the same as the likelihood ratio based on the marginal distribution (2.11), $L(\hat{\boldsymbol{\theta}})/L(\tilde{\boldsymbol{\theta}})$, if the two parameters $\boldsymbol{\theta}$ and $\boldsymbol{\gamma}$ are distinct (Rubin, 1976). Formally, distinctness of the two parameters is equivalent to the Cartesian product of the two parameter spaces, $\boldsymbol{\Omega} = \boldsymbol{\Theta} \times \boldsymbol{\Gamma}$, where $\boldsymbol{\Gamma}$ is the parameter space of $\boldsymbol{\gamma}$. Thus, $\boldsymbol{\Omega}$ is the set of all ordered pairs $\boldsymbol{\theta} \in \boldsymbol{\Theta}$ and $\boldsymbol{\gamma} \in \boldsymbol{\Gamma}$. The above statement about the likelihood ratio does not hold if the parameters $\boldsymbol{\theta}$ and $\boldsymbol{\gamma}$ are not distinct. However, distinctness of parameters is often considered to be a weak assumption and does hold in most situations. On the other hand, even if the parameters are not distinct, then estimators of scientific interest may still be (approximately) unbiased although (asymptotically) not efficient anymore. If the missing values are MNAR, then as is clear from (2.12), the above statements about the likelihood estimator do not hold because $g(\mathbf{r} \mid \mathbf{u}, \boldsymbol{\gamma})$ depends on $\mathbf{u}_{(0)}$.

The above results can also be justified based on the log-likelihood function. If the missing values are MAR, then the appropriate log-likelihood function is

$$l(\boldsymbol{\theta}, \boldsymbol{\gamma}) = \log f(\mathbf{u}_{(1)} \mid \boldsymbol{\theta}) + \log g(\mathbf{r} \mid \mathbf{u}_{(1)}, \boldsymbol{\gamma})\ .$$

Maximizing this log-likelihood function with respect to $\boldsymbol{\theta}$ leads to the same MLE $\hat{\boldsymbol{\theta}}$, as maximizing the (marginal) log-likelihood function $l(\boldsymbol{\theta}) = \log f(\mathbf{u}_{(1)} \mid \boldsymbol{\theta})$ ignoring the missing data mechanism, if $\boldsymbol{\theta}$ and $\boldsymbol{\gamma}$ are distinct. The same is true if the missing data are MCAR and the parameters are distinct. However, the log-likelihood function does not factorize in two additive terms if the missing values are MNAR.

Often likelihood inferences are evaluated from a frequentist point of view. Then the results from Sect. 2.4.1 apply and the missing data mechanism can be ignored if the missing values are MCAR and inferences are conditional on $\mathbf{r}$. If they are unconditional on $\mathbf{r}$ and the missing values are everywhere MCAR, then whatever function of $\mathbf{u}_{(1)}$ is considered, its distribution will depend on the missing data mechanism, although the impact of the missing data mechanism may diminish with increasing sample size. Similarly, if the missing values are MAR and inferences are unconditional or conditional on **r**, then in principle the missing data mechanism has to be taken into account. Again, however, the impact on the frequentist properties depends on sample size and the true data generating process, and inferences may be valid from a frequentist point of view even if missing values are MAR. If the missing values are assumed to be MAR then the standard errors should be calculated based on the observed information matrix, which can be calculated using minus the matrix of second derivatives of the log-likelihood function, and not on the expected information matrix (cf. Kenward & Molenberghs, 1998; Laird, 1988; Little, 1988; Seaman et al., 2013, see Appendix A.3.2). This is often the default in standard software packages, but it may be worth to check. If missing values are MNAR, then inferences can be expected to be invalid in most cases.

Example 2.6 (Conditional vs. Unconditional Inference) Suppose we are interested in the mean of a variable WAGE ($u_{i,2}$) but based on a sample of two variables, WAGE and reaction time ($u_{i,1}$: RT), where $i = 1, \ldots, n$. Sampling from the appropriate population we observe all reaction times but unfortunately not all wages. Hence, in addition to the two variables WAGE and RT, we observe the binary variable r which indicates whether WAGE is observed or not. The true data generating process, including a latent missing data mechanism, is assumed to follow a normal distribution such that

$$\begin{pmatrix} u_{i,1} \\ u_{i,2} \\ r_i^* \end{pmatrix} \sim N\left[\begin{pmatrix} 0 \\ \mu_2 \\ 0 \end{pmatrix}, \begin{pmatrix} 1 & \rho_{1,2} & \rho_{1,3} \\ \rho_{1,2} & 1 & \rho_{2,3} \\ \rho_{1,3} & \rho_{2,3} & 1 \end{pmatrix}\right],$$

where it is assumed that only μ_2 is unknown. Note that the other variables have expected value equal to zero and all variances are one.

The value of WAGE of unit i is observed if $r_i = 1$ and is not observed if $r_i = 0$, where $r_i = 1$ if $r_i^* \leq c$ and $r_i = 0$ otherwise. With these assumptions the unknown parameter μ_2 can be estimated by the method of maximum likelihood. The estimator $\hat{\mu}_2$ and its variance ignoring the missing data mechanism is given in Appendix A.3.2.1.

To illustrate the effect of inferences unconditional vs. conditional on **r** when the missing data mechanism is ignored, we simulated 100,000 data sets of size $n = 20$ and $n = 200$ each. We then generated missing values in WAGE by choosing c such that approximately 50% of the WAGE values are missing. Missing values are either MCAR or MAR. To generate values that are MCAR, we adopted

$$\mathbf{R} = \begin{pmatrix} 1 & 0.5 & 0 \\ 0.5 & 1 & 0 \\ 0 & 0 & 1 \end{pmatrix}$$

implying a correlation $\rho_{1,2} = 0.5$ only between $u_{i,1}$ and $u_{i,2}$, i.e., in a linear regression relationship $u_{i,1}$ and $u_{i,2}$ have no effect on r_i^* and hence on r_i. To generate missing values being MAR we used

$$\mathbf{R} = \begin{pmatrix} 1 & 0.5 & 0.8 \\ 0.5 & 1 & 0.4 \\ 0.8 & 0.4 & 1 \end{pmatrix}$$

which implies that

$$r_i^* = u_{i,1}\, 0.8 + \epsilon_i \quad \epsilon_i \sim N(0, 0.36)$$

and hence, that only $u_{i,1}$ has an effect on the probability of observing $u_{i,2}$. Thus, the missing values in the variables $u_{i,2}$ are MAR.

Table 2.1 presents the results of the simulation study with approximately 50% values missing completely at random (MCAR) or missing at random (MAR). In addition, inferences for μ_2 are unconditional or conditional on $\mathbf{r}$. The table shows the mean and standard deviation of the estimates over the 100,000 simulations, the square root of the (estimated) variances (standard error, se), the skewness, excess kurtosis and coverage of the true values ($\mu_2 = 0$) by 0.95-confidence intervals.

The results in Table 2.1 do not imply any bias in the ML estimator of μ_2 under all conditions. The standard deviations of the estimates over the simulation (sd) are very similar to the mean standard errors if inferences are not conditional on $\mathbf{r}$ or if $n = 200$. If inferences are conditional on $\mathbf{r}$ and the sample size is small, the differences in the variances and the mean estimated variances are slightly larger. However, the coverage rates are acceptable under all conditions. Note that each simulation is a binary experiment with possible outcomes being that the true value is covered by the confidence interval or not. With 100,000 trials and $\alpha = 0.05$, the coverage rates should be in the interval $0.95 \pm 1.96\sqrt{0.95 * 0.05/100{,}000}$, i.e.,

Table 2.1 ML estimation of μ_2: Mean (mean), standard deviation (sd), standard error (se), skewness (skew), excess kurtosis (exkurt) and coverage rates (cover) of true parameter values for μ_2

Inference	mdm	n	Miss	Mean	sd	se	Skew	Exkurt	Cover
Conditional	MCAR	20	0.500	0.0005	0.2731	0.2822	0.0007	−0.0014	0.9489
		200	0.500	−0.0002	0.0865	0.0869	0.0036	0.0061	0.9507
	MAR	20	0.500	0.0005	0.2732	0.2807	0.0014	0.0010	0.9484
		200	0.500	−0.0002	0.0865	0.0865	0.0039	0.0038	0.9495
Unconditional	MCAR	20	0.501	−0.0003	0.2814	0.2822	−0.0030	−0.1951	0.9496
		200	0.501	−0.0001	0.0868	0.0869	0.0200	−0.0341	0.9504
	MAR	20	0.497	−0.0002	0.2807	0.2807	0.0009	−0.2062	0.9493
		200	0.496	−0.0003	0.0864	0.0865	−0.0021	−0.0072	0.9503

Inferences conditional and unconditional on $\mathbf{r}$. Sample size n, missing data mechanism (mdm), fraction of missing values (miss). True value of $\mu_2 = 0$. See text for details

approximately [0.9486, 0.9514]. There are no conspicuities with respect to skewness under all conditions. In the small sample condition under the unconditional inference however, the excess kurtosis deviates negatively somewhat from zero, so the distributions of the estimates are slightly flatter than the normal distribution. However, this seems to have no effect on the coverage rates as they are still in the acceptable range. □

This example illustrates that ML based inferences may be valid even if the estimator is evaluated from a frequentist perspective conditional on **r** and the missing values are MAR or, unconditional, if they are everywhere MCAR or MAR. Note that although the fraction of missing values is high, the consequences with respect to the distribution of the estimator under the unconditional evaluation condition are not severe in this artificial example. This illustration should not carelessly be generalized, but it may imply that in many applications where the fraction of missing values is not too high and even if the distribution of the estimator of interest may deviate from the desired distribution, inferences may approximately be valid under a frequentist evaluation if the missing values are (everywhere) MCAR or MAR. The next example illustrates the effects of using the observed versus the expected information to estimate the variance of ML estimators.

Example 2.7 (Observed vs. Expected Information) Assume the same situation as in Example 2.6, but now μ_2 and $\rho_{1.2}$ are unknown and need to be estimated which will again be done by the method of maximum likelihood ignoring the missing data mechanism. First and second derivatives for maximum likelihood inferences are given in Appendix A.3.2.2.

To illustrate the effect of using the observed versus the expected information to calculate the standard errors, we simulated 10,000 data sets of size $n = 1000$ each. We then generated missing values in WAGE by choosing c such that approximately 50% of the WAGE values are missing. Missing values are either MCAR or MAR. To generate missing values we adopted the same correlation matrices **R** as in Example 2.6.

The results in Table 2.2 imply that the ML estimators seem to be approximately unbiased and that inferences using the observed information is valid if missing values are MCAR or MAR whether inferences are conditional on **r** or not. On the other hand, inferences using the expected information are valid only if the missing values are MCAR. If they are MAR, then the coverage rates are between approximately 90–92% percent. Two points should be noted, however. First, the sample size is large. This illustrates that the underestimation of the variance of the ML estimator using the expected information is not a small sample problem. In fact, we found the same result in smaller samples. Second, the fraction of missing values is around 50% which is large. Decreasing this fraction leads to better coverage rates. Thus, this phenomenon may not be a big problem in many real world applications, where the fraction of missing values is often smaller. □

Table 2.2 ML estimation: Mean (mean), standard deviation (sd), standard error based on observed (se.o) and expected (se.e) information and coverage rates (cover.o and cover.e) of true parameter values for μ_{WAGE} and $\rho_{1,2}$ (true)

			True	Mean	sd	se.o	Cover.o	se.e	Cover.e
Conditional	MCAR	μ_2	0	−0.0006	0.0388	0.0387	0.9467	0.0386	0.9464
		$\rho_{1,2}$	0.5	0.5009	0.0301	0.0311	0.9570	0.0311	0.9561
	MAR	μ_2	0	−0.0002	0.0450	0.0455	0.9497	0.0391	0.9097
		$\rho_{1,2}$	0.5	0.5011	0.0346	0.0363	0.9593	0.0311	0.9204
Unconditional	MCAR	μ_2	0	0.0000	0.0386	0.0388	0.9504	0.0387	0.9503
		$\rho_{1,2}$	0.5	0.5012	0.0302	0.0311	0.9530	0.0310	0.9526
	MAR	μ_2	0	0.0005	0.0445	0.0452	0.9543	0.0387	0.9104
		$\rho_{1,2}$	0.5	0.5005	0.0351	0.0365	0.9578	0.0314	0.9199

Inferences unconditional and conditional on **r**

2.4.3 *Bayesian Approach*

Within a Bayesian framework the posterior distribution of the parameter of interest $\boldsymbol{\theta}$ given the observed data is of major interest (see Sects. 1.5.2 and 1.8). Ignoring the missing data mechanism in a missing data context means to base inferences on

$$\int f(\mathbf{u} \mid \boldsymbol{\theta})\, d\mathbf{u}_{(0)}\; p(\boldsymbol{\theta}) ,$$

which is proportional to the posterior distribution of $\boldsymbol{\theta}$ given the observed values in $\mathbf{u}_{(1)}$ and where $p(\boldsymbol{\theta})$ is the prior distribution of $\boldsymbol{\theta}$.

However, in the presence of missing data, analyses are not only conditional on the observed values of $\mathbf{u}_{(1)}$ but also on the observed pattern in $\mathbf{r}$. Thus the correct joint posterior distribution of $\boldsymbol{\theta}$ and $\boldsymbol{\gamma}$ is proportional to

$$\int f(\mathbf{u} \mid \boldsymbol{\theta}) g(\mathbf{r} \mid \mathbf{u}, \boldsymbol{\gamma})\, d\mathbf{u}_{(0)}\; p(\boldsymbol{\theta}, \boldsymbol{\gamma}) ,$$

where $p(\boldsymbol{\theta}, \boldsymbol{\gamma})$ is the joint prior distribution of $\boldsymbol{\theta}$ and $\boldsymbol{\gamma}$.

Rubin (1976) shows that if the missing data are MAR and if $\boldsymbol{\theta}$ and $\boldsymbol{\gamma}$ are distinct, i.e., $p(\boldsymbol{\theta}, \boldsymbol{\gamma}) = p(\boldsymbol{\theta}) p(\boldsymbol{\gamma})$, then the missing data mechanism can be ignored for Bayesian non-frequentist analyses, because then the joint posterior distribution of $\boldsymbol{\theta}$ and $\boldsymbol{\gamma}$ is proportional to the simpler expression

$$[f(\mathbf{u}_{(1)} \mid \boldsymbol{\theta}) p(\boldsymbol{\theta})][g(\mathbf{r} \mid \mathbf{u}_{(1)}, \boldsymbol{\gamma}) p(\boldsymbol{\gamma})] ,$$

where only the left term in parentheses depends on $\boldsymbol{\theta}$ and thus inferences with respect to $\boldsymbol{\theta}$ do not depend on the missing data mechanism.

Similar to the likelihood case, if the missing data are MAR at all **r** and the parameters are distinct, then the missing data mechanism may be ignored in large samples even in frequentist analyses. To estimate variances, again, the observed instead of the expected information matrix should be adopted.

2.5 Supplementary Notes

Assumptions about the missing data mechanism are fundamental with respect to the further handling of the missing data problem. An important question is whether a missing data mechanism can be ignored. If a missing data mechanism is ignorable, then valid inferences are possible based on the variables whose values are observed and assumptions about their distributions. Otherwise, if the missing data mechanism is non-ignorable, then usually untestable explicit assumptions about the unknown missing data mechanism have to be made. Often, however, the situation is not so clear.

Firstly, one should be aware that the missing data mechanism may differ over variables and units even within one given data set. Hence for one variable it may be plausible to assume that the missing values are MCAR, for example, for a neutral question in a questionnaire, while for a delicate variable in the same data set they may be MNAR. Correspondingly, there may be groups of units whose response behaviour differs for the same variable. For example, the tendency of adolescents to answer embarrassing questions may, in contrast to adults, decrease with the intensity of the question, even after controlling for other variables.

Secondly, ignorability of the missing data mechanism does not mean that the standard analyses applied to the completely observed part of the data set can in general be adopted. For example, if the missing values in a data set are MAR, then all the relevant observed values in the data set should be used to allow valid inferences as ignoring those observed values which have an effect on the probability of observing values are then MNAR (for example, if μ_1 would have to be estimated in Example 2.6, all observed $u_{i,1}$ values would have to be used). This means that standard software can often not be used because the data set is not rectangular anymore. But even if all the missing values in a data set are MCAR, then using only the completely observed part, i.e., ignoring all the incompletely observed units, leads to a loss of information. On the other hand, if it is not clear what missing data technique to apply, it may be safer to just use the completely observed part of the data set, if all missing values are MCAR, as applying an improper technique may lead to invalid inferences.

Thirdly, whether or not a missing data mechanism is ignorable or not depends on the variables in the data set, their relationships and the intended analysis. For example, suppose a data set consists of two variables, mean hourly wage (u_i: WAGE) and number of children living in the household (v_i: NCHILD). Assume further, that only WAGE is affected by missing values. If the probability of observing or not observing WAGE depends on NCHILD but not in addition on WAGE itself, then the missing WAGE values are MAR if both variables are included in the intended analysis. Now suppose that the probability of observing or not observing WAGE values depends on NCHILD but WAGE and NCHILD are independent. Then, ignoring the variable NCHILD means that the marginal distribution of WAGE is considered, which in the presence of missing data with fixed **r**, leads to

$$\int\int \frac{f(\mathbf{u},\boldsymbol{\theta}_u)f(\mathbf{v},\boldsymbol{\theta}_v)g(\mathbf{r}\mid \mathbf{u}_{(1)},\mathbf{u}_{(0)},\mathbf{v},\boldsymbol{\gamma})}{\int\int f(\mathbf{u},\boldsymbol{\theta}_u)f(\mathbf{v},\boldsymbol{\theta}_v)g(\mathbf{r}\mid \mathbf{u},\mathbf{v},\boldsymbol{\gamma})\,d\mathbf{v}\,d\mathbf{u}}\,d\mathbf{v}\,d\mathbf{u}_{(0)} = f(\mathbf{u}_{(1)},\boldsymbol{\theta}_u)\,,$$

where $\mathbf{u} = (u_1,\ldots,u_n)^T$, $\mathbf{v} = (v_1,\ldots,v_n)^T$, $\boldsymbol{\theta}_u$ and $\boldsymbol{\theta}_v$ are the parameters governing the corresponding marginal distributions and $\boldsymbol{\gamma}$ is the parameter of the missing data mechanism, because $g(\mathbf{r}\mid \mathbf{u}_{(1)},\mathbf{u}_{(0)},\mathbf{v},\boldsymbol{\gamma}) = g(\mathbf{r}\mid \mathbf{u},\mathbf{v},\boldsymbol{\gamma}) = g(\mathbf{r}\mid \mathbf{v},\boldsymbol{\gamma})$ (Sect. 2.3.1). Thus, the missing data mechanism can be ignored.

A more realistic scenario is one in which we are interested in the regression of WAGE on NCHILD. If the probability of the observed pattern of observed and missing values in WAGE is assumed to depend on NCHILD but to be the same for all possible values of WAGE given NCHILD, then

$$\int \frac{f(\mathbf{u}\mid \mathbf{v},\boldsymbol{\theta})g(\mathbf{r}\mid \mathbf{u}_{(1)},\mathbf{u}_{(0)},\mathbf{v},\boldsymbol{\gamma})}{\int f(\mathbf{u}\mid \mathbf{v},\boldsymbol{\theta})g(\mathbf{r}\mid \mathbf{u},\mathbf{v},\boldsymbol{\gamma})\,d\mathbf{u}}\,d\mathbf{u}_{(0)} = f(\mathbf{u}_{(1)}\mid \mathbf{v},\boldsymbol{\theta})\,, \tag{2.13}$$

again because $g(\mathbf{r}\mid \mathbf{u}_{(1)},\mathbf{u}_{(0)},\mathbf{v},\boldsymbol{\gamma}) = g(\mathbf{r}\mid \mathbf{u},\mathbf{v},\boldsymbol{\gamma}) = g(\mathbf{r}\mid \mathbf{v},\boldsymbol{\gamma})$, where $\boldsymbol{\theta}$ is the parameter governing the conditional distribution of $\mathbf{u}\mid\mathbf{v}$. If we further assume that $f(\mathbf{u}\mid \mathbf{v},\boldsymbol{\theta})$ can be factorized into $\prod_{i=1}^{n} f(u_i\mid v_i,\boldsymbol{\theta})$ and that the distribution of $u_i\mid v_i$ is the same for all $i = 1,\ldots,n$, which is a standard assumption in regression analysis, then the missing data mechanism is ignorable in the typical regression context, i.e., analyses based on the completely observed part of the data set allow valid inferences. But (2.13) together with the independence assumption implies an even stronger result allowing missing values also in v_i. To see this, note that

$$\begin{aligned}
&\int f(\mathbf{u}\mid \mathbf{v},\boldsymbol{\theta})g(\mathbf{r}\mid \mathbf{u}_{(1)},\mathbf{u}_{(0)},\mathbf{v},\boldsymbol{\gamma})\,d\mathbf{u}_{(0)}\\
&= \Big[\prod_{i\in \mathrm{obs}(\mathbf{u})} f(u_i\mid v_i,\boldsymbol{\theta})\Big] g(\mathbf{r}\mid \mathbf{v},\boldsymbol{\gamma}) \int \prod_{i\in \mathrm{mis}(\mathbf{u})} f(u_i\mid v_i,\boldsymbol{\theta})\,du_i\\
&= \prod_{i\in \mathrm{obs}(\mathbf{u})} f(u_i\mid v_i,\boldsymbol{\theta})g(\mathbf{r}\mid \mathbf{v},\boldsymbol{\gamma})\,,
\end{aligned}$$

where $\mathrm{mis}(\mathbf{u})$ is the set of all i for which the value of u_i is missing and $\mathrm{obs}(\mathbf{u})$ is the set of all i for which the value of u_i is observed. Furthermore, $\int f(\mathbf{u}\mid \mathbf{v},\boldsymbol{\theta})g(\mathbf{r}\mid \mathbf{u},\mathbf{v},\boldsymbol{\gamma})\,d\mathbf{u} = g(\mathbf{r}\mid \mathbf{v},\boldsymbol{\gamma})$. Hence, (2.13) can be written as $\prod_{i\in \mathrm{obs}(\mathbf{u})} f(u_i\mid v_i,\boldsymbol{\theta})$. Note that in this case the missing values in v_i are even MNAR. Thus, if the probability of observing or not observing values in the dependent variable depends on the values of the independent variable, the values of the independent variable are completely observed if the dependent variable is observed, but some units are missing completely, then a standard regression analysis based only on the completely observed units still allows valid inferences, if the model is (approximately) correctly specified.

Fourthly, it seems worth noting that the missing data mechanism is conceptualized as a statistical model that creates binary outcomes. Thus it is a model like any other statistical model for binary outcomes. The model could be based on an underlying continuous variable or on classes, it could almost perfectly predict the observed pattern of observed and missing values or the binary variable could hardly be explained by other variables, in which case the missing values would be close to MCAR. The difference between models with a latent continuous variable and those based on latent classes seems to be only minor with respect to the consequences of the missing data mechanism. But a strong missing data mechanism with high predictive power may tend to create selective missing patterns in the incompletely observed variables.

Let us consider two variables, and assume that they are non-linearly related. For example, if a wage equation is estimated to assess the effect of experience on wage, the dependent variables in the corresponding regression model is usually the natural logarithm of wage and, in addition to other variables, experience as well as experience squared enter the model as predictors (e.g., Heckman, Lochner, & Todd, 2006).

Thus, the relationship between wage and experience is assumed to be non-linear. Suppose now that all wage values but not all values of experience are observed and that the missing values are missing at random. That is, the probability of observing experience depends on wage. Assume further, that the missing data mechanism is highly selective in that individuals with high wage do not respond to the experience question with high probability as compared to those with a lower wage. If the relationship between the two variables wage and experience is unknown and non-linear in that area or, more generally, if the missing data mechanism is highly selective and thins out certain regions in sample space of high curvature of the corresponding regression relationship then there may be not enough observations left to be used by a semi- or non-parametric method to compensate for missing data based on observed information. Therefore, in this region, information from outside the data set would be needed, like adopting a restrictive parametric model about the relationship of the two variables.

To illustrate this situation, we generated 100,000 data pairs $(u_i \;\; v_i)^T$ independently from each other according to a positive non-linear relationship and deleted approximately 30% of the values in v conditional on the observed values in u. The missing data mechanism is selective in that the probability of not observing v is high in the class of large u-values relative to the other u-values, but the missing values are MAR.

The framed white area in Fig. 2.4 is approximately the area where the completely observed data points are located. The grey area including the framed white area approximately represents the area populated by the realized data points. Note that the areas do not show densities of the variables and the bounds of the areas do not represent exact bounds. Since the true relationship between v and u is assumed to be unknown, we used spline regression and added the smoothed curves to the

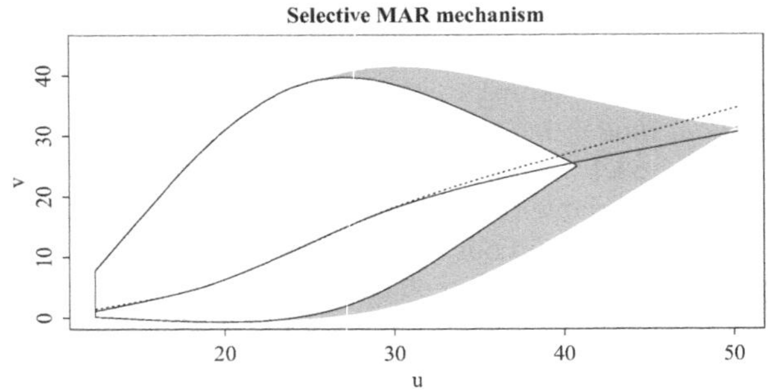

Fig. 2.4 Grey and white area: realized data points; framed white area: observed data points. Estimated non-linear regression function from v on u based on realized data (solid line) and completely observed pairs (dashed line)

graph. The solid line is calculated using all realized data points. The slope of this curve decreases at $u \approx 30$ as compared to the slope in the interval between approximately 22 and 30. At the same time the number of missing values starts to increase dramatically around this u-value. Hence, to calculate the non-linear smoothed regression line for the completely observed part of the data set, not much information is available beyond $u \approx 30$ and the dashed regression line calculated using the observed part of the sample differs from the solid line. Thus, the probability of observing values in that region may be so low that certain areas of the sample space are virtually not populated even in large samples. This may in extreme cases lead to invalid estimated relationships if information from the observed part drives the estimation of the relationship in the unobserved part. Therefore, outliers in the observed part of a sample may be valid observations from these areas and should therefore not be ignored unless the corresponding sub-population from which they are sampled is explicitly excluded from inferences.

Finally, there are two missing data situations that are worth taking a look at. In a first scenario, no values are observed at all in which case the missing values are either MCAR or MNAR. Because there are no observed values, the missing values cannot be MAR. Then, the sampling process can simply be repeated if the missing values are MCAR. If they are MNAR then the research question, the sampling process or the measurement instrument should probably be revised and a new sample should be selected. In a second scenario the sample is completely observed, but it is known that in exactly the same situation of data collection missing values can occur. Since there are no missing values, the actual missing data mechanism creates either missing values which are MCAR or MAR but not MNAR.

2.6 Diagnostic Tools

In this section we will introduce tools for displaying the frequencies, nonresponse patterns and possible clustering of binary response indicators. We will also discuss two techniques proposed to test the null hypothesis of missing values being MCAR. To illustrate the techniques, we generated a data set with four variables $(u_1, \ldots, u_4)^T$ for $n = 500$ units. Variables u_1 and u_4 are continuous variables, u_2 is a binary variable and u_3 is a count variable. Missing values being MAR are then generated in u_2, u_3 and u_4.

For a general overview, a first step in a descriptive analysis is to look at the marginal distributions of the variable values in the sample. In R (R Core Team, 2018) this can be accomplished by using the function `summary`, which gives the minimum, the maximum, the first and the third quartiles, the median or second quartile and the mean as well as the number of missing values for each variable in the data set.

These statistics give a first impression about the distribution of the observed values for each variable in the data set, including the response indicators. Note that the distribution suggested by these statistics refers to the distribution of the observed values only. If the missing data are not MCAR, then true distributions are likely to differ from those implied by the descriptive statistics. For example, a normally distributed variable may be transformed into a variable that follows a skewed distribution by applying the missing data mechanism and deleting values for which $r = 0$. Thus, the observed distribution in a data set should not be confused with the empirical distribution of the same variable one would get if there were no missing values.

The number of missing values gives an idea what a method to compensate for missing values is expected to manage: With an increasing number of missing values, the impact of the method to compensate for missing values on the final inferences of scientific interest increases relative to the method adopted to answer the scientifically interesting questions. This impact, however, should not get too strong because the methods to compensate for missing values often include assumptions which are less well justified as compared to assumptions needed for the applied-scientifically interesting model. If these assumptions are violated and the method to compensate for missing values has a strong impact, then the final inferences are likely to be invalid. As we will see in Chap. 4, however, the important criterion is the amount of missing information (see Sect. 4.3), which is only roughly approximated by the number of missing values.

Example 2.8 (Descriptive Statistics) Table 2.3 presents some basic statistics, created with the `summary` command in R (R Core Team, 2018), for each variable in the artificial data set.

Comparing the minimum with the maximum, the first quartile with the third quartile and the median with the mean of u_1 in Table 2.3 implies that the distribution of the values in the sample is rather symmetric. In fact, the values were generated from a normal distribution. Variable u_2 is a binary variable, the proportion of ones

Table 2.3 Minimum (Min.), first quartile (1st Qu.), median (Median), mean (Mean), third quartile (3rd Qu.), maximum (Max.) and number of missing values (NA's) for variables $u_1, \ldots, u_4$ in created data set with 500 units

	u_1	u_2	u_3	u_4
Min.	−12.2596	0.0000	0.0000	0.00008
1st Qu.	−0.8089	0.0000	0.0000	1.34573
Median	2.1138	0.0000	1.0000	3.05341
Mean	2.0025	0.2826	0.9258	4.88034
3rd Qu.	4.8370	1.0000	2.0000	6.24586
Max.	12.4866	1.0000	5.0000	31.91475
NA's	0	139	109	104

Table 2.4 Missing data pattern of simulated data set with $n = 500$

	$u.1$	u.4	u.3	u.2	
225	1	1	1	1	0
89	1	1	1	0	1
57	1	1	0	1	1
60	1	0	1	1	1
25	1	1	0	0	2
17	1	0	1	0	2
19	1	0	0	1	2
8	1	0	0	0	3
	0	104	109	139	352

First column: Number of units with the pattern given by 0's and 1's in column 2–5. Last column: Number of zeros in pattern. Last row: Number of missing values in the variables, with last entry being equal to the overall number of missing values

being 0.2826, with 139 missing values, which amounts to a proportion of 28.26%. Variable u_3 is a count variable and has 109 or 21.8% missing values, and u_4 is skewed to the right and has 104 or 20.8% missing values. Hence, the overall proportion of missing values is 17.6%. The proportions of missing values seem not to be too large so that handling the problem by some method to compensate for missing data may be appropriate. □

A second descriptive technique is the pattern of missing values (see Sect. 1.4). Since a monotone pattern simplifies the handling of missing values significantly, as will be seen in Chap. 4, it is worthwhile to have a look at the missing pattern. The package `mice` (van Buuren & Groothuis-Oudshoorn, 2011) in R (R Core Team, 2018) provides the function `md.pattern` to do the job. It displays for each pattern of missing values illustrated by a 0 for a missing value and 1 for an observed value, the number of units with this pattern. Additionally, for each variable the number of missing values is given as well as the overall number of missing values.

Example 2.9 (Descriptive Statistics: Missing Pattern (Example 2.8 Cont.)) Table 2.4 presents the output of the function `md.pattern` from the R-package `mice` (van Buuren & Groothuis-Oudshoorn, 2011) for the simulated data set. The number of occurrences of the pattern of observed and missing values in the data set is given in the first column and the number of zeros, i.e., the number of missing values in that particular pattern is given in the last column. The pattern spreads over the columns named after the variable names in the data set. The last line gives the number of missing values for the corresponding variables and the rightmost entry in the last line the number of missing values in the data set.

Table 2.4 reveals that the pattern of missing values is not monotone. Actually, if we would delete all observations that do not fit into a monotone missing pattern, we would have to delete 153 units. □

As a result of the discussion in the last section, it might be of interest whether missing values in one variable, say y, are MCAR or MAR and possibly clustered in a certain region of another variable, say x, with less or no missing values. If the distribution of missing values in y is proportional to the distribution of x-values, then they tend to be MCAR if it can be ruled out that they are MNAR. If the two variables y and x are related and if the missing values are not proportionally distributed relative to x, then missing values in y are MAR and if they are concentrated in certain regions of possible x-values, the missing data mechanism systematically tends to thin out regions in y. This can be visualized in R (R Core Team, 2018) by adding tick marks to the x-axis of a scatter plot for each missing value in y. Of course, one could also add corresponding tick marks to the y-axis to illustrate the missing values in x for which a y-values has been observed. Note, however, that if there are missing values in y and x, the corresponding data points will not be displayed. Hence, this graphic can, again, only give a rough idea about the relationship of y, x and the response indicator.

Example 2.10 (Descriptive Statistics: Clustered Missing Values (Example 2.8 Cont.)) Figure 2.5 shows scatter plots for two pairs of variables, $(u_4\ u_1)^T$ and

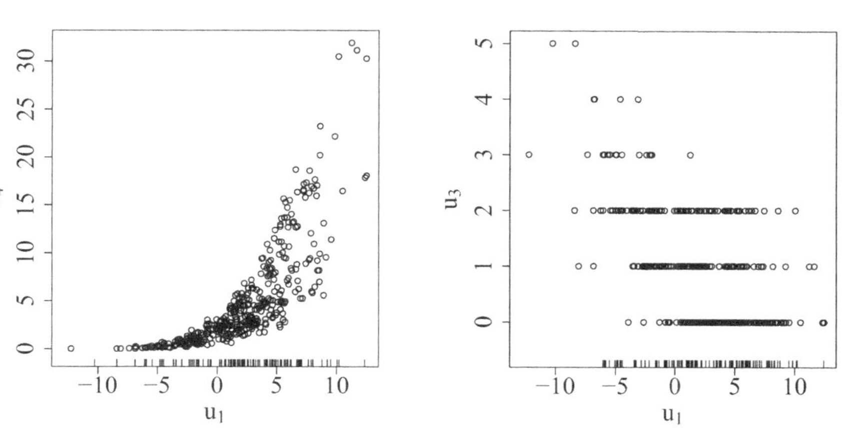

Fig. 2.5 Scatter plots for u_4 versus u_1 and u_3 versus u_1 for the simulated data set, $n = 500$. Completely observed pairs are represented by dots, observed x-values with unobserved y-values by extra tick marks at the x-axis

$(u_3\ u_1)^T$. Only completely observed pairs are represented by dots. Values observed for the x-variable but not for the y-variable are represented by tick marks on the x-axis pointing inwards the graph. These latter plots are also called rug plots. Note that there are no missing values in u_1.

Figure 2.5 implies that the observed values in u_4 and u_1 are non-linearly related and that missing values in u_4 are not clustered in the extreme regions of u_1. Missing values occur mainly in an area with high density of u_4-values. Assuming that the missing values are not MNAR, there is no evidence that the missing data mechanism is selective and thins out regions of high curvature. The results for u_3 versus u_1 are very similar. The observed data points imply a relationship but the missing values are not clustered in sparsely populated regions given that the missing values are not MNAR. It should be noted that the MAR assumption is crucial for the conclusions. In both cases missing values could be MNAR and the unobserved values could lie in a region where no u_3 or u_4 respectively is observed.

Figure 2.6 shows the same kind of scatter plots based on the same simulated data set. Again missing values are MAR, but now the missing data mechanism is highly selective. The left graphic implies that the probability of missing values in u_4 is very high for values in u_1 which are larger than approximately five, whereas this probability is low for smaller values. Similarly, the probability of not observing values in u_3 is large for values of u_1 below approximately one. In both cases the distribution of the response indicators is not proportional to the distribution of u_1.

□

Other techniques to describe possible relationships are easily available in R. For example, one could use the `plot` or `ggplot` statements to produce histograms of the proportions of missing values in y for a categorical variable x or classes of x,

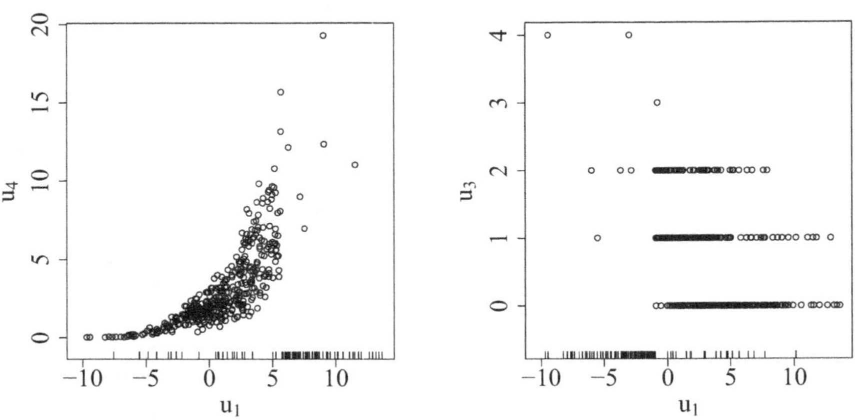

Fig. 2.6 Scatter plots for u_4 versus u_1 and u_3 versus u_1 for the simulated data set, $n = 500$. Completely observed pairs are represented by dots, observed x-values with unobserved y-values by extra tick marks at the x-axis

for example defined by its deciles. Such a graphic may give an idea of whether the missing values may not be MCAR with respect to the involved variable values in the data set.

Unfortunately, there is no general procedure that allows a distinction between missing values being MAR or MNAR. However, there are methods to test the null hypothesis that the missing values are MCAR. Little (1988) proposes a test statistic which is based on first identifying the missing data patterns, indexed by $j = 1, \ldots, J$, and then calculating the means $\bar{\mathbf{y}}_{(1),j}$ of the observed variables within each pattern. If the missing values in a data set are MCAR, then the expected values of the variables are the same for all observed missing data patterns and should be equal to the expected values of these variables over all possible missing data patterns. Therefore, in a further step, the mean $\boldsymbol{\mu}$ and the covariance matrix $\boldsymbol{\Sigma}$ of all variables over all missing data patterns under the assumption of ignorability and common normality are estimated. Let $\hat{\boldsymbol{\mu}}_{(1),j}$ and $\widehat{\boldsymbol{\Sigma}}_{(1),j}$ be those parts of the estimators $\hat{\boldsymbol{\mu}}$ and positive definite $\widehat{\boldsymbol{\Sigma}}$ which correspond to the variables observed in the jth group. Then the test statistic proposed by Little (1988) is

$$d^2 = \sum_{j=1}^{J} n_j (\bar{\mathbf{y}}_{(1),j} - \hat{\boldsymbol{\mu}}_{(1),j})^T \widehat{\boldsymbol{\Sigma}}_{(1),j}^{-1} (\bar{\mathbf{y}}_{(1),j} - \hat{\boldsymbol{\mu}}_{(1),j}) ,$$

where n_j is the number of observations in the jth group. Obviously, $d^2 \geq 0$ and if the missing values are MCAR then d^2 should be close to zero. Denote by p_j the number of variables observed in the jth group and p be the number of variables in the data set. Following Little (1988), if the covariance matrix can consistently be estimated then d^2 is approximately χ^2-distributed with $df = (\sum_j p_j) - p$ degrees of freedom in large samples even if the assumption of normality does not hold.

Under the normality assumption, Little (1988) derived the finite sample distribution of d^2 for the special case of a monotone missing pattern, which is still impracticable. In large samples, however, the normality assumption is not crucial. On the other hand, the test may only be appropriate if the variables are quantitative (see Little, 1988) or, depending on the sample size, at least a mixture of quantitative and binary variables. An additional assumption is that the covariance matrix does not differ over the missing data patterns and that the parameters of the missing data mechanism and the multivariate normal model are distinct. Consequences of violations of these assumptions might be a loss of power of the test, but may have only minor effects on the large sample results.

Example 2.11 (Diagnostic: Little's MCAR Test (Example 2.8 Cont.)) Little's MCAR test (Little, 1988) is realized in the `LittleMCAR` function of the R-package (R Core Team, 2018) `BaylorEdPsych` (Beaujean, 2012). Applying this test to the simulated data from example 2.8 gives $d^2 = 183.0216$ with $df = 16$ and a p-value close to zero. Hence, on a 0.05-alpha level one would reject the null hypothesis that the missing values are MCAR, which would, in this example, be a correct decision. □

2.7 Summary

The missing data mechanism is the process that generates the binary response variable indicating whether values of the variables in the data set are observed or not. The assumed missing data mechanism governed by an usually unknown parameter plays a central role in deciding how to deal with a missing data problem.

If the probability for the observed pattern of missing and not-missing values in a data set does not depend on any of the variables in the data set, then the missing values are said to be missing completely at random (MCAR). If the missing data are MCAR, then for the fixed response pattern any inferential analysis ignoring the missing data mechanism will allow valid inferences if all assumptions needed in case of no missing values are met.

If the observed pattern of the binary indicator is not considered to be fixed, usually in combination with a frequentist evaluation of the statistical inference tools, then some additional points have to be considered. The most important is that in small samples the distributions of statistics of interest are usually different from the distributions of the same statistics if the response pattern is fixed at the observed pattern. However, with increasing sample sizes, this problem may vanish in many situations of practical interest.

If missing values are MCAR, then one could simply ignore all the incompletely observed units and apply standard techniques for completely observed data sets, because the completely observed part of the data set is just a non-selective sub-sample. However, ignoring all incompletely observed cases is generally equivalent to ignoring a large amount of information. Thus a better choice would be to adopt a technique that uses all the information available in the data set, a strategy that usually precludes standard analysis tools. Going one step further, one could adopt a method that explicitly deals with the missing data problem and at the same time avoids ignoring information. This, however, calls for additional modeling assumptions which, if violated, may lead to invalid inferential results.

The missing values are called missing at random (MAR) if the probability for the observed pattern of missing and not-missing values in the data set, given the observed values, does not depend on the variables whose values have not been observed. If, in addition, the parameter of the model of scientific interest and the parameter of the missing data mechanism are not related to each other, i.e., if they are distinct, then statistical inferences are valid ignoring the missing data mechanism if a direct-likelihood or a Bayesian approach is adopted for a fixed pattern of observed and not-observed values. Note that this does not imply that in general the missing data or the incompletely observed part of the data set can be ignored. In fact, usually, more complex techniques have to be adopted that properly account for the non-rectangular data set and respect the relationships between variables. Usually in applications the MLE is calculated and its frequentist properties are utilized. For valid inferences in small samples this would require that the missing values are MCAR. However, in large samples MAR is generally sufficient if the observed information instead of the expected information is used to estimate the covariance matrix of the MLE. Most methods to compensate for missing values assume that the missing data are MAR.

Finally, if the missing values are neither MCAR nor MAR, they are missing not at random (MNAR), sometimes also denoted as not missing at random. Then the missing data mechanism is not ignorable in general and additional assumptions about the missing data mechanism and the process that generates the variables of interest are needed to allow valid inferences.

Several descriptive techniques to gain some insight in the relationship between observed values and the binary response indicators in the data set as well as a test on missing data being MCAR are available. Proportions of missing data for each variable may help to roughly access the amount of missing information. The higher the amount of missing information, the more weight is ascribed to the correctness of the assumptions with respect to the missing data mechanism and the method to compensate for the missing values. The missing data pattern helps to decide which compensation technique may be appropriate and graphics displaying the density of the binary indicator in relation to the relationship of observed variable values may indicate whether the missing data mechanism is selective or not. Besides these descriptive tools, a test on whether missing data are MCAR is discussed. However, this test assumes the variables to be quantitative. There is, however, neither a technique nor a test available that helps to decide whether the missing values are MAR or MNAR. This can only be decided based on available empirical results or on theoretical considerations.

References

Beaujean, A. A. (2012). BaylorEdPsych: R Package for Baylor University Educational Psychology Quantitative Courses. Computer software manual. https://CRAN.R-project.org/package=BaylorEdPsych (R package version 0.5).

Gonzalez, J. M., & Eltinge, J. L. (2007). Multiple matrix sampling: A review. In *Proceedings of the Section on Survey Research Methods* (pp. 3069–3075). Alexandria, VA: American Statistical Association.

Heckman, J. J., Lochner, L. J., & Todd, P. E. (2006). Earnings functions, rates of return and treatment effects: The Mincer equation and beyond. In E. Hanushek & F. Welch (Eds.), *Handbook of the economics of education* (Vol. 1, pp. 307–458). Amsterdam: Elsevier.

Kenward, M. G., & Molenberghs, G. (1998). Likelihood based frequentist inference when data are missing at random. *Statistical Science, 13*(3), 236–247.

Laird, N. M. (1988). Missing data in longitudinal studies. *Statistics in Medicine, 7*, 305–315.

Little, R. J. A. (1988). A test of missing completely at random for multivariate data with missing values. *Journal of the American Statistical Association, 83*(404), 1198–1202.

Little, R. J. A., & Rubin, D. B. (2002). *Statistical analysis with missing data* (2nd ed.). New Jersey, NJ: Wiley.

R Core Team. (2018). *R: A language and environment for statistical computing*. Vienna: R Foundation for Statistical Computing. https://www.R-project.org.

Rubin, D. B. (1976). Inference and missing data. *Biometrika, 63*(3), 581–590.

Rubin, D. B. (1987). *Multiple imputation for nonresponse in surveys*. New York, NY: Wiley.

Seaman, S., Galati, J., Jackson, D., & Carlin, J. (2013). What is meant by "missing at random"? *Statistical Science, 28*(2), 257–268.

van Buuren, S., & Groothuis-Oudshoorn, K. (2011). `mice`: Multivariate imputation by chained equations in R. *Journal of Statistical Software, 45*(3), 1–67.

Chapter 3
Missing Data Methods

3.1 Overview

In this chapter missing data procedures and techniques are reviewed and discussed. Among them are both, ad-hoc methods but also more sophisticated techniques including maximum likelihood estimation, weighting and imputation. We discuss pros and cons of the different approaches and techniques, and give practical advice which procedure might be suited best in a given scenario because valid inferences in applied research can only be expected based on informed decisions. A conclusion of this chapter will be that there is not the one method or technique that works best under every possible scenario.

3.2 Ad-hoc Methods

If a data set is affected by missing values, then standard software for completely observed data sets may either stop processing with an error message, or analyse only the completely observed units or cases, usually with a warning message. This is due to a feature of most analysis functions in standard software: They are not designed to handle incompletely observed data sets. To overcome this shortcoming, several ad-hoc methods have been proposed. Unfortunately, these ad-hoc methods usually lack a theoretical justification. That is, most of them are not justified by showing that inferences are still valid if they are applied to incompletely observed data sets. The motivation underlying these methods seems to be purely pragmatic, i.e., to allow statistical analyses with standard software tools. However, most of these methods lead to invalid inferences in the majority of cases. On the other hand, there are specific situations in which one or the other of these methods works.

K. Kleinke et al., *Applied Multiple Imputation*,
Statistics for Social and Behavioral Sciences,
https://doi.org/10.1007/978-3-030-38164-6_3

3.2.1 Complete Case and Available Case Analysis

One of the most common ad-hoc method is complete case analysis (CCA), where only the completely observed cases enter the analysis of interest. This is the method usually chosen by standard software if a data set with missing values is analysed. Corresponding programs simply ignore all incompletely observed cases and print a corresponding warning.

A related technique is available case analysis (ACA), which uses all cases for which the necessary values to calculate the statistic of interest have been observed. If, for example, a covariance matrix is to be calculated, the number of units to calculate variances and covariances can vary greatly. Thus, if various statistics have to be calculated, available case analysis avoids the problem of CCA of possibly ignoring a large amount of information by deleting all incompletely observed units. On the other hand, it may lead to technical problems. For example, if the entries of this matrix are calculated based on different numbers of observations, the resulting matrix may not be a positive (semi-)definite covariance matrix, which is, however, a requirement for various subsequent analyses processing covariance matrices, like, e.g., principal component analysis.

Both CCA and ACA allow valid inferences if the missing data are MCAR, because then the observed values are a simple random sample from the complete-data set, i.e., the set of observed and unobserved values. However, generally both methods lead to invalid inferences if the missing values are MAR or MNAR. The following artificial example illustrates the above points.

Example 3.1 (CCA and ACA) Suppose we are interested in three personality variables x_1, x_2 and x_3 for each of $i = 1, \ldots, n$ individuals. It is assumed that all $\mathbf{x}_i = \left(x_{i,1}\ x_{i,2}\ x_{i,3}\right)^T$ follow the same distribution. However, let us assume that after applying the corresponding personality scales to $n = 10$ individuals, we do not observe all values for every individual. The corresponding (simulated) data values are given in Table 3.1, where missing values are denoted by '·'.

Suppose we want to calculate the covariance matrix of the three scores in the data set. Then, first note that for each of the personality variables, we observe the values of seven out of the ten individuals only. The proportion of missing values is thus 0.3.

Table 3.1 Artificial data set of scores from three personality tests ($x_{i,1}$, $x_{i,2}$, $x_{i,3}$) for $i = 1, \ldots, 10$ individuals

i	$x_{i,1}$	$x_{i,2}$	$x_{i,3}$	i	$x_{i,1}$	$x_{i,2}$	$x_{i,3}$
1	26	56	·	6	20	43	134
2	25	·	158	7	·	50	161
3	20	40	·	8	·	48	·
4	·	49	158	9	21	·	134
5	24	·	164	10	25	53	169

Missing values: '·'

Following the CCA strategy, only two completely observed cases ($i = 6$ and $i = 10$) would enter the analysis. The number of cases considered is thus $n_{(1)} = 2$. For these two cases, the sample covariance matrix amounts to

$$\mathbf{S}_{\text{CCA}} = \begin{pmatrix} 12.5 & 25 & 87.5 \\ 25.0 & 50 & 175.0 \\ 87.5 & 175 & 612.5 \end{pmatrix}$$

(see Appendix A.2.1). A covariance matrix of a random vector $\mathbf{x}_i$ is positive semidefinite (see Appendix A.2.2), which means that the variance s^2 of every possible linear combination $\mathbf{a}^T\mathbf{x}_i$ is non-negative. For example, let $\mathbf{a} = \left(a_1\ a_2\ a_3\right)^T$ be a vector of fixed known real numbers. Then

$$\begin{aligned} s^2 &= \frac{1}{n-1}\sum_{i=1}^{n}\mathbf{a}^T(\mathbf{x}_i - \bar{\mathbf{x}})(\mathbf{x}_i - \bar{\mathbf{x}})^T\mathbf{a} \\ &= \frac{1}{n-1}\sum_{i=1}^{n}(a_1e_{i,1} + a_2e_{i,2} + a_3e_{i,3})^2 \geq 0\,, \end{aligned} \tag{3.1}$$

where $\mathbf{x}_i = \left(x_{i,1}\ x_{i,2}\ x_{i,3}\right)^T$, $\bar{\mathbf{x}} = \left(\bar{x}_1\ \bar{x}_2\ \bar{x}_3\right)^T$ and $e_{i,j} = x_{i,j} - \bar{x}_j$, $j = 1, 2, 3$.

Alternatively, if the ACA strategy is adopted, then different numbers of cases are used to calculate means, variances and covariances. In the example, for each mean and variance seven values are available (see Table 3.1). For the covariances of the first and the second variable and the second and the third variables, four pairs of values, and for the covariance of the first and the third variable, five pairs of values are observed. The sample covariance matrix rounded to two decimal places is

$$\mathbf{S}_{\text{ACA}} = \begin{pmatrix} 6.67 & -4.81 & -26.25 \\ -4.81 & 30.29 & 226.33 \\ -26.25 & 226.33 & 201.00 \end{pmatrix}.$$

However, this matrix is not positive (semi-)definite, which means that not all linear combinations of the variables in $\mathbf{x}_i$ have a non-negative variance. For example, if we choose $\mathbf{a} = \left(-1.9\ -1.9\ 0.14\right)^T$, we find that $\mathbf{a}^T\mathbf{S}_{\text{ACA}}\mathbf{a} = -3.80556$. Hence if, for example, we are interested in the variance of linear combinations of the three personality scores, we may end up with negative values for the variances. □

3.2.2 Completing Data Sets

Replacing missing values by somehow generated values is a strategy that avoids wasting available information by deleting incompletely observed cases. The validity of subsequent analyses, however, depends on the mechanism used to generate the plausible values and how it is accounted for the fact in subsequent analyses that the replacing values are just estimates for the unobserved values.

Many versions of the strategy of replacing each missing by just one somehow generated value, also called single imputation, have been used. The techniques adopted range from very simple ones, like replacing each missing value by a zero or another arbitrarily chosen value, the unconditional mean, median or mode, calculated based on the observed values of the incompletely observed relevant variable, to more elaborated versions, like using the mean, median or mode of the observed part conditional on observed variables or using the observed value of a (randomly selected) similar unit as an estimate.

If each missing value is replaced by the unconditional mean, median or mode and the missing values are MCAR, estimators of location will not be biased but, e.g., estimators of spread will very likely be downward biased. Hence not only standard errors as calculated by software for completely observed data sets, but also measures of dependence will be biased. If the missing values are not MCAR, this strategy will in general lead in addition to biased point estimators.

Using means, medians or modes conditional on other (fixed or random) variables to replace each missing value is a step in the right direction because this strategy takes into account relationships between the variable to be imputed and other variables in the data set. Hence, this strategy has the potential of allowing (asymptotically) unbiased inferences in specific settings, like estimating cell means.

In general, replacing each missing value by a conditional mean or any other single value, is equal to replacing unobserved independent information by an uncertain estimate based on information from the observed part of the data set. If these estimates are realizations of a biased estimator, then the estimator of scientific interest based on the completed data set will generally be biased as well. Furthermore, since every value in the data set is treated as being observed and thus the uncertainty in the predictions is ignored, the amount of information in the completed data set is systematically overestimated by standard software for completely observed data sets, and standard errors will be too small. This leads to a systematic underestimation of variances of estimators and thus to rejection rates of true null hypotheses being systematically too high and confidence intervals being too short. Thus, even if single imputations are properly generated, standard software cannot be used for inferences, but has to be adapted correspondingly. The main problem with ad-hoc methods is that an intuitive motivation replaces theoretical justification.

Example 3.2 (Single Imputation: Estimation of the Expected Value) Suppose we are interested in the mean of a variable μ_y, say income, and a simple random sample of $i = 1, \ldots, n$ units is selected. Unfortunately, not all y_i-values are observed. Therefore, we introduce an additional variable r^* which can be interpreted as a latent, unobserved 'response tendency'. We assume that n copies of $\left(y_i \; r_i^*\right)^T$ are surveyed, and that $\left(y_i \; r_i^*\right)^T$ is iid normally distributed for all i with mean and covariance matrix

$$\boldsymbol{\mu} = \begin{pmatrix} \mu_y \\ \mu_{r^*} \end{pmatrix} \quad \text{and} \quad \boldsymbol{\Sigma} = \begin{pmatrix} \sigma_y^2 & \sigma_{yr^*} \\ \sigma_{yr^*} & \sigma_{r^*}^2 \end{pmatrix} . \tag{3.2}$$

Instead of r_i^*, however, we observe a response indicator, r_i, which is related to r_i^* by the threshold relationship

$$r_i = \begin{cases} 1 \text{ if } r_i^* > c \\ 0 \text{ else,} \end{cases}$$

and indicates if the value of y_i is observed ($r_i = 1$) or not ($r_i = 0$). Thus, r_i is always observed, r_i^* is never observed and y_i is only observed if $r_i = 1$. The probability of observing y_i is determined by the missing data mechanism $g(r_i \mid y_i, \boldsymbol{\gamma})$, where $\boldsymbol{\gamma}$ is an unknown parameter vector. Replacing each missing value with the (marginal) mean of observed y_i-values, $\bar{y}_{(1)}$, and treating the imputed values as independently observed values, we may estimate μ_y by

$$\hat{\mu}_y = \frac{1}{n}\left[\sum_{i=1}^{n}(r_i y_i + (1 - r_i)\bar{y}_{(1)})\right] .$$

However, this estimator simplifies to $\hat{\mu}_y = (n_{(1)}\bar{y}_{(1)} + n_{(0)}\bar{y}_{(1)})/n = \bar{y}_{(1)}$, where $n_{(1)}$ and $n_{(0)}$ are the number of observed and unobserved y-values, respectively. Fixing the response indicator variable $\mathbf{r} = (r_1, \ldots, r_n)^T$ at the observed values, the expectation of $\hat{\mu}_y$ is

$$\begin{aligned} E(\hat{\mu}_y \mid \mathbf{r}) &= E\left[\frac{1}{n}\sum_{i=1}^{n}(r_i y_i + (1 - r_i)\bar{y}_{(1)})\Big|\mathbf{r}\right] = \frac{1}{n_{(1)}}\left[\sum_{i=1}^{n} r_i E(y_i \mid r_i)\right] \\ &= \mu_y + \frac{\sigma_{yr^*}}{\sigma_{r^*}}\frac{\phi(\tilde{r})}{1 - \Phi(\tilde{r})} , \end{aligned}$$

where $\tilde{r} = -\mu_{r^*}/\sigma_{r^*}$ (see Appendix A.2.6). Treating the imputed values $\bar{y}$ as independently observed data points implies adopting the variance estimator for $\hat{\mu}$ used for completely observed data sets,

$$\widehat{\text{var}}(\hat{\mu}_y) = \frac{1}{n(n-1)}\left[\sum_{i=1}^{n}(r_i y_i + (1 - r_i)\bar{y}_{(1)} - \hat{\mu}_y)^2\right]$$

to get the standard errors necessary for confidence intervals and hypothesis tests. Again fixing **r** and taking the expectation gives

$$E[\widehat{\text{var}}(\hat{\mu}_y) \mid \mathbf{r}] = \frac{1}{n(n-1)} \sum_{i=1}^{n} E(r_i(y_i - \bar{y}_{(1)})^2 \mid \mathbf{r}) = \frac{n_{(1)} - 1}{n(n-1)} \sigma^2_{y|r=1} ,$$

where

$$\sigma^2_{y|r=1} = \sigma^2_y + \frac{\sigma^2_{yr^*}}{\sigma^2_{r^*}} \left[\frac{\tilde{r}\,\phi(\tilde{r})}{\pi} - \left(\frac{\phi(\tilde{r})}{\pi} \right)^2 \right]$$

(see Appendix A.2.6). On the other hand, the true (conditional) variance of $\hat{\mu}_y$ is

$$\text{var}(\hat{\mu}_y \mid \mathbf{r}) = \text{var}(\bar{y}_{(1)}) = \frac{1}{n_{(1)}} \sigma^2_{y|r=1} ,$$

and obviously, $E[\widehat{\text{var}}(\hat{\mu}_y) \mid \mathbf{r}] < \text{var}(\hat{\mu}_y \mid \mathbf{r})$ if $n_{(1)} < n$. Hence, if observing income y is correlated with income itself and thus the missing values are MNAR, the estimator $\hat{\mu}_y$ will be biased. Only if both are uncorrelated, i.e., if $\sigma_{yr^*} = 0$, and the missing values are MCAR then this estimator will be unbiased. Note again that imputing $\bar{y}_{(1)}$ for each missing value leads to the same estimator for μ_y as CCA. However, suppose the missing values are MCAR. Then CCA allows valid inferences, but imputing $\bar{y}_{(1)}$ and treating these imputations as independent observations leads to a systematic underestimation of the variance of the estimator and thus to falsely rejecting true null hypotheses too often and to confidence intervals which are systematically too short. □

Obviously, a strategy that uses some arbitrarily chosen value, e.g., a zero or 999, for each unobserved value and treating this value as being observed leads to biased inferences in most cases, even if the missing values are MCAR.

Example 3.2 illustrates that replacing missing values by the mean of the observed values may lead to an unbiased estimator for the expected value, but with a standard error for this estimator which is systematically too small, even if the missing values are MCAR and standard estimation tools are used. The following example shows that imputing conditional means generally leads to biased estimators in the regression context, although it may allow consistent estimation in the context of estimating means as is illustrated in Example 3.5.

Example 3.3 (Single Imputation: Regression) Suppose we are interested in the regression of a variable y on another variable x but that not all x-values are observed. As in Example 3.2, we introduce an additional variable r^* which can be interpreted as a latent, unobserved response tendency. We assume that n copies of variables y, x and r^* are surveyed, and that $\left(y_i \; x_i \; r_i^*\right)^T$ is independently normally distributed for all $i = 1, \ldots, n$ with mean and covariance matrix

$$\boldsymbol{\mu} = \begin{pmatrix} \mu_y \\ \mu_x \\ \mu_{r^*} \end{pmatrix} \quad \text{and} \quad \boldsymbol{\Sigma} = \begin{pmatrix} \sigma_y^2 & \sigma_{yx} & \sigma_{yr^*} \\ \sigma_{yx} & \sigma_x^2 & \sigma_{xr^*} \\ \sigma_{yr^*} & \sigma_{xr^*} & \sigma_{r^*}^2 \end{pmatrix} . \tag{3.3}$$

Instead of r_i^*, however, we observe a response indicator, r_i, which is related to r_i^* by the threshold relationship

$$r_i = \begin{cases} 1 \text{ if } r_i^* > c \\ 0 \text{ else,} \end{cases}$$

indicating whether the value of x_i is observed ($r_i = 1$) or not ($r_i = 0$). Thus, y_i and r_i are always observed, r_i^* is never observed and x_i is observed only if $r_i = 1$. The probability of observing x_i, $\Pr(r_i = 1 \mid y_i, x_i)$, is determined by the missing data mechanism $g(r_i \mid y_i, x_i, \boldsymbol{\gamma})$, where $\boldsymbol{\gamma}$ is an unknown parameter vector.

The model of applied-scientific interest is a simple linear regression model,

$$y_i = \beta_0 + \beta_1 x_i + \epsilon_i \ , \quad \epsilon_i \sim N(0, \sigma_\epsilon^2) \tag{3.4}$$

for all $i = 1, \ldots, n$ which is usually estimated using the least squares method. The ordinary least squares (OLS) estimators for β_0 and β_1 are given by

$$\hat{\beta}_0 = \bar{y} - \frac{s_{yx}}{s_x^2}\,\bar{x} \quad \text{and} \quad \hat{\beta}_1 = \frac{s_{yx}}{s_x^2} ,$$

where $\bar{y}$ and $\bar{x}$ are the sample means of y and x, s_x^2 is the sample variance of x and s_{yx} is the sample covariance of y and x (cf. Appendix A.3.1). The theoretical versions of the OLS estimators are

$$\beta_0 = \mu_y - \beta_1 \mu_x \quad \text{and} \quad \beta_1 = \sigma_{yx}/\sigma_x^2 .$$

Given the normal distribution of $\left(y_i \ x_i \ r_i^*\right)^T$, the regression of r_i^* on the realized values of y_i and x_i is

$$r_i^* = \gamma_0 + y_i\gamma_1 + x_i\gamma_2 + v_i, \quad v_i \sim N(0, \sigma_v^2) \quad \text{for all} \quad i = 1, \ldots, n ,$$

$$\gamma_2 = \frac{\sigma_{xr^*}\sigma_y^2 - \sigma_{yx}\sigma_{yr^*}}{\sigma_y^2\sigma_x^2 - \sigma_{yx}^2}$$

and γ_0, γ_1 and σ_v^2 are easily derived from results given in Appendix A.2.5. For simplicity we will drop the index i if possible.

Assume further that $\sigma_{xr^*} = \sigma_{yx}\sigma_{yr^*}/\sigma_y^2$ which implies $\gamma_2 = 0$, so that given y, the probability of observing x does not depend on x itself, and the missing values are MAR. Note that if in addition $\sigma_{yr^*} = \sigma_{yx}\sigma_{xr^*}/\sigma_x^2$ (cf. Appendix A.2.5), then the missing values would be MCAR.

The response indicator divides the units into two groups: The completely and the incompletely observed part. The theoretical or model parameters β_0 and β_1 can be written as

$$\begin{aligned}\beta_0 &= (\pi\mu_{y,(1)} + (1-\pi)\mu_{y,(0)}) - \beta_1(\pi\mu_{x,(1)} + (1-\pi)\mu_{x,(0)}),\\ \beta_1 &= \frac{\pi(1-\pi)\Delta_y\Delta_x + \pi\sigma_{yx,(1)} + (1-\pi)\sigma_{yx,(0)}}{\pi(1-\pi)\Delta_x^2 + \pi\sigma_{x,(1)}^2 + (1-\pi)\sigma_{x,(0)}^2},\end{aligned} \tag{3.5}$$

where $\mu_{y,(1)}$ and $\mu_{x,(1)}$ are the means of y and x, $\sigma_{x,(1)}^2$ is the variance of x and $\sigma_{yx,(1)}$ is the covariance of y and x in the completely observed part, $\mu_{y,(0)}$, $\mu_{x,(0)}$, $\sigma_{x,(0)}^2$ and $\sigma_{yx,(0)}$ are their counterparts in the unobserved part, $\pi = \Pr(r = 1)$, $\Delta_y = \mu_{y,(1)} - \mu_{y,(0)}$ and $\Delta_x = \mu_{x,(1)} - \mu_{x,(0)}$.

To illustrate consequences of single imputation techniques with respect to the regression parameters in model (3.4), it is important to note that if the assumption of trivariate normality is correct, all the terms in (3.5) can be written as functions of the parameters given in (3.3), see Appendix A.2.6 for details.

Now, suppose that variables $(y_i\ x_i\ r_i^*)^T$, $i = 1, \ldots, n$, are normally distributed with

$$\boldsymbol{\mu} = \begin{pmatrix} -11 \\ 4 \\ 2 \end{pmatrix} \quad \text{and} \quad \boldsymbol{\Sigma} = \begin{pmatrix} 3 & 2.4 & 1.5 \\ 2.4 & 5 & 1.2 \\ 1.5 & 1.2 & 2 \end{pmatrix}$$

and let $c = 1.5$, which implies $\pi = 0.638$ (see Appendix A.2.6). Note that $\sigma_{xr^*} = \sigma_{yx}\sigma_{yr^*}/\sigma_y^2$ but $\sigma_{yr^*} \neq \sigma_{yx}\sigma_{xr^*}/\sigma_x^2$ as is easily verified, thus, the missing values are MAR. The true values of the regression parameters of interest are $\beta_0 = -12.92$ and $\beta_1 = 0.48$ (see Appendix A.2.4).

Table 3.2 presents the values of the theoretical parameters Δ_x, $\sigma_{x,(0)}^2$, $\sigma_{yx,(0)}$, β_0 and β_1 ('No missings') and, in all other cases, the corresponding implied theoretical parameter values when various single imputation techniques are adopted for the same population being separated by the response indicator into one completely and one incompletely observed part. For example, the technique 'Impute 0' denotes imputing zeros for missing x-values. This implies as parameter values $\tilde{\mu}_{x,(0)} = 0$, $\tilde{\sigma}_{x,(0)}^2 = 0$, $\tilde{\sigma}_{yx,(0)} = 0$ and thus $\beta_0 = -12.133$ and $\beta_1 = 0.395$. The technique 'Impute $\hat{\mu}_{x,(1)}$' is short for imputing the unconditional mean of the observed x-values. To impute conditional means, we can proceed as follows. First note that due to the normality assumption,

$$x_i = \theta_0 + y_i\theta_1 + u_i\,, \quad u_i \sim N(0, \sigma_u^2)$$

Table 3.2 True values of Δ_x, $\sigma^2_{x,(0)}$, $\sigma_{yx,(0)}$, β_0 and β_1 in the model and as implied by single imputation techniques (rounded to three decimal points)

	Δ_x	$\sigma^2_{x,(0)}$	$\sigma_{yx,(0)}$	β_0	β_1
No missings	1.377	4.491	1.764	−12.920	0.480
Imputation technique					
Impute 0	4.498	0	0	−12.133	0.395
Impute $\hat{\mu}_{x,(1)}$	0	0	0	−12.860	0.413
Impute $\hat{\mu}_{x\|y}$	1.377	1.411	1.764	−13.471	0.618

for all $i = 1, \ldots, n$. In addition, from Chap. 2 we know that if missing values are MAR, then the regression relationship of x on y is not distorted based on the completely observed cases. Thus imputations can be generated by estimating the above regression model, using the observed y values of the incompletely observed part and predict the x values. Imputing these predicted values conditional on y will be denoted as 'Impute $\hat{\mu}_{x|y}$'.

The results in Table 3.2 show that all the single imputation techniques considered do not in general imply the same population and true parameter values as if there were no missing values. Thus, estimators for β_0 and β_1 will be biased for the true parameters of interest. Even if conditional means are imputed, the regression relation of y on x is distorted (see Table 3.2). The explanation is that the implied variance of x-values in the incompletely observed part, $\sigma^2_{x,(0)}$, is too small because the true regression model for x on y would explicitly include an error variance, σ^2_u, which is ignored when (conditional) means are imputed. The parameters Δ_x and $\sigma_{yx,(0)}$ are not affected because the errors u_i have expectation zero and are independent from y. □

Other single imputation techniques have been proposed for specific analysis models. For example, in linear multiple regression models with missing predictor values, proposed techniques include response indicator variables as additional predictors together with interaction terms of incompletely observed variables and the corresponding response indicators. However, although these proposals are appealingly simple and therefore may be an attractive procedure for a seemingly easy handling of missing data problems, they all have their pitfalls and lead to invalid inferences under most scenarios. A discussion of these and related techniques as well as references to further work can be found, e.g., in Jones (1996).

Most of the proposed single imputation methods are attractive due to their simplicity. Unfortunately, as they usually lack theoretical justification, they lead to invalid inferences in most cases. And although the consequences depend on the amount of missing information which is usually unknown—for example, if only very few observations in a large data set are missing and the true values are close to the (unconditional) expected value, then no severe consequences for the downstream analyses may be expected if the mean of the observed values is imputed—these techniques cannot be recommended as standard strategies. It should further be noted that instead of the number of missing values, the amount of missing information is crucial, as we will see later in Chap. 4. On the other hand, there are theoretically justified or at least more sophisticated approaches for single imputation that do allow valid inferences under specific conditions, which will be considered in Sects. 3.3.2 and 3.5.1.

3.3 Maximum Likelihood Estimation

The general idea of maximum likelihood (ML) estimation is the same whether or not there are missing values. The difference between analysing a completely observed and an incompletely observed data set is that in the latter case the binary response indicator has to be considered as an additional variable, either treated as random or as a variable to be conditioned upon. This implies that the joint density or probability function of all the observed random variables conditional on all observed variables considered to be fixed has to be correctly specified. Like in the case of completely observed data sets, the value of the estimator maximizing the log-likelihood function has to be found.

3.3.1 Introduction

Suppose we are interested in the effect of variable $\mathbf{v}$ on another variable $\mathbf{u}$ and thus in the parameter $\boldsymbol{\theta}$ that governs the conditional distribution of $\mathbf{u} \mid \mathbf{v}$. Then we could select a simple random sample of variables $\mathbf{u}_i$ and $\mathbf{v}_i$, $i = 1, \ldots, n$, to estimate this parameter. Given that all variables $\left(\mathbf{u}_i^T \; \mathbf{v}_i^T\right)$ are independently distributed as $\left(\mathbf{u}^T \; \mathbf{v}^T\right)$, and assuming the distribution of $\mathbf{u} \mid \mathbf{v}$, $f(\mathbf{u} \mid \mathbf{v})$, to be known up to the unknown parameter $\boldsymbol{\theta}$, the likelihood function can be written as

$$L(\boldsymbol{\theta}) = \prod_{i=1}^{n} L_i(\boldsymbol{\theta}) = \prod_{i=1}^{n} f(\mathbf{u}_i \mid \mathbf{v}_i, \boldsymbol{\theta}) ,$$

where $L_i(\boldsymbol{\theta}) = f(\mathbf{u}_i \mid \mathbf{v}_i, \boldsymbol{\theta})$ is the contribution of the ith unit. The log-likelihood function is given by

$$l(\boldsymbol{\theta}) = \sum_{i=1}^{n} \log f(\mathbf{u}_i \mid \mathbf{v}_i, \boldsymbol{\theta})$$

and has to be maximized with respect to $\boldsymbol{\theta}$. The value $\hat{\boldsymbol{\theta}}$ that uniquely maximizes this function is, if it exists, the maximum likelihood estimator (ML estimator). In general, if all modeling assumptions are met and under some regularity conditions, the ML estimator is asymptotically normally distributed, consistent and asymptotically efficient, i.e., allows relatively precise statements. The variance of an ML estimator can be estimated using the (estimated) expected information matrix or via the observed information (see Appendix A.3.2). For a more detailed discussion see, e.g., Wooldridge (2002a), Lehmann (1998), Lehmann and Casella (1998), Newey and McFadden (1994) or Serfling (1980).

If in addition to the variables **u** and **v**, a vector of binary response indicator variables, **r**, is observed that selects the statistical units with regard to each variable into one of two groups, then the individual contributions to the likelihood function can be written as

$$L_i(\boldsymbol{\vartheta}_1, \boldsymbol{\vartheta}_2) = f(\mathbf{u}_i \mid \mathbf{r}_i, \mathbf{v}_i, \boldsymbol{\vartheta}_1)g(\mathbf{r}_i \mid \mathbf{v}_i, \boldsymbol{\vartheta}_2)\,, \tag{3.6}$$

where $\boldsymbol{\vartheta}_1$ is the parameter governing the conditional distribution of $\mathbf{u} \mid \mathbf{r}, \mathbf{v}$, and $\boldsymbol{\vartheta}_2$ is the parameter governing the conditional distribution of $\mathbf{r} \mid \mathbf{v}$. This formulation is also called a *pattern-mixture model* (e.g., Little & Rubin, 2002), because the first term after the equal sign describes the distribution of **u** in the strata defined by different values of **r** (and **v**), and the second term models the incidence of the different strata given **v**.

However, the individual distributions can also be written as

$$L_i(\boldsymbol{\theta}, \boldsymbol{\gamma}) = f(\mathbf{u}_i \mid \mathbf{v}_i, \boldsymbol{\theta})g(\mathbf{r}_i \mid \mathbf{u}_i, \mathbf{v}_i, \boldsymbol{\gamma})\,, \tag{3.7}$$

which is called a *selection model formulation*, because the second term models the incidence of the different patterns of missing and observed variables conditional on **u** and **v**, whereas the first term on the right-hand side models the conditional distribution of the dependent variable **u** given predictors **v**, which is often the model of applied-scientific interest. The term *selection model formulation* as it is used here is similar to the term *sample selection model* in econometrics which goes back to Heckman (1979). In that context, sample selection models are usually adopted to estimate the parameter of a regression model of interest in the presence of nonignorable unit nonresponse using a selection model but not necessarily based on a likelihood function. An example would be a model where one is interested in the effects of predictors on the dependent variable hourly wage offer, but only those individuals in the corresponding age span that participate in the job market can be observed. Hence, selection into work may have to be modeled as well. We will discuss this approach in more detail in Sect. 3.3.3 (see also Wooldridge, 2002a, Chapter 17.4).

If **r** denotes a binary response indicator variable and not all values of **u** and **v** are observed, then neither (3.6) nor (3.7) can be used to estimate the parameters of interest. Therefore, we have to consider the likelihood function based only on the observed part of the data set. The strategy to derive this likelihood is also used in other contexts, e.g., in latent variable modeling: Derive the marginal probability or probability density function by integrating out the unobserved (random) variables if they are continuous or by summing up the corresponding probability functions if they are discrete.

To keep the presentation simple, we will assume that all the variables with missing values are random continuous variables and that all units $i = 1, \ldots, n$

are mutually independent. Further, (1), if used as an index for a variable, denotes the observed part of this variable. Correspondingly, (0) denotes the unobserved part. Then, treating the binary response indicator as a random variable, the individual contribution of the ith unit to the marginal likelihood in a pattern-mixture formulation can be written as

$$L_i(\boldsymbol{\vartheta}_1, \boldsymbol{\vartheta}_2, \boldsymbol{\vartheta}_3) = \int\int f(\mathbf{u}_i \mid \mathbf{r}_i, \mathbf{v}_i, \boldsymbol{\vartheta}_1) g(\mathbf{r}_i \mid \mathbf{v}_i, \boldsymbol{\vartheta}_2) f(\mathbf{v}_{i,(0)} \mid \mathbf{v}_{i,(1)}, \boldsymbol{\vartheta}_3)\, d\mathbf{u}_{i,(0)}\, d\mathbf{v}_{i,(0)} \tag{3.8}$$

and in a model selection formulation

$$L_i(\boldsymbol{\theta}, \boldsymbol{\gamma}, \boldsymbol{\vartheta}_3) = \int\int f(\mathbf{u}_i \mid \mathbf{v}_i, \boldsymbol{\theta}) g(\mathbf{r}_i \mid \mathbf{u}_i, \mathbf{v}_i, \boldsymbol{\gamma}) f(\mathbf{v}_{i,(0)} \mid \mathbf{v}_{i,(1)}, \boldsymbol{\vartheta}_3)\, d\mathbf{u}_{i,(0)}\, d\mathbf{v}_{i,(0)}\,, \tag{3.9}$$

where each integral sign is short for integration over a domain corresponding to the two variables $\mathbf{u}_{i,(0)}$ and $\mathbf{v}_{i,(0)}$, and $\boldsymbol{\vartheta}_1, \boldsymbol{\vartheta}_2, \boldsymbol{\vartheta}_3, \boldsymbol{\theta}_1$ and $\boldsymbol{\gamma}$ are the parameters governing the corresponding distributions. Note that although the predictors $\mathbf{v}$ are usually treated as fixed, here the unobserved part is considered to be random, following a distribution which is known up to the parameter $\boldsymbol{\vartheta}_3$.

A closer look at (3.9) reveals that without simplifying assumptions, estimation of the parameters of interest is hardly feasible: We would have to derive the integrand and then integrate out $\mathbf{u}_{i,(0)}$ and $\mathbf{v}_{i,(0)}$. However, in most applications, the only model that is justified is $f(\mathbf{u} \mid \mathbf{v}, \boldsymbol{\theta})$, for example, a cross-sectional regression model or a multilevel model. Modeling $g(\mathbf{r} \mid \mathbf{u}, \mathbf{v}, \boldsymbol{\gamma})$ and $f(\mathbf{v}_{(0)} \mid \mathbf{v}_{(1)}, \boldsymbol{\vartheta}_3)$ becomes necessary only if the data set at hand is affected by missing values and usually the corresponding models are formulated not before analyses are carried out. Since these models are not of applied-scientific interest, they may not be well justified. For example, $\mathbf{r}$ may depend on $\mathbf{u}$ and $\mathbf{v}$ in a highly non-linear way, but neither a theory nor empirical findings are available for this model and the specific research question given the surveyed variables $\mathbf{u}$ and $\mathbf{v}$.

On the other hand, the pattern-mixture formulation (3.8) becomes relevant if one is interested in the phenomenon of nonresponse and thus in learning about response behaviour in certain situations. In this case, models $f(\mathbf{u} \mid \mathbf{r}, \mathbf{v}, \boldsymbol{\vartheta}_1)$ and $g(\mathbf{r} \mid \mathbf{v}, \boldsymbol{\vartheta}_2)$ are subjects of scientific interest and should be well justified. However, the pattern-mixture formulation may also be relevant if the derivation of the marginal likelihood is simpler via (3.8) than via the selection formulation in the presence of missing data (e.g., Little, 1993). In any case, deriving the function $f(\mathbf{u}, \mathbf{r}, \mathbf{v}_{(0)} \mid \mathbf{v}_{(1)}, \boldsymbol{\vartheta})$ and integrating out $\mathbf{u}_{(0)}$ and $\mathbf{v}_{(0)}$ is not an easy task in general. Therefore, software implementations are available only for specific models, often based on strong underlying assumptions.

3.3.2 The Ignorable Case

Likelihood inference is comparatively simple if the missing data mechanism is ignorable, the likelihood can be factored into easy-to-handle components and the parameters of these components are distinct. For example, assume that we are interested in a parameter $\boldsymbol{\theta}$, e.g., the parameter of a conditional model or unconditional means, variances and correlations in a marginal model, but a given data set is affected by nonresponse in several variables. In case of a regression model, the dependent variable $\mathbf{u}$ is treated as random, whereas the predictors $\mathbf{v}$ are usually considered to be fixed. For simplicity assume that variables affected by missing values are continuous.

Given that missing values are MAR,

$$g(\mathbf{r}_i \mid \mathbf{u}_i, \mathbf{v}_i, \boldsymbol{\gamma}) = g(\mathbf{r}_i \mid \mathbf{u}_{i,(1)}, \mathbf{v}_{i,(1)}, \boldsymbol{\gamma}) ,$$

and the distinctness of the parameters in a selection model formulation, $\left(\boldsymbol{\theta}^T \ \boldsymbol{\vartheta}_3^T\right)^T$ and $\boldsymbol{\gamma}$, i.e., ignorability of the missing data mechanism in case of the direct-likelihood approach, the marginal likelihood function starting with selection formulation (3.9) and based on the observed sample can be written as

$$L(\boldsymbol{\theta}, \boldsymbol{\vartheta}_3, \boldsymbol{\gamma}) = \prod_{i=1}^{n} f(\mathbf{u}_{i,(1)} \mid \mathbf{v}_{i,(1)}, \boldsymbol{\theta}, \boldsymbol{\vartheta}_3) g(\mathbf{r}_i \mid \mathbf{u}_{i,(1)}, \mathbf{v}_{i,(1)}, \boldsymbol{\gamma}) .$$

The log-likelihood is then

$$l(\boldsymbol{\theta}, \boldsymbol{\vartheta}_3, \boldsymbol{\gamma}) = \sum_{i=1}^{n} \log f(\mathbf{u}_{i,(1)} \mid \mathbf{v}_{i,(1)}, \boldsymbol{\theta}, \boldsymbol{\vartheta}_3) + \log g(\mathbf{r}_i \mid \mathbf{u}_{i,(1)}, \mathbf{v}_{i,(1)}, \boldsymbol{\gamma})$$

and, since $\left(\boldsymbol{\theta}^T \ \boldsymbol{\vartheta}_3^T\right)$ and $\boldsymbol{\gamma}$ are distinct, the first term on the right-hand side can be maximized with respect to $\left(\boldsymbol{\theta}^T \ \boldsymbol{\vartheta}_3^T\right)$ to get the ML estimate. Note that in the case of incompletely observed data sets, more parameters are involved as if there were no missing values.

Although maximizing $\sum_{i=1}^{n} \log f(\mathbf{u}_{i,(1)} \mid \mathbf{v}_{i,(1)}, \boldsymbol{\theta}, \boldsymbol{\vartheta}_3)$ may seem to be straightforward, it must be noted that $f(\mathbf{u}_{i,(1)} \mid \mathbf{v}_{i,(1)}, \boldsymbol{\theta}, \boldsymbol{\vartheta}_3)$ depends on the pattern of observed and missing values and is usually different from $f(\mathbf{u}_i \mid \mathbf{v}_i, \boldsymbol{\theta})$.

Example 3.4 (Normal Linear Regression) Consider Example 3.3 but assume for the moment that there are no missing values. Then the log-likelihood function to estimate the interesting parameter, $\boldsymbol{\theta} = \left(\beta_0 \ \beta_1 \ \sigma_\epsilon^2\right)^T$ would be given by

$$l(\boldsymbol{\theta}) = \sum_{i=1}^{n} \log f(y_i \mid x_i, \boldsymbol{\theta}) = -\frac{n}{2} \log(2\pi) - \frac{n}{2} \log \sigma_\epsilon^2 - \frac{1}{2} \sum_{i=1}^{n} \frac{(y_i - \beta_0 - x_i \beta_1)^2}{\sigma_\epsilon^2}$$

and the ML estimators would be

$$\hat{\beta}_1 = \frac{s_{yx}}{s_x^2}\,, \qquad \hat{\beta}_0 = \bar{y} - \bar{x}\hat{\beta}_1 \quad \text{and} \quad \hat{\sigma}_\epsilon^2 = \frac{1}{n}\sum_{i=1}^{n}[y_i - (\hat{\beta}_0 + x_i\hat{\beta}_1)]^2\,,$$

where $\bar{y}$, $\bar{x}$ and s_x^2 are the sample means of y and x and the variance of x, respectively, and s_{yx} is the sample covariance of y and x. Assume now missing values in x, and r being a response variable indicating whether x is observed ($r = 1$) or not ($r = 0$). We will assume that the probability distribution of r depends on y but not additionally on x. Thus the missing values are MAR. Then, to derive the log-likelihood function for $\boldsymbol{\theta}$, we could start with (3.9) and, since $r \mid y$ does not depend on x, first note that $g(r \mid y, x, \boldsymbol{\gamma}) = g(r \mid y, \boldsymbol{\gamma})$. Since for each unit there is only one predictor x which is either observed or missing, we have to model $f(y \mid x, \boldsymbol{\theta})$ if x is observed and $f(y \mid x, \boldsymbol{\theta})f(x, \boldsymbol{\vartheta}_3)$ if x is not observed. However, we have to integrate $x_{(0)}$ only out of the latter term. Thus,

$$l(\boldsymbol{\theta}, \boldsymbol{\xi}, \boldsymbol{\gamma}) = \sum_{i=1}^{n} r_i \log f(y_i \mid x_i, \boldsymbol{\theta}) + (1 - r_i) \log f(y_i, \boldsymbol{\xi}) + \log g(r_i \mid y_i, \boldsymbol{\gamma})\,, \tag{3.10}$$

where $\boldsymbol{\xi}$ is the parameter of the marginal distribution of y. It is not sufficient to maximize $r_i \log f(y_i \mid x_i, \boldsymbol{\theta})$ with respect to $\boldsymbol{\theta}$. The corresponding estimator will be biased as we would only consider the observed part of the sample. Put differently, we would ignore y values for which x was not observed. These values would, however, be MNAR. Thus, instead of the marginal distribution $f(x_{(0)}, \boldsymbol{\vartheta}_3)$, we now have to model $f(y_i, \boldsymbol{\xi})$ in addition to $f(y_i \mid x_i, \boldsymbol{\theta})$. This implies that we have to estimate two parameters of the marginal distribution of y, i.e., the mean and the variance, and three parameters of the conditional distribution of $y \mid x$, the constant, the slope and the variance. What is important for the next step, however, is that $\left(\boldsymbol{\theta}^T \; \boldsymbol{\xi}^T\right)^T$ and $\boldsymbol{\gamma}$ are distinct. Then, $\log g(r_i \mid y_i, \boldsymbol{\gamma})$ can be ignored when $l(\boldsymbol{\theta}, \boldsymbol{\xi}, \boldsymbol{\gamma})$ is maximized with respect to $\boldsymbol{\theta}$.

Finding the ML estimator for $\boldsymbol{\theta}$ based on (3.10) is not easy. It is easier to maximize the log-likelihood function

$$l(\boldsymbol{\zeta}, \boldsymbol{\xi}) = \sum_{i=1}^{n}[r_i \log f(x_i \mid y_i, \boldsymbol{\zeta}) + \log f(y_i, \boldsymbol{\xi})] \tag{3.11}$$

with respect to $\boldsymbol{\zeta}$ and $\boldsymbol{\xi}$, where $\boldsymbol{\zeta}$ is the parameter governing the distribution of $x_i \mid y_i$, and then find the transformation to the parameter of interest $\boldsymbol{\theta}$. Given consistent and asymptotically normally distributed ML estimators $\hat{\boldsymbol{\zeta}}$ and $\hat{\boldsymbol{\xi}}$, the function $\hat{\boldsymbol{\theta}}$ of $\hat{\boldsymbol{\zeta}}$ and $\hat{\boldsymbol{\xi}}$ is an ML estimator which is consistent and asymptotically normally distributed under weak conditions on the transformation (e.g., Serfling, 1980, p. 149). Sections 2.3.1 and 2.3.2 show that if the missing data are MCAR or MAR, the conditional distribution of $x \mid y$ does not depend on the response indicator. Thus, ML estimators based on (3.11) are

$$\hat{\zeta}_1 = \frac{s_{yx,(1)}}{s^2_{y,(1)}} , \qquad \hat{\zeta}_0 = \bar{x}_{(1)} - \bar{y}_{(1)}\hat{\zeta}_1, \qquad \hat{\sigma}^2_u = \frac{1}{n_{(1)}} \sum_{i=1}^{n} r_i [x_i - (\hat{\zeta}_0 + y_i\hat{\zeta}_1)]^2 ,$$

$$\hat{\boldsymbol{\xi}} = \left(\hat{\mu}_y \ \hat{\sigma}^2_y\right)^T , \qquad \hat{\mu}_y = \bar{y} = \frac{1}{n}\sum_{i=1}^{n} y_i \quad \text{and} \quad \hat{\sigma}^2_y = s^2_y = \frac{1}{n}\sum_{i=1}^{n}(y_i - \hat{\mu}_y)^2 ,$$

where index (1) is used to indicate that the corresponding function is evaluated using the completely observed subsample and σ^2_u is the error variance from the regression of x on y. The parameters of interest are then given by

$$\hat{\beta}_1 = \frac{\hat{\zeta}_1\hat{\sigma}^2_y}{\hat{\sigma}^2_u + \hat{\zeta}^2_1\hat{\sigma}^2_y} , \qquad \hat{\beta}_0 = \hat{\mu}_y - (\hat{\zeta}_0 + \hat{\mu}_y\hat{\zeta}_1)\hat{\beta}_1 \quad \text{and} \quad \hat{\sigma}^2_\epsilon = \hat{\sigma}^2_y - \hat{\beta}^2_1(\hat{\sigma}^2_u + \hat{\zeta}^2_1\hat{\sigma}^2_y) .$$

As an estimator of the variance of $\hat{\boldsymbol{\theta}} = \left(\hat{\beta}_1 \ \hat{\beta}_0 \ \hat{\sigma}^2_\epsilon\right)^T$, the negative inverse of the matrix of second derivatives of the log-likelihood function with respect to $\boldsymbol{\theta}$ can be used. □

Example 3.4 shows that in the case of missing data being not MCAR, ML estimation of the parameters may become cumbersome even in problems which are easily handled if all values were observed. In addition, strong assumptions are usually needed: In the example, if the assumption of a linear regression relationship of y on x with homoscedastic errors is correct, then the reverse regression of x on y can only be linear if y and x are bivariate normally distributed (Spanos, 1995). Thus, the assumption of bivariate normality, which is not necessary in case of ML estimators for $\boldsymbol{\theta}$ if there are no missing values, is crucial here. If this assumption is violated, inferences may be misleading.

There are additional subtleties that should be considered if not all values are observed, some of which already discussed in Chap. 2. One point is that the estimator of the variance should be based on the observed information and not on the expected information. Furthermore, since additional distributional assumptions in the presence of missing data are necessary when the ML method is adopted, inferences may be more sensitive with respect to model misspecification.

In Example 3.4, one variable is completely observed, but the other is not. This is the simplest version of a monotone missing pattern (see Sect. 1.4). Since the parameters $\boldsymbol{\zeta}$ and $\boldsymbol{\xi}$ of the two likelihood components are distinct, we can maximize the first part to get an estimate for $\boldsymbol{\zeta}$ using the completely observed part of the sample and, separately, the second component to get an estimate for $\boldsymbol{\xi}$ based on all n units. Factorizing the likelihood into terms which can separately be maximized is a strategy that may be applied to situations with more than two variables. An example is a linear panel or longitudinal model where units are observed at least at the first time and may drop out later. If the missing data mechanism is ignorable, which gains plausibility if drop out is an absorbing state, then ML estimation is possible based only on the observed variable values for each unit and assuming multivariate normality of the dependent variables by simply factorizing the likelihood similar to the bivariate case considered above.

Given distinctness of parameters and a decomposition of the log-likelihood into easy-to-maximize log-likelihood terms also allows simple calculation of a variance estimator for the ML estimators, so that likelihood or Bayes inference can easily be carried out. In applications this requires, however, that corresponding software is available being able to combine and transform the estimation results properly. Otherwise, standard software may be used and results need to be combined with additional programming effort.

In the context of structural equation modeling, ML estimation with incompletely observed units is often called full information maximum likelihood (FIML) estimation. The difference between FIML and ML as sometimes used in the context of structural equation modeling is that in the latter case only the completely observed units are included, corresponding to what would be denoted CCA here based on a misspecified likelihood function if the missing values are not MCAR.

Example 3.5 (ML Estimation of the Mean) Consider again Example 3.4 but assume now that we want to estimate μ_x. Thus, only the first term on the right-hand side of (3.11) is needed. Again we will make use of the binary response indicator r, where $r = 1$ if x is observed and $r = 0$ if it is not. We assume the same missing data mechanism as in Example 3.4. Note that

$$\zeta_1 = \frac{\sigma_{yx}}{\sigma_y^2}, \qquad \zeta_0 = \mu_x - \mu_y \zeta_1, \quad \text{and} \quad \sigma_u^2 = \sigma_x^2 - \sigma_{yx}^2/\sigma_y^2 .$$

The ML estimator for μ_x is the solution to the estimating equations

$$0 = \bar{x}_{(1)} - (\mu_x - \hat{\mu}_y \hat{\zeta}_1 + \bar{y}_{(1)} \hat{\zeta}_1) ,$$

which is given by

$$\hat{\mu}_x = \frac{1}{n_{(1)}} \sum_{i=1}^{n} r_i [x_i - \hat{\zeta}_1 (y_i - \hat{\mu}_y)] , \quad \hat{\zeta}_1 = \frac{s_{yx,(1)}}{s_{y,(1)}^2} \quad \text{and} \quad \hat{\mu}_y = \frac{1}{n} \sum_{i=1}^{n} y_i .$$

Thus, μ_y can be estimated using the n observed y values, and μ_x can be estimated from the completely observed part of the sample plus a correction term. Using the fact that under missing data being MAR, the conditional mean of $x \mid y$ can be consistently estimated using the completely observed subsample only, $\hat{\mu}_x$ can be rewritten as

$$\hat{\mu}_x = \frac{1}{n} \sum_{i=1}^{n} [r_i x_i + (1 - r_i)(\hat{\zeta}_0 + \hat{\zeta}_1 y_i)] ,$$

where the last term in brackets is the conditional mean of $x_i \mid y_i$. Thus, to calculate $\hat{\mu}_x$, each missing value in x is implicitly replaced by the (estimated) conditional mean of $x_i \mid y_i$. If it would be known that $\mu_y = \mu_x$, then the parameters of the two terms in (3.11) would not be distinct. In this case, we would have to maximize the log-likelihood function (3.11) using both terms on the right-hand side. □

If a missing pattern is non-monotone, but close to being monotone, then one might adopt the strategy of creating a monotone missing pattern by either deleting (a few) values or by imputing (a few) values based on some simple imputation method. Both versions may be adopted if the number of units to be deleted or values to be imputed or, more precisely, the amount of missing information is small so that the problem of applying possibly inadequate techniques is minimized. A better solution, however, is to apply the expectation maximization (EM) algorithm offered by some software packages.

The EM algorithm (Dempster, Laird, & Rubin, 1977) and its further developments simplify ML estimation in otherwise complicated problems by deconstructing a difficult task into a sequence of simpler tasks, the solution of which converges to the solution of the difficult task. Thus the EM algorithm is particularly suited to deal with general missing data problems, but the field of applications is remarkably broader than standard missing data situations.

The underlying idea is as follows. Let $\mathbf{u}$ be a vector of continuous variables, where $\mathbf{u}_{(1)}$ is the observed part and $\mathbf{u}_{(0)}$ is the unobserved part. The density function of $\mathbf{u}$ can be written as

$$f(\mathbf{u}, \boldsymbol{\vartheta}) = f(\mathbf{u}_{(1)}, \boldsymbol{\vartheta}_1) f(\mathbf{u}_{(0)} \mid \mathbf{u}_{(1)}, \boldsymbol{\vartheta}_2) ,$$

where $\boldsymbol{\vartheta}$, $\boldsymbol{\vartheta}_1$ and $\boldsymbol{\vartheta}_2$ are unknown parameters. Taking the logarithm and rearranging terms leads to

$$l(\boldsymbol{\vartheta}_1, \mathbf{u}_{(1)}) = l(\boldsymbol{\vartheta}, \mathbf{u}) - \log f(\mathbf{u}_{(0)} \mid \mathbf{u}_{(1)}, \boldsymbol{\vartheta}_2) .$$

Based on starting values for the unknown parameters, the EM algorithm iterates over two steps, the expectation or E-step, and the maximization or M-Step.

In the E-step, the expectation of the log-likelihood is taken with respect to the variables with missing values, conditional on the observed values $\mathbf{u}_{(0)} \mid \mathbf{u}_{(1)}$ at the parameter value $\hat{\boldsymbol{\vartheta}}_2^{(j-1)}$ from the $(j-1)$th step,

$$Q(\hat{\boldsymbol{\vartheta}}^{(j)} \mid \hat{\boldsymbol{\vartheta}}^{(j-1)}) = \int l(\hat{\boldsymbol{\vartheta}}^{(j)}, \mathbf{u}) f(\mathbf{u}_{(0)} \mid \mathbf{u}_{(1)}, \hat{\boldsymbol{\vartheta}}_2^{(j-1)}) \, d\mathbf{u}_{(0)}$$

and

$$H(\hat{\boldsymbol{\vartheta}}_2^{(j)} \mid \hat{\boldsymbol{\vartheta}}_2^{(j-1)}) = \int \log f(\mathbf{u}_{(0)} \mid \mathbf{u}_{(1)}, \hat{\boldsymbol{\vartheta}}_2^{(j)}) f(\mathbf{u}_{(0)} \mid \mathbf{u}_{(1)}, \hat{\boldsymbol{\vartheta}}_2^{(j-1)}) \, d\mathbf{u}_{(0)} .$$

Since $l(\hat{\boldsymbol{\vartheta}}_1^{(j)}, \mathbf{u}_{(1)})$ is not a function of $\mathbf{u}_{(0)}$,

$$l(\hat{\boldsymbol{\vartheta}}^{(j)}, \mathbf{u}_{(1)}) = Q(\hat{\boldsymbol{\vartheta}}^{(j)} \mid \hat{\boldsymbol{\vartheta}}^{(j-1)}) - H(\hat{\boldsymbol{\vartheta}}^{(j)} \mid \hat{\boldsymbol{\vartheta}}^{(j-1)}) .$$

In this step, missing values are replaced by estimated values or, in more general problems, missing sufficient statistics or even the log-likelihood is estimated.

In the M-step, $Q(\hat{\boldsymbol{\vartheta}}^{(j)} \mid \hat{\boldsymbol{\vartheta}}^{(j-1)})$ resulting from the E-step is maximized with respect to $\boldsymbol{\vartheta}$, leading to a new estimate $\hat{\boldsymbol{\vartheta}}^{(j+1)}$. Repeating these steps generates a sequence of estimates $\hat{\boldsymbol{\vartheta}}^{(j)}$, $j = 1, 2, \ldots$, for which

$$l(\hat{\boldsymbol{\vartheta}}_1^{(j+1)}, \mathbf{u}_{(1)}) \geq l(\hat{\boldsymbol{\vartheta}}_1^{(j)}, \mathbf{u}_{(1)}) .$$

For a proof, see e.g., Lehmann and Casella (1998) and for a detailed presentation, see Little and Rubin (2002). However, some additional assumptions are necessary for this sequence to converge to an ML estimator, which are met in many standard cases, if the sample size is not too small and the proportion of missing information is not too large. For a discussion of this and related points, but also how to overcome some technical shortfalls of the EM algorithm, like further simplifications in complicated situations or increasing the speed of convergence and how to overcome the problem that standard errors are not automatically calculated, see, e.g., Lehmann and Casella (1998) or Little and Rubin (2002), Rubin (1987), Meng and Rubin (1991, 1993), Meng and van Dyk (1997), Liu and Rubin (1994), Oakes (1999) or Jamshidian and Jennrich (2000). An example of how the EM algorithm works is presented in the next section.

Often the terms to be imputed in the E-step can analytically be derived. Then the E-step simplifies considerably. Similarly, maximization of $Q(\hat{\boldsymbol{\vartheta}}^{(j)} \mid \hat{\boldsymbol{\vartheta}}^{(j-1)})$ is often not more complicated than maximizing the log-likelihood function of the completely observed sample. This makes the EM algorithm, if available for the specific problem at hand, a very attractive method for the analysis of incompletely observed data sets even in situations that seem to be hardly tractable with standard methods. But it should be noted that as for ML estimators in general, strong assumptions beyond those that are necessary if there were no missing values are required to hold for valid inferences.

3.3.3 The Nonignorable Case

If missing values are nonignorable, then the relationship between $(\mathbf{u}_{(1)}^T \;\; \mathbf{v}_{(1)}^T)^T$, $\mathbf{r}$ and $(\mathbf{u}_{(0)}^T \;\; \mathbf{v}_{(0)}^T)^T$ need to be considered and modeled explicitly for likelihood inferences in general. The likelihood function can either be written in form of the pattern-mixture model formulation (3.8) or in a selection model formulation (3.9) (e.g.,

Schafer, 2003). One way to get ML estimates in this case is via the EM algorithm. The approach of iterating over the E- and the M-step is in principle the same as in the case of an ignorable missing data mechanism, but now the parameter of the missing data mechanism has to be estimated as well.

Example 3.6 (ML Estimation of the Mean: EM Algorithm) Suppose that random variables y_i $(i = 1, \dots, n)$ are independently normally distributed as $y \sim N(\mu, 1)$, and y is observed if $y \leq c + \mu$ and is not observed otherwise. Then the missing values are MNAR, and $\Pr(r_i = 1) = \Pr(y_i \leq c + \mu) = \Phi(c)$ where $\Phi(\cdot)$ is the standard normal distribution function. Let the data be ordered such that the first $n_{(1)}$ values are observed, and the last $n_{(0)} = n - n_{(1)}$ values are not observed. If there were no missing values, then the likelihood function using the n observations would be

$$L(\mu) = \prod_{i=1}^{n} (2\pi)^{-1/2} \exp\left\{-\frac{(y_i - \mu)^2}{2}\right\} .$$

For the incompletely observed data set we get

$$L_{(1)}(\mu) = \left[\prod_{i=1}^{n_{(1)}} \frac{(2\pi)^{-1/2} \exp\left\{-\frac{(y_i-\mu)^2}{2}\right\}}{\Phi(c)}\right] \left[\Phi(c)^{n_{(1)}} (1 - \Phi(c))^{n_{(0)}}\right] .$$

The conditional density of the variables whose values have not been observed, given the observed values is

$$f(\mathbf{y}_{(0)} \mid \mathbf{y}_{(1)}, \mu) = f(\mathbf{y}_{(0)} \mid \mu) = \prod_{i=n_{(1)}+1}^{n} \frac{(2\pi)^{-1/2} \exp\left\{-\frac{(y_i-\mu)^2}{2}\right\}}{1 - \Phi(c)} ,$$

where $\mathbf{y}_{(1)}$ denotes the vector of variables y_i whose values have been observed and $\mathbf{y}_{(0)}$ denotes the vector of variables y_i whose values have not been observed. Taking the logarithm of $L(\mu)$ and then the expectation with respect to $f(\mathbf{y}_{(0)} \mid \hat{\mu}^{(j)}) = f(\mathbf{y}_{(0)} \mid \mathbf{y}_{(1)}, \hat{\mu}^{(j)})$ results in

$$Q(\mu \mid \hat{\mu}^{(j)}) = -\frac{n}{2} \ln(2\pi) - \frac{1}{2} \sum_{i=1}^{n_{(1)}} (y_i - \mu)^2$$
$$- \frac{1}{2} \sum_{i=n_{(1)}+1}^{n} \int (y_i - \mu)^2 f(y_i \mid r_i = 0, \hat{\mu}^{(j)})\, dy_i .$$

Taking the derivative with respect to μ and setting the result equal to zero leads to

$$\sum_{i=1}^{n_{(1)}} (y_i - \mu) + \int \sum_{i=n_{(1)}+1}^{n} (y_i - \mu) f(y_i \mid r_i = 0, n_{(0)}, \hat{\mu}^{(j)})\, dy_i = 0 .$$

Since the variables whose values have not been observed are all independently distributed according to the same distribution, they all have the same expectation, which will be denoted as $E(y_{(0)} \mid \hat{\mu}^{(j)})$ at a given parameter value $\hat{\mu}^{(j)}$. Solving the above estimating equations for $\hat{\mu}^{(j+1)}$ gives

$$\hat{\mu}^{(j+1)} = n^{-1}(n_{(1)}\bar{y}_{(1)} + n_{(0)}E(y_{(0)} \mid \hat{\mu}^{(j)})) . \tag{3.12}$$

In the E-step we therefore have to calculate $E(y_{(0)} \mid \hat{\mu}^{(j)})$, which is the expectation of a truncated normally distributed variable (see Appendix A.2.6)

$$E(y_{(0)} \mid \hat{\mu}^{(j)}) = \hat{\mu}^{(j)} + \frac{\varphi(c)}{1 - \Phi(c)} ,$$

where $\varphi(c)$ is the standard normal density function. In the M-step $\hat{\mu}^{(j+1)}$ has to be calculated according to (3.12).

To illustrate the calculation of the estimate via the EM algorithm, we simulated data for $n = 100$ units and c such that values for $n_{(1)} = 68$ units were observed and values for $n_{(0)} = 32$ units were missing, and calculated the EM estimates for successive iteration steps of the EM algorithm. The true value was $\mu = 0$ and the starting value was $\hat{\mu}^{(0)} = 1$. The results are presented in Table 3.3, also including the differences of successively generated estimates. The algorithm stopped when the absolute value of the difference between $\hat{\mu}^{(j)}$ and $\hat{\mu}^{(j+1)}$ was below 10^{-6} , which was reached after seven iterations.

We generated not only one artificial data set, but performed the process of generating a data set and then estimating μ_y 1000 times. The mean over the 1000 estimates of μ calculated via the EM algorithm was $\bar{\hat{\mu}}_{EM} = 0.001928$. The mean over estimates of μ based on the data sets before any values were deleted, was $\bar{\hat{\mu}}_{com} = 0.001736$. Both are close to the true value zero. □

If nonignorable missing units have to be compensated, then one might adopt a sample selection model. In a cross-sectional data set, this amounts usually to

Table 3.3 Successive estimates $\hat{\mu}^{(j)}$ and differences $\hat{\mu}^{(j)} - \hat{\mu}^{(j-1)}$ for $j = 1, \ldots$ using the EM-algorithm to estimate the expectation of a truncated normally distributed variable given missing values being MNAR

j	$\hat{\mu}^{(j)}$	$\hat{\mu}^{(j)} - \hat{\mu}^{(j-1)}$
1	0.1160033	−0.8839967
2	0.0085419	−0.1074614
3	−0.0010473	−0.0095893
4	−0.0018731	−0.0008257
5	−0.0019439	−0.0000709
6	−0.0019500	−0.0000061
7	−0.0019505	−0.0000005

Starting value $\hat{\mu}^{(0)} = 1$, $n = 100$, $n_{(1)} = 68$ and true value $\mu_0 = 0$
Estimate for complete-data set $\hat{\mu}_{com} = -0.0281$

estimating a two-equation model: The first equation models the probability of observing the unit and the second model equation is the model of applied-scientific interest. Assuming the model of applied-scientific interest to be linear and ignoring the index i, the two-equation model is given by

$$r^* = \mathbf{z}^T \boldsymbol{\gamma} + \upsilon \ , \qquad \text{where} \qquad r = \begin{cases} 1, \text{ if } & r^* > 0, \\ 0 \text{ else}, \end{cases}$$

and

$$y = \mathbf{x}^T \boldsymbol{\beta} + \epsilon \ ,$$

where $(\upsilon \ \epsilon)$ is iid, $E(\epsilon) = E(\upsilon) = 0$ and independent from $\mathbf{z}$ and $\mathbf{x}$. Both predictor vectors, $\mathbf{z}$ and $\mathbf{x}$, include a constant term and may have variables in common. Note that from these assumptions it follows that $y \mid \mathbf{x}$ does not additionally depend on $\mathbf{z}$ and, vice versa, that $r^* \mid \mathbf{z}$ does not additionally depend on $\mathbf{x}$. The variable of interest, y, is observed, if $r = 1$ and is not observed, otherwise. Further note that r^* is never observed, r and $\mathbf{z}$ are always observed and $\mathbf{x}$ is observed if $r = 1$ and may not be observed when $r = 0$.

Let us assume that we completely observe the first $n_{(1)}$ units but not the remaining $n_{(0)} = n - n_{(1)}$. Thus, estimating the parameter of interest, $\boldsymbol{\beta}$, would be based only on the first $n_{(1)}$ observed units if the missing data mechanism would be ignored. Depending on the missing data mechanism, this might lead to a biased estimator: If υ is not independent from ϵ, then r^* depends not only on $\mathbf{z}$ and the independent error υ but in addition on unobserved variables that have an effect on y. Correspondingly, y would depend on υ even after conditioning on $\mathbf{x}$ and ϵ. Thus, the missing values would be MNAR.

Usually the parameter of interest $\boldsymbol{\beta}$ is estimated based on a model selection formulation, either using the maximum likelihood method or adopting a two-step approach (e.g., Heckman, 1979). To illustrate the consequences of the above assumptions about the missing data mechanism and the model of applied-scientific interest, however, a pattern-mixture formulation is adopted.

Given the above assumptions and ignoring dependence on parameters for the moment, we can write

$$f(y \mid \mathbf{x}, \mathbf{z})^r g(r \mid y, \mathbf{x}, \mathbf{z}) = f(y \mid \mathbf{x})^r g(r \mid y, \mathbf{z}) \ .$$

If we are willing to assume that $(\upsilon \ \epsilon)$ is bivariate normally distributed with variances $\sigma_\upsilon^2, \sigma_\epsilon^2$ and covariance $\sigma_{\upsilon\epsilon}$, then $\upsilon = \sigma_{\upsilon\epsilon}/\sigma_\epsilon^2\,(y - \mathbf{x}^T\boldsymbol{\beta}) + u$, where $u \sim N(0, \sigma_\upsilon^2 - \sigma_{\upsilon\epsilon}^2/\sigma_\epsilon^2)$ (see Appendix A.2.5), and

$$\begin{aligned} g(r = 1 \mid y, \mathbf{z}) = g(r = 1 \mid \epsilon, \mathbf{z}) &= \Pr(r^* > 0 \mid \epsilon, \mathbf{z}) \\ &= \Pr(\mathbf{z}^T \boldsymbol{\gamma} + \sigma_{\upsilon\epsilon}/\sigma_\epsilon^2 (y - \mathbf{x}^T \boldsymbol{\beta}) + u > 0) \end{aligned}$$

$$= \Pr\{u > -[\mathbf{z}^T \boldsymbol{\gamma} + \sigma_{\upsilon\epsilon}/\sigma_\epsilon^2 (y - \mathbf{x}^T \boldsymbol{\beta})]\}$$

$$= 1 - \Phi \left\{ [\mathbf{z}^T \boldsymbol{\gamma} + \sigma_{\upsilon\epsilon}/\sigma_\epsilon^2 (y - \mathbf{x}^T \boldsymbol{\beta})] / \sqrt{\sigma_\upsilon^2 - \sigma_{\upsilon\epsilon}^2/\sigma_\epsilon^2} \right\} ,$$

where $\Phi(\cdot)$ denotes the standard normal distribution function. Let $\tilde{\boldsymbol{\gamma}} = \left(\boldsymbol{\gamma}^T \ \sigma_{\upsilon\epsilon}/\sigma_\epsilon^2\right)^T / \sqrt{\sigma_\upsilon^2 - \sigma_{\upsilon\epsilon}^2/\sigma_\epsilon^2}$ and $\boldsymbol{\theta} = \left(\boldsymbol{\beta}^T \ \sigma_\epsilon^2\right)^T$, then the log-likelihood function is

$$l(\tilde{\boldsymbol{\gamma}}, \boldsymbol{\beta}) = \sum_{i=1}^{n} \log g(r_i \mid \mathbf{z}_i, y_i, \tilde{\boldsymbol{\gamma}}, \boldsymbol{\theta}) + r_i \log f(y_i \mid \mathbf{x}_i, \boldsymbol{\theta}) .$$

Note that $g(r_i \mid \mathbf{z}_i, y_i, \tilde{\boldsymbol{\gamma}}, \boldsymbol{\theta})$ is, given the normality assumption, a binary Probit model.

Obviously, the response mechanism cannot be ignored when $\sigma_{\upsilon\epsilon} \neq 0$, i.e., when the response probability depends on variables $\mathbf{z}$ and additionally on unobserved variables that have an effect on y. In that case, the missing values are MNAR and the missing data mechanism has to be explicitly modeled and included into the log-likelihood function to estimate $\boldsymbol{\theta}$. Note that whether inferences about $\boldsymbol{\beta}$ are valid depends not only on assumptions underlying the model of applied-scientific interest being met but also whether the assumptions about the missing data mechanism and the relationship between the model for r and y are met.

As an illustration assume we were interested in a wage equation and in addition to variables like age, years of schooling which we include in our model as predictor variables $\mathbf{x}$, an unobserved variable 'social competence' plays an important role with respect to wage. Even without missing values, we would have to assume that social competence is not correlated with $\mathbf{x}$. Otherwise, if social competence were correlated with years of schooling, say, then years of schooling would not be exogenous and the above ML estimator of $\boldsymbol{\beta}$ would be biased. If social competence were uncorrelated with $\mathbf{x}$, however, but had an effect on y and on r^*, then missing units would be MNAR and we could adopt the above modeling approach, if we were willing to make the distributional assumption of bivariate normality. If social competence had no effect on y additional to $\mathbf{x}$, but only on r^*, it would simply be part of υ. However, since the response mechanism as part of the log-likelihood function involves $\boldsymbol{\beta}$ if $\sigma_{\upsilon\epsilon} \neq 0$, it has to be correctly specified for consistent estimation of $\boldsymbol{\beta}$. Hence, the normality assumption for the response mechanism is one crucial assumption with respect to consistent estimation of $\boldsymbol{\beta}$. Another important point is to include all relevant variables into both models. Usually $\mathbf{z}$ includes at least parts of $\mathbf{x}$ and additional variables thought to be relevant for r. Note that variables included in $\mathbf{z}$ have to be observed for all units.

Adopting a selection formulation approach, one would specify a binary model for the missing data mechanism, $g(r \mid \mathbf{z})$, and the regression model of applied-scientific interest including a term that corrects for systematic differences between the incompletely and the completely observed group if $\sigma_{\upsilon\epsilon} \neq 0$, $f(y \mid \mathbf{x}, r = 1)$.

Finally, it should be noted that non-ML approaches to estimate sample selection models have been proposed as well. For example, Heckman (1979) describes a two-step approach which leads to less efficient but simple estimators (for the basic idea, see Appendix A.2.5). Generalizations of sample selection models to panel data have also been described, e.g., by Hausman and Wise (1979), Ridder (1990), Vella (1998) or Spiess and Kroh (2010). For further discussion, see Little and Rubin (2002), Wooldridge (2002a), Cameron and Trivedi (2005) or Pagan and Ullah (1999).

3.4 Weighting

Weighting to compensate for unequal probabilities of observing units is well known in frequentist survey statistics, since at least Horvitz and Thompson (1952) proposed a weighted estimator to adjust for unequal selection probabilities. The rough idea is to attach higher weights to units that are expected to be observed with lower probability as compared to units with higher expected probability of being observed. A simple example illustrates the idea.

Example 3.7 (Weighted Estimation of the Mean) Suppose we select a sample from a finite dichotomous population, where only a small portion of units have a certain characteristic, e.g., disease A. Based on this sample, it is intended to estimate models for this specific population, but inferences are also intended for the whole population, for example, the population mean of a metric depression scale. To allow inferences for the small subpopulation with disease A, units from this subpopulation are selected with higher probability than from the other part of the population, so that the corresponding subsample is large enough for the analyses of interest. Let π_A be the probability of selecting a unit from the subpopulation with disease A and $\pi_{\bar{A}}$ be the probability of selecting a unit from the subpopulation without the disease. Let j index the population elements and N be the size of the population, such that $j = 1, \ldots, N$. Assume we select a sample with n elements and use $i = 1, \ldots, n$ as the index for these elements. Let s_j be a selection indicator such that if $s_j = 1$, then y_j, the metric depression score of the jth population unit is selected. Otherwise, if $s_j = 0$, then y_j is not selected from the population. Given a sample where units are selected with probability $\pi_j = \pi_A$ if unit j is from the subpopulation with disease A and $\pi_j = \pi_{\bar{A}}$ if not, respectively, the estimator of the mean depression score in the whole population is

$$\hat{m}(y) = \frac{1}{N} \sum_{i=1}^{n} \frac{y_i}{\pi_i} = \frac{1}{N} \sum_{j=1}^{N} \frac{s_j}{\pi_j} y_j .$$

Note that N is a fixed number, but $n = \sum_{j=1}^{N} s_j$ is random. Treating the depression scores as fixed numbers, which is a common strategy in survey statistics where statements about finite populations are of interest, the expectation of this estimator is

$$E(\hat{m}(y)) = \frac{1}{N}\sum_{j=1}^{N}\frac{E(s_j)}{\pi_j}y_j = \frac{1}{N}\sum_{j=1}^{N}\frac{\pi_j}{\pi_j}y_= \frac{1}{N}\sum_{j=1}^{N}y_j = m(y)\,.$$

Thus, by weighting each selected unit by its inverse selection probability, we obtain an unbiased estimator. For an extensive discussion of these kind of estimators and alternatives, see, e.g., Särndal et al. (1992). □

The process of arriving at an observed sample of units can be interpreted as a two-stage selection process: Selection into the gross or intended sample and selection into the observed part or net sample. Unlike the probabilities of selecting units into the gross sample, the probabilities of selection into the net sample, the response probabilities, are usually unknown. The use of weighted estimators to account for unit nonresponse thus requires that the response probabilities are estimated. This has been proposed in the context of survey statistics (Särndal et al., 1992), but has been transferred to frequentist model-based statistics to account for unit nonresponse when one is interested in aspects of theoretical distributions, like regression parameters, e.g., by Robins, Rotnitzky, and Zhao (1995), Wooldridge (2002a, 2002b, 2007).

Therefore, in a first step, the parameters of the response model $g(r \mid \mathbf{z}, \boldsymbol{y})$ have to be estimated assuming that all necessary predictors are included. Instead of a fully parametric model, like a Logit- or Probit model, semi- or even nonparametric models may be adopted as well (see McCaffrey, Ridgeway, & Morral, 2004, for an example). The predicted response probabilities from this step are then used in a weighted analysis. For example, let $\hat{\pi}_i$, $i = 1, \ldots, n$, be the estimated response probabilities of a sample of observed units, then the contribution of each unit to the estimation of the parameters of interest and its variance is weighted by the inverse of this estimated probability, $1/\hat{\pi}_i$. In general regression problems as described in Robins et al. (1995) or Wooldridge (2002a), the estimator of the variance of the parameters of interest ignores the fact that $\hat{\pi}_i$ are estimates. However, it turns out that this strategy leads to slightly conservative inferences, i.e., the actual rejection level of true null hypothesis is below the nominal level and confidence intervals are slightly too large, but at the same time to more efficient estimators, as compared to estimators that would use the true response probabilities because, e.g., the nominal confidence intervals are shorter if estimated response probabilities are used (Robins et al., 1995). Hence although variances are slightly overestimated, the estimators tend to be slightly more precise.

The need to estimate the response probabilities makes an explicit modeling of the response mechanism necessary. This is usually done by adopting binary regression models, like Logit- or Probit models, the dependent variable being a binary variable indicating whether the corresponding unit was observed or not and assuming that the missing units are MAR. Since we are not interested in the parameter governing the response model, but in the predicted probabilities, it is wise to include as many predictors and functions of them as possible into the estimation model. In fact, Robins et al. (1995) show that including additional variables and functions thereof tends to lead to more efficient estimators of applied scientific of interest. Of course, these predictors need to be observed for all units.

Although statistical software often allows weighted analyses, it is important to note that these weights are estimated inverse probability weights and should not be confused with frequency weights, which would lead to severely biased standard errors. If this is not anyway the default, a robust estimator should be chosen to estimate the variance of the estimators of interest. Furthermore, standard software is often not able to deal with weights that vary within units, like in panel models when there is attrition. In the latter case units drop out at a certain point in time. However, this leads to varying observation probabilities over time for those participating. The variation may even become more pronounced when attrition is not an absorbing state, i.e., if some units that dropped out at time point t are again observed at time point $t + k$. These units will receive relatively small probabilities of being observed—although for these cases, response probability models may be hard to justify and estimate.

On the other hand, if estimated probabilities are close to zero, the consequence may be exorbitant weights. This may lead to very large standard errors and possibly even biased estimators (e.g., Freedman and Berk 2008; but see also Kang and Schafer 2007 and the subsequent discussion in the same volume). In applications one might thus compare results of weighted analyses including all units and including all but those x percent with the highest weights, x depending on the sample distribution of the weights. If inferences do not change substantially, then large weights or even outliers have no substantial effect. However, if there is a substantial change, then one should inspect the sample distribution of the weights more closely, possibly change the response model, for example, by adding additional variables and/or functions thereof. If this does not reduce the effect of extreme weights, other compensation methods may be considered, like selection models (see Sect. 3.3.3) or multiple imputation (see Sect. 3.5.2).

Since weighted estimation may lead to larger standard errors, an interesting question is whether or not weights should be used in a certain application. If totals, means or proportions in a finite population have to be estimated, then weighting is necessary to adjust for different probabilities of observing the units. If aspects of statistical models have to be estimated, things are more complicated (Wooldridge, 2007).

Of course, weighting is unnecessary when missing units are MCAR. If aspects of an unconditional distribution are of interest, then unweighted estimation leads to consistent estimators only if the missing units are MCAR. In this case the unweighted estimator is preferred since generating weights is a potential source of misspecification, in which case the parameter estimator of interest may be biased. If aspects of conditional distributions are of interest, like regression parameters, then whether or not the parameters of interest are consistent, depends on several aspects.

Throughout we will consider the case of a correctly specified model of applied-scientific interest if not stated otherwise. That is, if a regression model is to be estimated, we presuppose that this model or the interesting aspects of this model and all the assumptions necessary for consistent estimation of this model or its interesting aspects are met if there were no missing units. For a detailed discussion, see Wooldridge (2007).

If selection into the observed part of the sample depends only on predictors included into the model of applied-scientific interest, then unweighted estimation allows consistent estimation of the interesting parameters. Note that in this scenario the predictors need not be observed for all units. Weighted estimation may or may not lead to consistent estimators. If the functional form of the response probability is misspecified or predictors are not completely observed and therefore cannot be included into the response model, then weighting may not lead to consistent estimators of applied-scientific interest. This latter situation arises if, for example, panel data are analysed and drop out of units at time $t + 1$ depends on time varying variables not observed at time t and which are not independent from the dependent variables in the model of applied-scientific interest. Only if the predictors in the model of interest are always observed and included into the response model, then weighted estimation allows consistent estimation of the parameters of interest (Wooldridge, 2007). Note that weighting is not necessary in this case.

However, if there are variables relevant for the probability of responding that are not part of the predictor vector in the model of interest and which are not independent from the dependent variable of the conditional model of interest, are always observed and included into the model for the response probabilities, then weighted estimation allows consistent estimation, whereas unweighted estimation does not.

In situations in which weighting is not necessary for consistent estimation, unweighted estimators tend to be more efficient as compared to weighted estimators. Hence weighting as a strategy to compensate for unit nonresponse may be adopted, for example, when the database producer has access to variables that explain response behaviour but that cannot be passed to the analyst due to data protection laws, these variables are observed for all units and are relevant for estimating the response probabilities. Similarly, good candidates for predictors in models to generate weights are variables explaining response but which are usually not considered as predictors in models of applied-scientific interest and are observed for all units. In face-to-face interviews where units are interviewed at home, examples of the variables are interviewer- or other external information about the neighbourhood of units or meteorological or geographical variables that can be linked with the units to be observed.

3.5 Imputation Methods

Imputation methods are methods that generate one or more predictions for each missing value. In principle, imputation methods can be adopted whether missing data are MCAR, MAR or MNAR. In the latter case, however, strong assumptions are necessary or external information needs to be available to allow valid inferences. Software packages that provide imputation tools usually presuppose that missing values are MAR.

Given that missing values are MAR, important questions are how to generate these predictions and how to deal with the fact that these predictions are not deterministically derived but uncertain estimates used to complete an incompletely observed data set. Thus, these predicted values usually do not convey new information but are mainly made up of information already available in the observed part of the sample in addition to some modeling assumptions. Thus, treating these predictions as observed values would lead to an overestimation of information carried by the completed sample.

It is not difficult to somehow generate imputations. It is much harder to justify an imputation method that allows valid inferences. Correspondingly, the most important question is how to generate imputations such that inferences of scientific interest tend to be valid even in the presence of missing data.

3.5.1 Single Imputation

Many ad-hoc methods generate imputations to complete-data sets, with one prediction for each missing value. Some of these techniques are described in Sect. 3.2.2. Usually they are not theoretically justified and allow valid inference only under very restrictive conditions. Often the general problems are not tackled: How to generate the imputations such that the final applied-scientific analyses are valid. An example not mentioned in Sect. 3.2.2 is, e.g., the technique denoted as 'last observation carried forward' that replaces an unobserved value at a certain point in time t by the value observed for that same unit from the last observed time point $t - k$, $k > 0$. There are several refinements of this technique available that take into account neighbouring information from the same unit and/or other units in the same data sets. The major drawback of most of these techniques, however, is that there is no theoretical justification. This is easiest seen if the simplest version is considered: First, if values from $t - k$ are used to estimate the value at time t, this may lead to a severe underestimation of the dynamics in the data. More sophisticated techniques include time dependent information from other variables to predict the unobserved values at t. Then underestimation of the dynamics may be less severe. Second, if these predictions are treated as being observed values carrying independent information, then standard errors will be too small. As a consequence, the proportion of falsely rejecting null hypotheses will be too high and confidence intervals will be too small.

On the other hand, single imputation methods which allow valid inferences have been discussed, e.g., in a very general regression context by Wang and Robins (1998) and Robins and Wang (2000). However, their approach is a solution for specific regression problems, which requires a good knowledge of statistics and good programming skills of the data analyst. Generating single imputations that allow valid inferences is costly, but once such a technique is implemented, the additional effort of generating multiple imputations mainly requires computing time. Thus, we will not describe single imputation methods at length. Instead, in the next section, we will give a brief introduction into the method of multiple imputation.

3.5.2 *Multiple Imputation*

The original idea of multiple imputation (MI) is that the database producer and the analyst are two different entities and it is assumed that the database producer has access to resources like time, statistical and programming skills and information being not available to the analyst. Hence, the main burden of generating the multiple imputations is on the database producer and not on the analyst. The database producer has access to many resources an applied researcher usually does not have, i.e., time, information and skills, to generate a multiply imputed data set that can be used for various analyses from different analysts.

MI is a method proposed to compensate for item nonresponse in situations with not more than 30–50% of missing information (Rubin, 1987, 1996). The idea is to generate multiple predictions or imputations for each missing datum, thereby generating multiple versions of an incompletely observed data set that can be analysed using standard methods. The multiple results are then combined according to some simple rules to allow inferences about statistical models of applied-scientific interest. MI is developed based on a Bayesian approach and if the imputation method is proper in a sense defined by Rubin (1987) and extended by Rubin (1996), the final inferences will in general be valid in a frequentist sense.

Let the data set not being affected by missing data be denoted as the complete-data set, and the (unknown) parameter estimates of the parameter of scientific interest and its variance be denoted as complete-data set statistics. Basically, for an MI method to be proper, the estimator of the parameter of scientific interest and its variance based on a multiply imputed data set must be approximately unbiased for the corresponding complete-data statistics, and an estimator of the variance of the estimator of scientific interest across imputations must also be approximately unbiased. If the multiple imputation method is proper and the inference based on the complete-data set is valid, then the analysis using the multiply imputed data set tends to be valid for the unknown population parameters.

The advantage of MI over other methods is that it allows various different analyses in a rather easy way once a data set is multiply imputed. Further, theoretical justification for the method is given, e.g., by Rubin (1987, 1996), Meng (1994) and Tsiatis (2006). Although several tools are available to generate imputations, it is not straightforward to generate imputations according to a proper method. For example, as mentioned in Sect. 3.3.2, a linear imputation regression model for some variable treated as a predictor in a homoscedastic linear regression model of applied-scientific interest is a correctly specified imputation model only if both, the variable treated as the dependent variable and this covariate, are bivariate normally distributed (Spanos, 1995). On the other hand, if a continuous variable needs to be imputed, most software packages that allow generating multiple imputations propose a homoscedastic normal linear regression model which might thus be a misspecified imputation model in many cases. Additionally, if important variables are not included into the imputation model, it may be misspecified and the imputation method would not be proper, in which case the estimator of applied-scientific interest may not have the desired properties. A detailed treatment of the MI method is given in Chap. 4.

3.6 Summary

In this chapter various approaches to deal with missing units and/or values were discussed. Most of the simple ad-hoc methods allow valid inferences at best in very specific situations and if software for downstream analyses is adapted correspondingly. The problem with these methods is that they have been proposed mainly for pragmatic reasons without a theoretical justification.

For specific models and situations if the missing data mechanism is ignorable, maximum likelihood methods are available, probably based on the EM-algorithm. If one is willing to make all necessary, usually rather strong assumptions, then this is the method of choice.

As also discussed in this chapter, in specific situations methods for nonignorable missing data mechanisms are available, as well. However, it should be noted that in that case strong additional assumptions about the missing data mechanism and its relationship to the model of interest are necessary to justify inferences for the model of applied-scientific interest. If at least one of these assumptions is violated, then the validity of the inferences is questionable.

Another technique is weighting based on estimated response probabilities, which has been proposed to compensate for missing units if they are MAR. If this strategy is adopted, not only the model of applied-scientific interest but also a model of the missing data mechanism has to be specified. Beside an introduction into the general idea, we therefore discussed situations where, in the presence of missing units, weighting is appropriate and others in which it can safely be avoided. Although weighting has also been proposed to account for missing items, we are not aware of any publicly available analysis software that can be applied to general missing item problems.

Finally, imputation approaches were presented. Single imputation methods can either be ad-hoc methods, like imputing the mean of the observed values of an incompletely observed variable for each missing value, or more sophisticated methods which, at least in principle, allow valid inferences. Single imputation strategies always require adapting standard errors if analysis software for completely observed data sets is adopted. A strategy that requires only slightly more effort than an appropriate single imputation method and is theoretically justified is the method of multiple imputation, where each missing value is replaced by several plausible values. The method of multiple imputation is introduced and discussed in the next chapter.

References

Cameron, A. C., & Trivedi, P. K. (2005). *Microeconometrics: Methods and applications*. Cambridge, UK: University Press.

Dempster, A. P., Laird, N. M., & Rubin, D. B. (1977). Maximum likelihood from incomplete data via the *EM* algorithm. *Journal of the Royal Statistical Society. Series B, 39*(1), 1–22.

Freedman, D. A., & Berk, R. A. (2008). Weighting regressions by propensity scores. *Evaluation Review, 32*(4), 392–409.

Hausman, J. A., & Wise, D. A. (1979). Attrition bias in experimental and panel data: The Gary income maintenance experiment. *Econometrica, 47*(2), 455–473.

Heckman, J. J. (1979). Sample selection bias as a specification error. *Econometrica, 47*(1), 153–161.

Horvitz, D. G. & Thompson, D. J. (1952). A generalization of sampling without replacement from a finite universe. *Journal of the American Statistical Association, 47* (260), 663–685.

Jamshidian, M., & Jennrich, R. I. (2000). Standard errors for *EM* estimation. *Journal of the Royal Statistical Society, Series B, 62*(2), 257–270.

Jones, M. P. (1996). Indicator and stratification methods for missing explanatory variables in multiple linear regression. *Journal of the American Association, 91*(433), 222–230.

Kang, J. D. Y., & Schafer, J. L. (2007). Demystifying double robustness: A comparison of alternative strategies for estimating a population mean from incomplete data. *Statistical Science, 22*(4), 523–539.

Lehmann, E. L. (1998). *Elements of large-sample theory*. New York, NY: Springer.

Lehmann, E. L., & Casella, G. (1998). *Theory of point estimation* (2nd ed.). New York, NY: Springer.

Little, R. J. A. (1993). Pattern-mixture models for multivariate incomplete data. *Journal of the American Statistical Association, 88*(421), 125–134.

Little, R. J. A., & Rubin, D. B. (2002). *Statistical analysis with missing data* (2nd ed.). New Jersey, NJ: Wiley.

Liu, C., & Rubin, D. B. (1994). The *ECME* algorithm: A simple extension of *EM* and *ECM* with faster monotone convergence. *Biometrika, 81*(4), 633–648.

McCaffrey, D. F., Ridgeway, G., & Morral, A. R. (2004). Propensity score estimation with boosted regression for evaluating causal effects in observational studies. *Psychological Methods, 9*(4), 403–425.

Meng, X.-L. (1994). Multiple-imputation inferences with uncongenial sources of input. *Statistical Science, 9*(4), 538–558.

Meng, X.-L., & Rubin, D. B. (1991). Using *EM* to obtain asymptotic variance-covariance matrices: The SEM algorithm. *Journal of the American Statistical Association, 86*(416), 899–909.

Meng, X.-L., & Rubin, D. B. (1993). Maximum likelihood estimation via the *ECM* algorithm: A general framework. *Biometrika, 80*(2), 267–278.

Meng, X.-L., & van Dyk, D. (1997). The *EM* algorithm—an old folk-song sung to a fast new tune. *Journal of the Royal Statistical Society, 59*(3), 511–540.

Newey, W. K., & McFadden, D. L. (1994). Large sample estimation and hypothesis testing. In R. F. Engle & D. L. McFadden (Eds.), *Handbook of econometrics* (Vol. IV, pp. 2111–2245). Amsterdam: Elsevier.

Oakes, D. (1999). Direct calculation of the information matrix via the *EM* algorithm. *Journal of the Royal Statistical Society, Series B, 61*(2), 479–482.

Pagan, A., & Ullah, A. (1999). *Nonparametric econometrics*. Cambridge, UK: Cambridge University Press.

Ridder, G. (1990). Attrition in multi-wave panel data. In J. Hartog, G. Ridder, & J. Theeuwes (Eds.), *Panel data and labor market studies* (pp. 45–67). Amsterdam: Elsevier.

Robins, J. M., Rotnitzky, A., & Zhao, L. (1995). Analysis of semiparametric regression models for repeated outcomes in the presence of missing data. *Journal of the American Statistical Association, 90*(429), 106–121.

Robins, J. M., & Wang, N. (2000). Inference for imputation estimators. *Biometrika, 87*(1), 113–124.

Rubin, D. B. (1987). *Multiple imputation for nonresponse in surveys*. New York, NY: Wiley.

Rubin, D. B. (1996). Multiple imputation after 18+ years. *Journal of the American Statistical Association, 91*(434), 473–489.

Särndal, C.-E., Swensson, B., & Wretman, J. (1992). *Model assisted survey sampling*. New York, NY: Springer.

Schafer, J. L. (2003). Multiple imputation in multivariate problems when the imputation and analysis models differ. *Statistica Neerlandica, 57*(1), 19–35.

Serfling, R. J. (1980). *Approximation theorems of mathematical statistics*. New York, NY: Wiley.

Spanos, A. (1995). On normality and the linear regression model. *Econometric Reviews, 14*(2), 195–203.

Spiess, M., & Kroh, M. (2010). A selection model for panel data: The prospects of green party support. *Political Analysis, 18*(2), 172–188.

Tsiatis, A. A. (2006). *Semiparametric theory and missing data*. New York, NY: Springer.

Vella, F. (1998). Estimating models with sample selection bias: A survey. *The Journal of Human Resources, 33*(1), 127–169.

Wang, N., & Robins, J. M. (1998). Large-sample theory for parametric multiple imputation procedures. *Biometrika, 85*(4), 935–948.

Wooldridge, J. M. (2002a). *Econometric analysis of cross section and panel data*. Cambridge, MA: MIT Press.

Wooldridge, J. M. (2002b). Inverse probability weighted *M*-estimators for sample selection, attrition and stratification. *Portuguese Economic Journal, 1*(2), 117–139.

Wooldridge, J. M. (2007). Inverse probability weighted estimation for general missing data problems. *Journal of Econometrics, 141*(2), 1281–1301.

Chapter 4
Multiple Imputation: Theory

4.1 Overview

In this chapter, we provide an overview over the theory of multiple imputation. Topics covered are justification of multiple imputation strategies based on monotone and non-monotone missing patterns, the approach based on joint modeling of all variables with missing values and the fully conditional modeling approach, where only univariate marginal models are used to generate imputations. Additional topics are rounding, how to deal with restrictions and how to treat interaction or higher polynomial terms.

4.2 Multiple Imputation: Introduction

Functions to multiply impute incompletely observed data sets are widely available and most software packages provide the possibility to generate imputations. Chapter 3 shows that completing data sets with arbitrarily generated imputations may lead in general to invalid inferences. This implies that for valid inferences about models of scientific interest, the method to generate imputations has to meet some requirements.

In this chapter, we will give an introduction into the theory of multiple imputation proposed by Rubin (1987, 1996). Since a full treatment of the theory would be beyond the scope of this book, we will focus on key aspects of the theory and the process of generating multiple imputations which are relevant for valid conclusions.

K. Kleinke et al., *Applied Multiple Imputation*,
Statistics for Social and Behavioral Sciences,
https://doi.org/10.1007/978-3-030-38164-6_4

4.3 Theoretical Background

Before considering the theory of multiple imputation and discussing the concept of a proper imputation method, it has to be clarified what 'valid inferences' means. We then give a short overview over the theory of multiple imputation (Rubin, 1987, 1996) and describe conditions under which inferences based on multiple imputations tend to be valid.

4.3.1 Valid Inferences

The goal associated with the application of a statistical technique depends on the population, often approximated by a model, and on the specific aspects of the problem. For example, if a sample is not completely observed and missing values are replaced by imputations, a first step could be to apply descriptive techniques to this completed sample. Thus the finite complete sample would be the population of interest and its description would be the goal of the analysis. With histograms or frequency tables in mind, one objective in this case could be to impute only values that are possible to observe, probably in addition restricted to the observed range of values, like non-negative integers below some observed maximum for the number of children living in a household. Yet another goal could be to generate predictions for new cases or possible future values for the same cases. Then one might be interested in predictions which are as close as possible to the true but unobserved values ignoring any uncertainty in the predictions ('hit-rate' criterion).

In many scientific analyses, however, interest is in inferences about finite population statistics, model parameters or, more generally, aspects of statistical models. These inferences are based on functions of random variables, like estimators or test statistics, and are therefore afflicted with uncertainty. In these cases the criteria for valid inferences depend on the statistical approach (see Chap. 2) and are geared towards the properties of the scientifically interesting estimators, test statistics and confidence intervals in specific applications. The evaluation of imputation methods in Rubin (1987, 1996) does not cover the performance of descriptive analyses based on imputed data sets. Hence, imputed values need neither necessarily be plausible or realistic nor need they be as close as possible to the true but unobserved values.

The former statement is not an exclusive concept of multiple imputation. For example, for the χ^2-independence test the expected number of observations needs to be calculated as an intermediate result, rarely resulting in (non-negative) integers. Imputed values can be considered as intermediate results in the same sense, generated to allow inferences about finite but not completely observed populations or models approximating abstract populations. See de Jong, van Buuren, and Spiess (2016) for an example where inferences are valid although imputations for a count variable were generated from a continuous distribution, whereas inferences are invalid when imputations for the same variable were sampled from a restrictive

Poisson distribution, although the latter produced possible values. In that example the imputed count variable entered the model of scientific interest as a metric predictor variable and therefore there was no need to generate integer values as imputations. Nonetheless, in applications there may be the requirement that only values that could be observed, i.e., values from the set of possible realizations of this variable should be generated because the imputed variables enter the corresponding model of applied-scientific interest as the dependent variable. Therefore, under the primacy of finally valid inferences about the model of scientific interest, the models to generate imputations should generate values from this set whenever possible. Of course, nominal or ordered variables should be generated using imputation models appropriate for these measurement levels.

Since the method of multiple imputation is designed to solve problems within a design- or model-based approach evaluated from a frequentist perspective, see (Rubin, 1996, p. 474) and (Meng, 1994, p. 547), and since the model-based approach combined with a frequentist evaluation is adopted in much of the applied-scientific work, we will focus on the latter for the rest of the book. The Bayesian approach, however, will still be needed to motivate the method of multiple imputation.

Under a classical frequentist evaluation scheme assuming parameters of interest to be fixed, a minimum requirement for inferences to be valid is that in large samples the actual coverage of the true value by a confidence interval for that parameter (or statistic) is at least approximately $1 - \alpha$ with α being a predefined value or, in terms of testing true null hypotheses, that falsely rejecting the null hypothesis is not larger than approximately α. Note that this statement covers not only the situation in which the actual coverage rate of confidence intervals is approximately equal to the nominal coverage and the actual rejection rate is approximately equal to the nominal rejection rate, but also that the actual coverage rate is not below and the actual rejection rate is not higher than (approximately) the corresponding nominal rates. This latter situation is denoted as 'confidence valid' by Rubin (1996) and if actual coverage or non-rejection rates are larger than $1 - \alpha$, inferences are often called conservative.

A further criterion is that the estimator of scientific interest is (approximately) unbiased or consistent, i.e., approximately unbiased in finite samples. An estimator of scientific interest is, for example, the regression parameter in the model intended to estimate. The variance estimator of this estimator is usually not of primary interest. It is needed to calculate confidence intervals or conduct hypothesis tests. If this estimator overestimates the true variance of the parameter of scientific interest, then inferences will be conservative but inferences will still be valid: Confidence intervals that cover the true value more often than expected by the predefined $1 - \alpha$ level or hypothesis tests that falsely reject a true null hypotheses less often than expected by α still lead to correct inferences, although the precision of confidence intervals and the power of hypothesis tests are lower.

Although the criteria mentioned at the beginning of this section, i.e., plausibility of values and the hit-rate criterion, are sometimes adopted to evaluate multiple imputation techniques, they are not theoretically justified and may favour techniques that do not lead to valid inferences based on the method of multiple imputation developed by Rubin (1987, 1996). In Sect. 4.3.4.1 we will pick up again the hit-rate criterion as an example of a criterion that may favour imputation methods whose relationship to valid inferences are not known. The relevant criteria adopted in what follows to evaluate imputation methods will therefore be those aimed at properties of estimators, statistics, confidence intervals and hypothesis tests of scientific interest and finally those that allow valid statistical inferences about models or populations beyond the selected data set.

4.3.2 Bayesian Motivation

The basic idea of multiple imputation is to generate for each missing value several plausible values from an appropriate predictive model in such a way that the predictions are not systematically biased and the variation in these values reflects the uncertainty inherent in the predictions. Specifically the latter point deserves more attention, because it is the only source reflecting the uncertainty in the predictions in Rubins multiple imputation theory (Rubin, 1987, 1996) which is not easily captured otherwise in many situations (cf. Robins & Wang, 2000). However, this information is important to get the variance estimator for the estimator or statistic of scientific interest and thus the standard error by the combining rules proposed by Rubin (1987) correctly.

For a more in-depth treatment, we need the vector of response indicators $\mathbf{r}$ and the vector of all collected variables $\mathbf{u}$. In the most general case, we would in addition need the selection indicator for each population unit. However, in most scientific surveys the sampling design, which is also called sampling mechanism (e.g., Rubin, 1987), is known and ignorable. A sampling mechanism is ignorable if the probability of the observed pattern of selected and non-selected units into the sample does not depend on variables of units not selected or on variables in $\mathbf{u}$ whose values are not observed, conditional on the observed values in $\mathbf{u}$ and the response indicators whose values are observed in the sample (cf. the definition of ignorability of the missing data mechanism in Sect. 2.4; see Rubin 1987, p. 50, Result 2.1). Furthermore, the sampling design often does not depend on unknown parameters. So, for example, the sampling design would be ignorable at the observed values, if the probability of selecting units would possibly depend on observed characteristics of the residential area observed for all units in the population, but not on unobserved educational levels if, conditional on the observed values, this variable is associated with the random variable of scientific interest in $\mathbf{u}$, for example, wage. In a model-based approach it is usually assumed that the sampling design is ignorable.

If the sampling design is ignorable at the observed values, then the actual posterior distribution of a parameter or statistic of interest, $\boldsymbol{\theta}$, in the presence of missing data is

$$\int p(\boldsymbol{\theta} \mid \mathbf{u}_{(1)}, \mathbf{u}_{(0)}, \mathbf{r}) f(\mathbf{u}_{(0)} \mid \mathbf{u}_{(1)}, \mathbf{r})\, d\mathbf{u}_{(0)}\ , \tag{4.1}$$

(Rubin 1987, p. 50, result 2.1 and p. 82, result 3.1; Rubin 1996, p. 476; cf. Sect. 2.4.3), where in case of discrete variables in $\mathbf{u}_{(0)}$ integration reduces to summation for these components. Note that (4.1) is the marginal posterior distribution $\int p(\boldsymbol{\theta}, \boldsymbol{\gamma} \mid \mathbf{u}_{(1)}, \mathbf{r})\, d\boldsymbol{\gamma}$, where $p(\boldsymbol{\theta}, \boldsymbol{\gamma} \mid \mathbf{u}_{(1)}, \mathbf{r})$ is the joint posterior distribution of $\boldsymbol{\theta}$ and $\boldsymbol{\gamma}$ conditional on the observed values (cf. Sect. 2.4.3) and $\boldsymbol{\gamma}$ governs the missing data mechanism.

Unfortunately, the posterior distribution of $\boldsymbol{\theta}$ is often complicated, particularly if different types of variables, like continuous, ordered and count variables, are incompletely observed, or if the pattern of missing values is arbitrary. A central theme in multiple imputation is thus to break down a complicated problem into easier to solve tasks, like in (4.1).

The idea how to generate imputations seems now evident: Generate values from $f(\mathbf{u}_{(0)} \mid \mathbf{u}_{(1)}, \mathbf{r})$ for all those variables in $\mathbf{u}$ whose values are not observed and insert these values in the model for $\boldsymbol{\theta}$ based on the completed data set $p(\boldsymbol{\theta} \mid \mathbf{u}_{(1)}, \mathbf{u}_{(0)}, \mathbf{r})$, to get a value for the parameter of interest $\boldsymbol{\theta}$. Repeating these steps many times creates values for $\boldsymbol{\theta}$ from the desired distribution if all modeling assumptions are met. However, the two distributions under the integral are often not easily available. Even more, they still depend on $\mathbf{r}$. Before returning to this topic and considering a more feasible way of generating imputations, the combining rules derived by Rubin (1987) will be introduced.

4.3.3 The Combining Rules

Suppose we were able to generate $m = 1, \ldots, M$ plausible values for $\mathbf{u}_{(0)}$ from $f(\mathbf{u}_{(0)} \mid \mathbf{u}_{(1)}, \mathbf{r})$ independently over the M steps as described above. Letting $M \to \infty$, the above described procedure would generate values from the joint distribution of $\boldsymbol{\theta}$ and $\mathbf{u}_{(0)}$. For inferences we could use only the $\boldsymbol{\theta}$ values, their distribution being equal to the desired posterior distribution (4.1).

However, valid non-frequentist Bayesian inferences formally require that the distributions in (4.1) are correctly specified. This assumption is stronger than assumptions needed for valid frequentist-based inferences (cf. Rubin, 1996, pp. 474, 477). Since in addition many inferences are evaluated from a frequentist point of view, this is the strategy to evaluate inferences based on the method of multiple imputation. Hence, the combining rules refer not to the entire actual posterior distribution of $\boldsymbol{\theta}$, (4.1), but only to its expectation and variance

$$E(\boldsymbol{\theta} \mid \mathbf{u}_{(1)}, \mathbf{r}) = E(E(\boldsymbol{\theta} \mid \mathbf{u}, \mathbf{r}) \mid \mathbf{u}_{(1)}, \mathbf{r})$$

$$\mathrm{Var}(\boldsymbol{\theta} \mid \mathbf{u}_{(1)}, \mathbf{r}) = E(\mathrm{Var}(\boldsymbol{\theta} \mid \mathbf{u}, \mathbf{r}) \mid \mathbf{u}_{(1)}, \mathbf{r}) + \mathrm{Var}(E(\boldsymbol{\theta} \mid \mathbf{u}, \mathbf{r}) \mid \mathbf{u}_{(1)}, \mathbf{r})\,.$$

Let $\hat{\boldsymbol{\theta}}_m$ and $\widehat{\text{Var}}(\hat{\boldsymbol{\theta}}_m)$ be an estimator for the parameter of scientific interest $\boldsymbol{\theta}$ and an estimator of its variance for the mth completed data set, respectively, both for completely observed data sets. The combining rules are

$$\bar{\boldsymbol{\theta}} = M^{-1} \sum_{m=1}^{M} \hat{\boldsymbol{\theta}}_m \quad \text{and} \quad \widehat{\text{Var}}(\bar{\boldsymbol{\theta}}) = \overline{\mathbf{W}} + (1 + M^{-1})\hat{\mathbf{B}} , \tag{4.2}$$

where $\overline{\mathbf{W}} = M^{-1} \sum_{m=1}^{M} \widehat{\text{Var}}(\hat{\boldsymbol{\theta}}_m)$ is the so-called 'within variance' and $\hat{\mathbf{B}} = (M - 1)^{-1} \sum_{m=1}^{M} (\hat{\boldsymbol{\theta}}_m - \bar{\boldsymbol{\theta}})(\hat{\boldsymbol{\theta}}_m - \bar{\boldsymbol{\theta}})^T$ is the 'between variance' (see Rubin, 1987, p. 76).

The between variance can be interpreted as reflecting the amount of missing information with respect to $\boldsymbol{\theta}$: The less information available to predict the unobserved values, the higher the uncertainty in the imputations and the larger the between variance. On the other hand, if the missing values could be predicted without any uncertainty, then the estimator $\hat{\boldsymbol{\theta}}_m$ would not vary over the imputed data sets and the between variance would be zero. As a measure of the fraction of missing information for infinite M, (Rubin, 1987, pp. 85–86) defines the eigenvalues of the matrix

$$\boldsymbol{\Gamma}_\infty = (\overline{\mathbf{W}} + \tilde{\mathbf{B}})^{-1/2} \tilde{\mathbf{B}} (\overline{\mathbf{W}} + \tilde{\mathbf{B}})^{-1/2} ,$$

where $\tilde{\mathbf{B}} = (M - 1)/M \hat{\mathbf{B}}$ which is practically identical to $\hat{\mathbf{B}}$ if $M \rightarrow \infty$, and $\mathbf{A}^{1/2}$ denotes the symmetric square root of a positive definite matrix $\mathbf{A}$ (see Appendix A.1.3). Note that the trace of matrix $\boldsymbol{\Gamma}_\infty$, $\text{tr}(\boldsymbol{\Gamma}_\infty)$ is equal to the sum of its eigenvalues and $\text{tr}(\boldsymbol{\Gamma}_\infty) = \text{tr}[(\overline{\mathbf{W}} + \tilde{\mathbf{B}})^{-1}\tilde{\mathbf{B}}] = \text{tr}[(\overline{\mathbf{W}} + \tilde{\mathbf{B}})^{-1/2}\tilde{\mathbf{B}}(\overline{\mathbf{W}} + \tilde{\mathbf{B}})^{-1/2}]$ (see Appendix A.1). In this respect it makes sense to interpret $\text{tr}(\boldsymbol{\Gamma}_\infty)$ as the overall fraction of missing information. For a scalar parameter θ, this measure simplifies to

$$\gamma_\infty = \tilde{b}/(\bar{w} + \tilde{b}) , \tag{4.3}$$

where $\overline{w}$ and $\tilde{b}$ are the scalar versions of $\overline{\mathbf{W}}$ and $\tilde{\mathbf{B}}$. Hence, γ_∞ can be interpreted as the portion of variation due to missing information relative to the total variation.

4.3.4 *Frequentist Evaluation*

The last subsection described how to combine estimation results based on multiple imputations. It is, however, important that the imputations are generated in a way that allows valid inferences if these combining rules are applied. For example, the combining rule for $\widehat{\text{Var}}(\bar{\boldsymbol{\theta}})$ in (4.2) assumes that the estimators $\hat{\boldsymbol{\theta}}_m$ given the observed values are uncorrelated over $m = 1, \ldots, M$. Imputations generated in some way may lead to valid inferences as well, but generally not based on the above combining rules (see, e.g., Robins & Wang, 2000). Thus, the process of generating multiple imputations cannot be arbitrary for valid inferences based on (4.2). But according to which guidelines should imputations be generated to allow valid inferences in a frequentist sense? Actually (4.1) points towards a way to generate imputations. However, does an imputation method based on the Bayesian-motivated posterior distribution (4.1) allow frequentist valid inferences? And are there probably other, non-Bayesian imputation methods that allow valid inferences? In this section we will discuss criteria for a multiple imputation method to allow frequentist (confidence) valid inferences.

4.3.4.1 Accuracy of Imputations: The Hit-Rate Criterion

An intuitive criterion is derived from the following idea: Since the best value to impute would be the true but unobserved value, a 'good' imputation method should try to generate values as close as possible to the true values. This leads to what has been called the 'hit-rate'-criterion and was considered to be one important aspect of data quality in the context of official statistical agencies and other public data providers (see Kuchler & Spiess 2009 and the literature cited therein). The same idea still plays an important role in various disciplines and is adopted to evaluate imputation methods, for example, in the context of traffic flow data, monthly rainfall data, microarray gene expression or other biological or medical laboratory data (see Salfrán, Jordan, and Spiess 2016 and the literature cited therein).

For continuous variables, this evaluation criterion is realized by considering a function of the distance between the true but unobserved and the imputed values. In the case of categorical data, often the proportion of correct predictions ('hits') is considered. A popular measure for continuous variables is the positive square root of the mean of the squared differences between imputed and true values (Root Mean Squared Error, RMSE). Imputation methods are then evaluated based on this or a related distance measure using simulated data. The imputation method with the lowest RMSE is then considered to be the most accurate or precise (e.g., Templ, Kowarik, & Filzmoser, 2011 or Troyanskaya et al. 2001).

Unfortunately, these measures are not informative with respect to the validity of downstream analyses as is illustrated by Rubin (1996). The point is that there is no theoretical connection between the accuracy or precision of an imputation method, in the sense realized in the different 'hit-rate' measures, and valid inferences in the analyses of interest. The following example illustrates the problem and its possible consequences.

Example 4.1 (Imputation of an Incompletely Observed Binary Variable) A simple example illustrating that the hit-rate criterion may even favour biased over unbiased estimators is given by Rubin (1996, p. 475) (see also Salfrán et al., 2016). Here we will adapt this example assuming a binary variable x (1 : 'male' vs. 0 : 'not male' in a certain profession) being affected by missing values which are MCAR. Further assume that from official statistics it is known that the fraction of males in this profession is $p = 0.6$ in a certain population and we treat this as the true value in the model that approximates our population of interest. One strategy, say A, could be to impute the value one for each missing value because selecting a male is more likely ($p = 0.6$) than selecting not a male ($1 - 0.6 = 0.4$). For strategy B, we could try to mimic the random data generating process and generate an imputation for each missing value based on a Bernoulli distribution. This means that for each missing value a '1' is generated with probability 0.6 and a '0' is generated with probability 0.4.

The true hit-rate for strategy A is $0.4 \times 0 + 0.6 \times 1 = 0.6$. Strategy B implies $0.4 \times 0.4 + 0.6 \times 0.6 = 0.52$. Thus, strategy A would be superior to strategy B if the hit-rate criterion would be adopted. On the other hand, if we are interested in estimating the expected value of the binary variable x, then the mean would be an estimator which is upward biased for strategy A but would be unbiased under strategy B. To see this, let $\pi = \Pr(x_i = 1)$, n be the sample size, $n_{(1)}$ and $n_{(0)}$ be the sizes of the observed and the unobserved subsamples, respectively, and assume the observations to be sorted such that the first $n_{(1)}$ are observed. Let $\hat{\pi}$ be the estimator for the unknown probability. Then, under strategy A with fixed n, $n_{(0)} > 0$ and $\pi < 1$,

$$E(\hat{\pi}_A) = \frac{1}{n}\left(\sum_{i=1}^{n_{(1)}} E(x_i) + n_{(0)}\right) = \frac{n_{(1)}}{n}\pi + \frac{n_{(0)}}{n} > \frac{n_{(1)}}{n}\pi + \frac{n_{(0)}}{n}\pi = \pi$$

and under strategy B,

$$E(\hat{\pi}_B) = \frac{1}{n}\left(\sum_{i=1}^{n_{(1)}} E(x_i) + \sum_{i=n_{(1)}+1}^{n} E(x_i)\right) = \frac{1}{n}(n_{(1)}\pi + n_{(0)}\pi) = \pi \; .$$

□

The above example illustrates that the hit-rate criterion does not say anything about whether an imputation method allows valid inferences or not, a property this criterion shares with many other strategies that lack theoretical justification. Thus this criterion may foster imputation methods that lead to invalid inferences while penalizing imputation methods that would allow valid inferences. A good strategy is therefore to check whether the imputation technique provided by the software in use has been shown to allow valid inferences in principal. This could have been done either theoretically usually under restrictive assumptions or, for specific situations, by means of simulations. The latter case is very common since a theoretical justification under rather general, often mostly unknown conditions, is often not possible. In both cases it is worth to check under which conditions the imputation method in question has been shown to work. In the case of simulations, attention should be paid to reported biases and coverage rates of multiple-imputation-based estimators instead of the RMSE or similar measures.

4.3.4.2 Proper and Confidence Proper Imputation

Rubin (1987) gives conditions, generalized by Rubin (1996), for final inferences based on multiple imputations and combining rules (4.2) to allow valid inferences. Because the method of multiple imputation is not intended to correct shortcomings of the scientifically interesting analysis, it is assumed that this analysis would lead to (confidence) valid inferences if applied to the data set not affected by missing values ('complete-data inference'). Then, a multiply imputed data set allows (confidence) valid inferences if the method used to create the multiple imputations is (confidence) proper for the complete-data estimates $\bar{\boldsymbol{\theta}}$ and $\widehat{\text{Var}}(\bar{\boldsymbol{\theta}})$ (cf. Rubin, 1987, 1996; Tsiatis 2006).

Apart from some technical conditions, the definition of a proper imputation method treats the complete-data set as the population and the observed part as a random sample from that population. The following definitions rest on an hypothetically infinite number of imputations, i.e., $M = \infty$. Hence, $\bar{\boldsymbol{\theta}}_\infty$, $\overline{\mathbf{W}}_\infty$ and $\hat{\mathbf{B}}_\infty$ denote $\bar{\boldsymbol{\theta}}$, $\overline{\mathbf{W}}$ and $\hat{\mathbf{B}}$ for $M = \infty$. The imputed values are considered to be independent random draws from a model assumed to approximate the true mechanism that generated the unobserved values. The unobserved estimate of scientific interest $\hat{\boldsymbol{\theta}}$ and its variance estimate $\widehat{\text{Var}}(\hat{\boldsymbol{\theta}})$ that could have been observed without missing values are treated as fixed but unknown statistics to be estimated based on the multiply imputed data set.

The first condition for an imputation method to be proper is that the estimator $\bar{\boldsymbol{\theta}}_\infty$ is approximately unbiased for $\hat{\boldsymbol{\theta}}$ in the given complete-data sample and normally distributed with variance $\mathbf{B}$ over repeated sampling from the complete-data set under the assumed missing data mechanism. A second condition is that the estimator $\overline{\mathbf{W}}_\infty$ is approximately unbiased for $\widehat{\text{Var}}(\hat{\boldsymbol{\theta}})$. Note that here $\mathbf{r}$ is the only variable treated as random, selecting values from the complete-data set into the observed part of the samples. The third condition is that under the assumed missing data mechanism the estimator $\hat{\mathbf{B}}_\infty$ of the variance of $\bar{\boldsymbol{\theta}}_\infty$ conditional on the complete-data set is approximately unbiased for $\mathbf{B}$, again treating $\mathbf{r}$ as random.[1]

A more general definition is that of a confidence proper imputation method that accounts for situations in which the information used differs between the imputation step and the applied-scientifically interesting statistical analysis. In this case $\bar{\boldsymbol{\theta}}_\infty$ and $\overline{\mathbf{W}}_\infty$ are not directly compared with the complete case estimates $\hat{\boldsymbol{\theta}}$ and $\widehat{\text{Var}}(\hat{\boldsymbol{\theta}})$, respectively. Instead, an imputation method is confidence proper if $\bar{\boldsymbol{\theta}}_\infty$ and $\overline{\mathbf{W}}_\infty$ are approximately unbiased for the expectation of $\hat{\boldsymbol{\theta}}$ and $\widehat{\text{Var}}(\hat{\boldsymbol{\theta}})$, denoted as $\boldsymbol{\theta}_0$ and $\text{Var}(\hat{\boldsymbol{\theta}})$, over the missing and the sampling mechanism, respectively, and if the expected value of $\hat{\mathbf{B}}_\infty$ is larger than or equal to the variance of $\bar{\boldsymbol{\theta}}_\infty$ due to the variation of the imputations, i.e., the excess variance in $\bar{\boldsymbol{\theta}}_\infty$ over $\hat{\boldsymbol{\theta}}$ (Rubin, 1996).

[1] The technical conditions mentioned at the beginning of the second paragraph above refer to the variability of estimators $\overline{\mathbf{W}}_\infty$ and $\hat{\mathbf{B}}_\infty$. The assumptions are that their variability is lower than the variability of $\bar{\boldsymbol{\theta}}_\infty$. In addition, the variability of $\mathbf{B}$ over repeated sampling and under random $\mathbf{r}$ is presupposed to be lower than $\text{Var}(\hat{\boldsymbol{\theta}})$ (cf. Rubin, 1987).

Assuming all assumptions are met, the inequality of this last condition allows for conservative inferences, i.e., confidence intervals which are possibly too wide and hypotheses tests leading to a rejection rate of true null hypotheses which are below or equal to the predefined α (Rubin, 1996).

If a multiple imputation method is proper for $\bar{\boldsymbol{\theta}}$ and $\widehat{\text{Var}}(\hat{\boldsymbol{\theta}})$, then it is confidence proper for $\bar{\boldsymbol{\theta}}$ and $\widehat{\text{Var}}(\hat{\boldsymbol{\theta}})$. If the complete-data inference is valid and if the multiple imputation method with $M = \infty$ is proper, then the resulting inference is valid in the sense that $\bar{\boldsymbol{\theta}}_\infty$ is approximately unbiased for $E(\hat{\boldsymbol{\theta}})$ and $\widehat{\text{Var}}(\bar{\boldsymbol{\theta}}_\infty)$ is approximately unbiased for the variance of $\bar{\boldsymbol{\theta}}_\infty$. If the complete-data inference is (confidence) valid and if the multiple imputation method with $M = \infty$ is (confidence) proper, then the resulting inference is confidence valid in the sense that $\bar{\boldsymbol{\theta}}_\infty$ is approximately unbiased for $E(\hat{\boldsymbol{\theta}})$ and $\widehat{\text{Var}}(\bar{\boldsymbol{\theta}}_\infty)$ is (approximately) not smaller than the variance of $\bar{\boldsymbol{\theta}}_\infty$. Hence, in this latter case, inferences may be conservative. For a more detailed treatment and discussions see Rubin (1987, 1996, 2003), Tsiatis (2006), Nielsen (2003) and Robins and Wang (2000).

Furthermore, inferences about $\boldsymbol{\theta}$ from large samples using the complete-data estimator $\hat{\boldsymbol{\theta}}$ can often be based on the normal distribution. In many practical cases, the distribution of the mean of iid random variables, $\hat{\boldsymbol{\theta}}_m$, conditional on the observed values, converges to a normal distribution by the central limit theorem. Thus in large samples, the above results imply that inferences about $\boldsymbol{\theta}$ using $\bar{\boldsymbol{\theta}}_\infty$ can often also be based on the normal distribution replacing the unknown variance by its estimator $\widehat{\text{Var}}(\bar{\boldsymbol{\theta}}_\infty)$.

In some cases it is straightforward to decide whether an imputation method is (confidence) proper or not. For instance, imputing unconditional means is not a (confidence) proper imputation method (cf. Example 3.3 in Chap. 3): Imputing the unconditional mean of the observed x-values for unobserved x-values in a regression context usually violates the requirement that $\bar{\boldsymbol{\theta}}_\infty$, which in this case would be equal to $\hat{\boldsymbol{\beta}}_\infty$ based on the imputed data set, should approximately be unbiased for $\hat{\boldsymbol{\theta}}$ or $\boldsymbol{\theta}_0$. The main reason is that by replacing all missing data points by one fixed value reduces almost always the variance of x-values and—if the unconditional mean is used—also reduces the covariance of x- and y-values in the sample. Thus, $\bar{\boldsymbol{\theta}}_\infty$ will be biased for $\hat{\boldsymbol{\theta}}$ and $\boldsymbol{\theta}_0$ in general. Note that, additionally, replacing missing x-values by the mean of observed x-values implies that $\bar{\boldsymbol{\theta}}_m$ does not vary over imputations, so that this method is actually a single imputation method. Thus, there is no between variance and the amount of information in the completed data set is overestimated by the combining rule for the variance estimator given in Eq. (4.2) leading to standard errors which are systematically too small if the variance estimator for $\bar{\boldsymbol{\theta}}_m$ is not adapted correspondingly.

More often, however, it may not be easy to decide whether a chosen imputation method is (confidence) valid or not. Following Rubin (1987) and Rubin (1996, p. 478, 482), an imputation method tends to be (confidence) proper in large samples under the assumed missing data mechanism if the imputations approximate independent draws from a Bayesian posterior distribution derived under a carefully chosen model for the variables whose values are not observed (cf. (4.1)). We will revisit this discussion in Sect. 4.4 but will illustrate some of the ideas in the next simulation examples.

Example 4.2 (Proper, Confidence Proper and Improper Multiple Imputation) In this example, we illustrate possible consequences of a proper, confidence proper and improper multiple imputation method via simulations. Simulations are used because the analysis of a single data set can hardly tell anything about the statistical properties of estimators and test statistics. Each of the reported results is based on 500 simulations. Evaluation criteria will be the mean of the estimates over the simulations (mean) compared with the true values, the mean standard error (actually the positive square root of the mean of the estimated variances; se), the standard deviation of the estimates over the simulations (sd), the average confidence interval width (delta) and the portion of simulations in which the $1-\alpha$-confidence intervals cover the true value (cover; $\alpha = 0.05$).

Let us consider three variables y, x and z and assume that the regression of y on x and z is of applied-scientific interest. The underlying assumptions are: The $i = 1, \ldots, n$ variables $(y_i\ x_i\ z_i)^T$ are independent and follow the same distribution as $(y\ x\ z)^T$. This distribution is such that $y \mid x, z$ is normally distributed with mean zero and variance σ^2. In addition, a linear regression of y on x, z is assumed to be (approximately) correct. Assume further that the predictor variable x is affected by missing values with the fraction of missing values being approximately 0.3. In addition, the missing values are assumed to be missing at random such that whether missing values occur in x depends only on y. The sample size is $n = 500$.

The true data generating process in the simulations is in agreement with the above standard assumptions. However, to simulate data more aspects have to be defined: The true regression parameter from y on the constant, x and z is $\boldsymbol{\beta} = (0\ 1\ \ -1)^T$, the error variance is $\sigma^2 = 1$. Further, also the missing data mechanism has to be made more precise: We generated four response classes with decreasing response probabilities as y increases. The response probabilities are 0.95, 0.85, 0.75 and 0.10. The missing data mechanism is based on true values $\boldsymbol{\gamma} = (0.5\ 0\ 0)^T$ weighting y, x and z as the predictor variables in the missing data mechanism.

Under each of the scenarios, the data are generated in a first step and the regression y on x and z is estimated. This analysis based on the complete-data set, denoted as com in the following tables, will be the benchmark for the other results. If all assumptions are met, then the mean of the estimates over the simulations should be close to the true value, se should be close to sd, delta should be small and the coverage rate, calculated under the normal assumption, should approximately be 0.95. In a second step, missing values are generated and the regression model is estimated using the completely observed cases only (complete case analysis; CCA) in the same way as it is done in the complete-data case. In a next step, multiple imputations ($M = 20$) are generated assuming that the missing data mechanism is ignorable and adopting a Bayesian model with an uninformative (or flat) prior distribution (see Rubin, 1987, pp. 166–167). To generate the imputations, a normal linear model of x, the variable to be imputed, on y and z is adopted (cf. Sect. 4.4.2), for each imputation the unknown parameters are either randomly drawn from their posterior distribution or known parameter values are used, and the M imputations are generated as M independent draws from the corresponding conditional distribution. Then, in the last step, the regression of interest is estimated based on the multiply imputed data sets, results are combined as described in Sect. 4.3.3 and confidence intervals are calculated assuming normality (imp).

The values for the predictor variables x and z are generated from different distributions. In the first scenario, $(x\ z)^T$ is from a multivariate normal distribution with mean zero, variances equal to one and covariance 0.6. Hence, $x \mid y, z$ follows a known normal distribution. The only difference between the first and the second scenario is that in the latter the true parameter values for the imputation of $x \mid y, z$ are used, which can easily be calculated from the true means, variances and covariances if $(y\ x\ z)^T$ is multivariate normally distributed (see Appendix A.2.5).

In general, using (correct) knowledge in generating the imputations not used at the analysis stage, like the true parameter values of the imputation model, leads to superefficient imputations. Estimators of scientific interest based on strongly superefficient imputations are at least as efficient as the complete-data estimator, but at the same time variances tend to be overestimated. Still, superefficient and strongly superefficient estimators are approximately unbiased for the same statistic or parameter of scientific interest. The concept of superefficient and strongly superefficient imputations is discussed in Rubin (1996) and Meng (1994).

Finally, in the third scenario, we generated both x and z independently from a χ^2-distribution with three degrees of freedom ($df = 3$). Once the x- and z-values are generated they are fixed over the 500 simulations. Like the y-values, missing values were generated new in every simulation loop. Results under the different scenarios are presented in Tables 4.1, 4.2, and 4.3.

In the first scenario the imputation method is proper: The true distribution of $x \mid y, z$ is normal with a fixed variance, the imputation model is thus correctly specified, all relevant variables are included in the imputation model and the uncertainty is properly accounted for. Thus the imputations are (independent) draws from their posterior distribution. Since the analysis based on the complete-data set is valid and the imputation method is proper, the analysis should be valid.

The results in Table 4.1 illustrate the validity of the imputation-based estimator: The mean of the estimates over the 500 simulations for the constant (β_0), the

Table 4.1 Variables x and z are generated from a normal distribution

	$\beta_0 = 0$			$\beta_1 = 1$			$\beta_2 = -1$		
	com	cca	imp	com	cca	imp	com	cca	imp
Mean	−0.003	−0.301	0.008	1.002	0.792	1.009	−1.001	−0.793	−1.010
se	0.045	0.055	0.052	0.053	0.070	0.062	0.055	0.071	0.062
sd	0.044	0.052	0.052	0.052	0.063	0.059	0.053	0.066	0.060
Delta	0.176	0.216	0.202	0.209	0.274	0.243	0.217	0.280	0.242
Cover	0.960	0.000	0.946	0.960	0.138	0.956	0.956	0.158	0.950

Parameters of the imputation model are estimated (for abbreviations see text)

Table 4.2 Variables x and z are generated from a normal distribution

	$\beta_0 = 0$			$\beta_1 = 1$			$\beta_2 = -1$		
	com	cca	imp	com	cca	imp	com	cca	imp
Mean	0.001	−0.295	0.021	1.002	0.792	1.015	−1.002	−0.796	−1.020
se	0.045	0.055	0.048	0.053	0.070	0.060	0.055	0.071	0.061
sd	0.043	0.050	0.039	0.052	0.065	0.050	0.054	0.068	0.051
Delta	0.176	0.216	0.189	0.209	0.275	0.237	0.217	0.279	0.238
Cover	0.956	0.000	0.966	0.948	0.110	0.976	0.964	0.176	0.980

Parameters of the imputation model are known (for abbreviations see text)

Table 4.3 Variables x and z are generated from a χ^2-distribution with $df = 3$

	$\beta_0 = 0$			$\beta_1 = 1$			$\beta_2 = -1$		
	com	cca	imp	com	cca	imp	com	cca	imp
Mean	0.002	−0.088	−0.168	1.000	0.954	1.101	−1.001	−0.974	−1.009
se	0.088	0.106	0.108	0.019	0.032	0.031	0.018	0.021	0.022
sd	0.094	0.107	0.110	0.020	0.033	0.036	0.018	0.021	0.021
Delta	0.347	0.417	0.424	0.073	0.126	0.119	0.071	0.082	0.085
Cover	0.930	0.864	0.646	0.940	0.680	0.112	0.962	0.764	0.934

Parameters of the imputation model are estimated (for abbreviations see text)

parameters weighting x (β_1) and z (β_2) are close to the true vales, the average standard errors are close to the standard deviations and the coverage rates are within acceptable intervals of approximately 0.93 and 0.97.[2]

As expected, the analysis based on the complete-data set leads to valid inferences as well but, considering delta, with shorter intervals than for the imputation-based estimators. This latter result is explained by the fact that more information is available allowing more precise inferences in case of the complete-data set analyses. Complete case analysis is invalid. The estimator based on the completely observed part of the data set seems to be biased for all three parameters, leading to unacceptably low coverage rates.

The results in Table 4.2 are generated according to the same data generating process underlying the results in Table 4.1 but now imputations for x are generated using the true parameters. Thus, in this case not only the functional form of the model for the regression of x on y, z but also the regression parameters and the error variance of the errors are known.

With respect to the analyses based on the complete-data set and the completely observed part of the data set, the results are similar to those in Table 4.1 but there is an interesting effect on the estimator for $\boldsymbol{\beta}$: The standard deviations (sd) of its

[2]Each simulation is a binary experiment: Either the confidence interval covers the true value or not. Hence a 0.95-symmetric probability interval for the coverage rates can be calculated. If all assumptions are met, the coverage rates should be approximately between 0.93 and 0.97 for 500 simulations using the normal approximation.

elements are slightly smaller than those of the complete-data set estimator, but the mean standard errors are larger. Thus the variances of the estimators seem to be overestimated leading to confidence intervals that cover the true values slightly too often—at least for β_1 and β_2. This case is an example of a confidence proper multiple imputation method which generates superefficient imputations. Note that the confidence intervals are slightly smaller than in the first scenario.

In a third scenario instead of generating values for x and z from a common normal distribution, values were generated independently from a χ^2-distribution with three degrees of freedom. This χ^2-distribution is positively skewed which, together with the strong missing data mechanism may lead to deleting values in x in a highly selective way. In addition, the relationship of x conditional on y and z which is needed at least approximately to generate imputations for x is not linear anymore.

Table 4.3 illustrates what may happen if the imputation method is improper. Note that the imputation method assumes a linear relationship of x on y, z, which does not hold in this case (e.g., Spanos, 1995). As expected, the inferences based on the complete-data set are valid, whereas those from CCA are invalid. Results for imputation-based inferences are mixed: Inferences seem to be valid for β_2 but not for β_0 and β_1. Notably the estimator for β_1 seems to be biased and the coverage rate is much too low. □

The above example illustrates that the method of multiple imputation allows (confidence) valid inferences if all assumptions are met but that using an improper imputation method may lead to severely biased inferences. Although this latter statement seems to be trivial, it should be noted that the imputation model used in the third scenario is the default model in many software packages to generate imputations for continuous variables.

4.3.5 Inferences Based on Finite M

The efficiency and thus the precision of estimators depends on the number of imputations. The loss of efficiency due to using a finite number of imputations is generally rather small in large samples for a moderate amount of missing information (Rubin, 1987, 1996). Hence the proposed number of imputations ranges from $M = 2$ or 3 (e.g., Rubin, 1987, p. 114) if only a small amount of information is missing to $M = 5$ or 10 if the amount of missing information is not unusually high (e.g., below 30%; cf. Rubin 1996; Schafer 1999a) but can be 100 or even more if small effects are of interest (e.g., Graham, Olchowski, & Gilreath, 2007) and for estimates of variances of estimators to remain stable. As the amount of missing information can usually only be estimated ex post, one imputation strategy would be to successively increase the number of imputations starting with 5 or 10 with step lengths of 10 or 15 (cf. Graham et al., 2007), compare—depending on the research interest—test statistics, confidence intervals or point estimates and their standard errors and stop if changes are below a predefined threshold in two or three successive steps. Alternatively, one may adopt a two stage procedure to identify the appropriate number of imputations as proposed by von Hippel (2018).

For finite M and if the imputation method is proper, Rubin (1987, 1996) justifies the approximation of the distribution of q-dimensional $\bar{\boldsymbol{\theta}}$ over repeated sampling and treating the response indicator as random by

$$\bar{\boldsymbol{\theta}} \sim N(\boldsymbol{\theta}_0, \mathrm{Var}(\bar{\boldsymbol{\theta}}))$$

for inferences about $\boldsymbol{\theta}$. Since in finite samples a t-distribution is usually more appropriate, Barnard and Rubin (1999) propose

$$\widehat{\mathrm{Var}}(\bar{\boldsymbol{\theta}})^{-1/2}(\bar{\boldsymbol{\theta}} - \boldsymbol{\theta}_0) \sim t_{\breve{\nu}_M} ,$$

where $t_{\breve{\nu}_M}$ denotes the multivariate (here: q-dimensional) t-distribution with estimated degrees of freedom given by

$$\breve{\nu}_M = \left(\frac{1}{\nu_M} + \frac{1}{\hat{\nu}_{\mathrm{obs}}}\right)^{-1} ,$$

where

$$\nu_M = (M-1)\hat{\gamma}_M^{-2} , \quad \hat{\gamma}_M = q^{-1}(1+M^{-1})\,\mathrm{tr}(\hat{\mathbf{B}}\widehat{\mathrm{Var}}(\bar{\boldsymbol{\theta}})^{-1}) ,$$

$$\hat{\nu}_{\mathrm{obs}} = \lambda(\nu_{\mathrm{com}})\,\nu_{\mathrm{com}}\,(1-\hat{\gamma}_M) , \quad \lambda(\nu_{\mathrm{com}}) = (\nu_{\mathrm{com}}+1)(\nu_{\mathrm{com}}+3)^{-1} ,$$

ν_M is the degrees of freedom proposed by Rubin (1987) to be adjusted for small data sets, $\hat{\nu}_{\mathrm{obs}}$ is the estimated degrees of freedom based on the observed data set and ν_{com} is the complete-data set degrees of freedom. It can be shown that $\breve{\nu}_M$ is always less than the complete-data degrees of freedom ν_{com} but also less than the estimated degrees of freedom ν_M (see Rubin, 1987) which can even be larger than ν_{com}. Note that $\hat{\gamma}_M$ can be interpreted as (approximately) the estimated mean fraction of missing information with respect to the elements in $\bar{\boldsymbol{\theta}}$. For a scalar estimator, it simplifies to an estimator for γ_∞ (cf. 4.3). Simulation results in Barnard and Rubin (1999) suggest that $\breve{\nu}_M$ leads to confidence intervals which are closer in average to the nominal level than confidence intervals based on ν_M in most scenarios.

Inferences about a q-dimensional parameter $\boldsymbol{\theta}$ or subvectors thereof can be based on the test statistic

$$D_M = q^{-1}(\bar{\boldsymbol{\theta}} - \boldsymbol{\theta}_0)^T \widehat{\mathrm{Var}}(\bar{\boldsymbol{\theta}})^{-1}(\bar{\boldsymbol{\theta}} - \boldsymbol{\theta}_0) \sim F_{q,\bar{\nu}_M} ,$$

where $F_{q,\bar{\nu}_M}$ is the F-distribution with q and $\bar{\nu}_M$ degrees of freedom, where

$$\bar{\nu}_M = (M-1)(1+r_M^{-1})^2 \quad \text{and} \quad r_M = q^{-1}(1+M^{-1})\mathrm{tr}(\hat{\mathbf{B}}\overline{\mathbf{W}}^{-1}) \tag{4.4}$$

(Rubin, 1987). The advantage of this statistic together with the $F_{q,\bar{\nu}_M}$ distribution is that it is rather insensitive against a varying fraction of missing information over the q elements in $\boldsymbol{\theta}$. On the other hand, for small M the matrix $\hat{\mathbf{B}}$ may be an unstable estimator and may even be close to being singular (cf. Li, Raghunathan, & Rubin, 1991). As a rule of thumb, M/q should be larger than 5 (see Rubin, 1987).

Another test statistic for q-dimensional $\bar{\boldsymbol{\theta}}$ also proposed by Rubin (1987) is

$$\tilde{D}_M = \frac{1}{q(1+r_M)}(\bar{\boldsymbol{\theta}} - \boldsymbol{\theta}_0)^T \overline{\mathbf{W}}^{-1}(\bar{\boldsymbol{\theta}} - \boldsymbol{\theta}_0) ,$$

where r_M is given in (4.4). As a reference distribution for this test statistic, Li et al. (1991) propose the $F_{q,\tilde{\nu}_M}$ distribution, where

$$\tilde{\nu}_M = \begin{cases} 4 + (q(M-1)-4)\left[1 + \frac{1-\frac{2}{q(M-1)}}{r_M}\right]^2 & \text{if} \quad q(M-1) > 4 \\ (M-1)\left(\frac{q+1}{2}\right)(1+r_M^{-1})^2 & \text{otherwise.} \end{cases}$$

Unlike D_M, $\tilde{D}_M$ was derived under the assumption of equal fractions of missing information for the elements in $\boldsymbol{\theta}$. Results presented in Li et al. (1991) imply that $\tilde{D}_M$ together with the estimated degrees of freedom $\tilde{\nu}_M$ leads to tests with actual rejection rates being close to the nominal rejection rate α in many situations even with small M and varying fractions of missing values. The power loss for small M as compared to $M = \infty$ was rather small. However, $\tilde{D}_M$ as well as D_M may not work well if $M = 2$, q is small and the fraction of missing values varies strongly over the elements of $\boldsymbol{\theta}$.

Note that the above results have been derived for proper imputation methods and valid complete-data inferences. In case of confidence proper imputation methods inferences based on the above statistics and their distributions will be conservative due to overestimated between variances.

4.4 How to Generate Multiple Imputations

4.4.1 General

Coming back to the question on how to generate imputations, it can be shown that the completed-data posterior distribution in (4.1), $p(\boldsymbol{\theta} \mid \mathbf{u}_{(1)}, \mathbf{u}_{(0)}, \mathbf{r})$, is equal to the complete-data posterior distribution $p(\boldsymbol{\theta} \mid \mathbf{u}_{(1)}, \mathbf{u}_{(0)})$ if the missing data mechanism is ignorable. It is close to $p(\boldsymbol{\theta} \mid \mathbf{u}_{(1)}, \mathbf{u}_{(0)})$ in many other cases of practical interest (see Rubin, 1987, p. 103, result 3.3). This is a useful result because it implies that, once $\mathbf{u}_{(0)}$ is generated, standard techniques to calculate possible values for $\boldsymbol{\theta}$ can be adopted and hence no additional assumptions due to nonresponse beyond the assumptions required for completely observed data sets are needed.

The second distribution under the integral in (4.1), $f(\mathbf{u}_{(0)} \mid \mathbf{u}_{(1)}, \mathbf{r})$, is the posterior predictive distribution of the missing values which, after simplification, can be written as

$$f(\mathbf{u}_{(0)} \mid \mathbf{u}_{(1)}, \mathbf{r}) = \frac{\int\int f(\mathbf{u} \mid \boldsymbol{\theta}) g(\mathbf{r} \mid \mathbf{u}, \boldsymbol{\gamma}) p(\boldsymbol{\theta}, \boldsymbol{\gamma})\, d\boldsymbol{\theta}\, d\boldsymbol{\gamma}}{\int\int\int f(\mathbf{u} \mid \boldsymbol{\theta}) g(\mathbf{r} \mid \mathbf{u}, \boldsymbol{\gamma}) p(\boldsymbol{\theta}, \boldsymbol{\gamma})\, d\boldsymbol{\theta}\, d\boldsymbol{\gamma}\, d\mathbf{u}_{(0)}}, \tag{4.5}$$

using that the distribution of $\mathbf{u} \mid \boldsymbol{\theta}$ does not depend on $\boldsymbol{\gamma}$ and the distribution of $\mathbf{r} \mid \mathbf{u}, \boldsymbol{\gamma}$ does not depend on $\boldsymbol{\theta}$. Given the missing data mechanism is ignorable for Bayesian inferences, then (4.5) simplifies to

$$f(\mathbf{u}_{(0)} \mid \mathbf{u}_{(1)}, \mathbf{r}) = \int f(\mathbf{u}_{(0)} \mid \mathbf{u}_{(1)}, \boldsymbol{\theta}) p(\boldsymbol{\theta} \mid \mathbf{u}_{(1)})\, d\boldsymbol{\theta} \tag{4.6}$$

(see Appendix A.4), where $p(\boldsymbol{\theta} \mid \mathbf{u}_{(1)})$ is the observed-data posterior distribution of $\boldsymbol{\theta}$,

$$p(\boldsymbol{\theta} \mid \mathbf{u}_{(1)}) = \frac{\int f(\mathbf{u} \mid \boldsymbol{\theta}) p(\boldsymbol{\theta})\, d\mathbf{u}_{(0)}}{\int\int f(\mathbf{u} \mid \boldsymbol{\theta}) p(\boldsymbol{\theta})\, d\mathbf{u}_{(0)}\, d\boldsymbol{\theta}} = \frac{f(\mathbf{u}_{(1)} \mid \boldsymbol{\theta})}{f(\mathbf{u}_{(1)})}\, p(\boldsymbol{\theta})\,. \tag{4.7}$$

Although (4.6) does not depend on the observed $\mathbf{r}$, $f(\mathbf{u}_{(0)} \mid \mathbf{u}_{(1)}, \boldsymbol{\theta})$ is still too complicated to be manageable in general. A first and obvious simplification is the standard assumption, also adopted here throughout, that $\mathbf{u}_i \mid \boldsymbol{\theta}$ is independent and identically distributed for all i, which leads to

$$f(\mathbf{u}_{(0)} \mid \mathbf{u}_{(1)}, \boldsymbol{\theta}) = \prod_{i \in \overline{\text{cob}}} f(\mathbf{u}_{i,(0)} \mid \mathbf{u}_{i,(1)}, \boldsymbol{\theta}), \tag{4.8}$$

where $\overline{\text{cob}}$ is short for the set of units for which at least one u is not observed. Further, the observed-data posterior distribution of $\boldsymbol{\theta}$, (4.7), simplifies to

$$p(\boldsymbol{\theta} \mid \mathbf{u}_{(1)}) = \frac{\prod_{i \in \text{pob}} f(\mathbf{u}_{i,(1)} \mid \boldsymbol{\theta})}{f(\mathbf{u}_{(1)})}\, p(\boldsymbol{\theta})\,, \tag{4.9}$$

where pob denotes the set of units with at least one u observed. For a justification of both, (4.8) and (4.9), see Appendix A.4.

For easier readability we used a simplified notation above. Therefore, it is worth to point out some subtleties that may not immediately be obvious. First note that although we used $f(\cdot)$ to denote the distributions of subvectors of $\mathbf{u}$, the various distributions can be very different from each other. The same is true for $p(\cdot)$. It should also be noted that the parameters governing the different distributions are usually different functions of $\boldsymbol{\theta}$, the parameter of the joint distribution of all components in $\mathbf{u}$, which is notationally only implied by the arguments of $f(\cdot)$. In addition, the parameter of applied-scientific interest may not be $\boldsymbol{\theta}$ but some function of $\boldsymbol{\theta}$. For example, we might be interested in the linear regression of u_1 on u_2 which are assumed to be jointly normally distributed. Then the parameters of interest are the regression coefficients of this regression relationship. For confidence intervals and hypothesis tests the error variance is needed as well. If u_2 is not completely observed but the missing data mechanism is ignorable for Bayesian analysis, we need the regression coefficients and the error variance of the regression of u_2 on u_1 to generate imputations. Both sets of parameters, i.e., the parameters governing the regression from u_1 on u_2 and those of the reverse regression of u_2 on u_1, are functions of $\boldsymbol{\theta}$ but are in general not identical. Moreover, $\boldsymbol{\theta}$ may include parameters not used in the analysis of scientific interest if, for example, additional variables are used to generate imputations which are not assumed to be relevant at the analysis stage. Finally, in addition to $\mathbf{u}$, Rubin (1987, Section 5.2) considers variables $\mathbf{x}$ which are assumed to be always observed. Then the additional assumption of prior independence of parameters $\boldsymbol{\theta}_{\mathbf{u}|\mathbf{x}}$ and $\boldsymbol{\theta}_{\mathbf{x}}$ governing $f(\mathbf{u} \mid \mathbf{x}, \boldsymbol{\theta}_{\mathbf{u}|\mathbf{x}})$ and $f(\mathbf{x} \mid \boldsymbol{\theta}_{\mathbf{x}})$, respectively, is needed for corresponding simplifications. With this assumption $f(\mathbf{x} \mid \boldsymbol{\theta}_{\mathbf{x}})$ and $p(\boldsymbol{\theta}_{\mathbf{x}})$ can be ignored if the missing data mechanism is ignorable (Rubin, 1987, pp. 165–166).

Despite the above simplifications, generating imputations is still not straightforward because the distributions in (4.8) and (4.9) are generally difficult to specify, particularly if the pattern of missing values is arbitrary and if $\mathbf{u}_{(0)}$ comprises different types of variables, like income, age and level of education. In these cases $f(\mathbf{u}_{i,(0)} \mid \mathbf{u}_{i,(1)}, \boldsymbol{\theta})$ and $f(\mathbf{u}_{i,(1)} \mid \boldsymbol{\theta})$ may for some units be univariate (conditional) distributions of different types, depending on which variable is affected by missing values, and multivariate (conditional) distributions for different types of variables and varying dimensions for other units.

4.4.2 Monotone-Distinct Structure

The distribution of $\mathbf{u}_1, \ldots, \mathbf{u}_q$, $\mathbf{u}_l = (u_{1,l}, \ldots, u_{n,l})^T$, where $l = 1, \ldots, q$, conditional on $\boldsymbol{\theta}$ can always be written as

$$f(\mathbf{u}_1, \ldots, \mathbf{u}_q \mid \boldsymbol{\theta}) = f(\mathbf{u}_1 \mid \boldsymbol{\theta}_1) f(\mathbf{u}_2 \mid \mathbf{u}_1, \boldsymbol{\theta}_2) \cdots f(\mathbf{u}_q \mid \mathbf{u}_{q-1}, \ldots, \mathbf{u}_1, \boldsymbol{\theta}_q), \tag{4.10}$$

where $\boldsymbol{\theta}_q$ are different functions of $\boldsymbol{\theta}$ and the conditional distributions may differ depending on their arguments. If, as we assume throughout, the $\mathbf{u}_i \mid \boldsymbol{\theta}$ are iid, each factor in (4.10) is a univariate regression model based on n independent contributions. For example, $f(\mathbf{u}_1 \mid \boldsymbol{\theta}_1)$ could be a logit model for binary $\mathbf{u}_1$ with θ_1 the probability that $u_{i,1} = 1$ and $f(\mathbf{u}_2 \mid \mathbf{u}_1, \boldsymbol{\theta}_2)$ could be a standard normal linear regression model for continuous $\mathbf{u}_2$ with $\boldsymbol{\theta}_2 = (\boldsymbol{\beta}_2^T, \log \sigma_2)^T$, where $\boldsymbol{\beta}_2$ includes the intercept and the slope parameter of the assumed regression and σ_2 is the standard deviation of the error.

A situation that is relatively easy to handle when the missing data mechanism is ignorable is the case of a monotone-distinct structure. As an example, consider variables $\mathbf{u}_1, \ldots, \mathbf{u}_q$ where $\mathbf{u}_1$ is completely observed but $\mathbf{u}_2, \ldots, \mathbf{u}_q$ are not and are sorted according to an increasing amount of missing values. This would be called a monotone-distinct structure if the missing pattern is monotone (cf. Fig. 1.1 in Sect. 1.4) and, in combination with factorization (4.10), parameters $\boldsymbol{\theta}_l, l = 1, \ldots, q$ are distinct (see Sect. 2.4).

If the parameters are a priori distinct and if the missing data pattern is monotone, then the parameters $\boldsymbol{\theta}_l$ are a posteriori distinct. This means that (4.9) simplifies to a product of q univariate conditional distributions with dependent variables $u_{i,l}$. Together with (4.10) this implies that drawing values for $\boldsymbol{\theta}_l$, $l > 1$ and plausible values for unobserved $\mathbf{u}_l$ requires only univariate conditional models based on observed values of $\mathbf{u}_1, \ldots, \mathbf{u}_{l-1}$ (if $l = 1$, a model with an intercept only is adopted). Furthermore in this case, generating imputations is also based on q univariate conditional models where for all variables $u_{i,l}$ with unobserved values these conditional models are equal to the corresponding models for $u_{i,l}$ with observed values. The imputation models for missing $u_{i,l}$ as the dependent variable use observed or already imputed values for $u_{i,1}, \ldots, u_{i,l-1}$ as predictors, which is justified by the ignorability assumption (cf. (2.13) in Chap. 2) and the fact that the posterior predictive distribution is the same whether or not the variable values are observed or not (cf. (4.6) which does not depend on $\mathbf{r}$). With these results, creating imputations for monotone-distinct structures simplifies to the sequential application of techniques for univariate imputation problems (Rubin, 1987, pp. 174–178).

It should be noted that if prior independence is not justified, then posterior independence cannot be claimed and the observed-data posterior distribution $p(\boldsymbol{\theta} \mid \mathbf{u}_{(1)})$ does not simplify accordingly. It is also worth noting that an observed pattern of missing and observed values in $\mathbf{u}$ may be the result of one out of a large number of missing data mechanisms. But if ignorability of the missing data mechanism is assumed, it seems plausible that if $u_{i,l-1}$ is not observed then $u_{i,l}, \ldots, u_{i,q}$ are not observed with probability one, so not observing $u_{i,l-1}$ is an absorbing state, but if $u_{i,l-1}$ is observed then observing $u_{i,l}$ may depend on $u_{i,1}, \ldots, u_{i,l-1}$.

Assuming reasonable prior distributions $p(\boldsymbol{\theta}_l)$, an algorithm to create imputations could proceed as follows:

Algorithm 4.1 Generate multiple imputations: monotone-distinct structure and ignorable missing data mechanism

---

For $l = 1, \ldots, q$

1. Define a reasonable prior distribution for $\boldsymbol{\theta}_l$,
2. Specify a sensible observed-data likelihood function for the regression of $u_{i,l}$ on $u_{i,l-1}, \ldots, u_{i,1}$ using those units for which the values of $u_{i,1}, \ldots, u_{i,l}$ are observed, where a regression of $u_{i,1}$ on a constant is adopted if $l = 1$, and derive the posterior distribution for $\boldsymbol{\theta}_l$,
3. Randomly select a value for $\boldsymbol{\theta}_l$ from its observed-data posterior distribution,
4. Plug the selected value for $\boldsymbol{\theta}_l$ into the regression model for those units with unobserved values for $u_{i,l}$ and observed or imputed values for $u_{i,l-1}, \ldots, u_{i,1}$ to generate plausible values for the unobserved values $u_{i,l}$.

Perform steps 3–4 $m = 1, \ldots, M$ times or, alternatively, perform each of these steps M times to generate M imputations.

Example 4.3 (Monotone-Distinct Structure) Suppose we have a data set with $i = 1, \ldots, n$ units and three variables $u_{i,1}$, $u_{i,2}$ and $u_{i,3}$. Whereas $u_{i,1}$ is observed for all units, $u_{i,2}$ is a continuous variable and observed only for $n_2 < n$ units. Finally, $u_{i,3}$ is a binary variable observed only for $n_3 \leq n_2$ units and such that if $u_{i,2}$ is missing then $u_{i,3}$ is missing too (cf. Fig. 1.1). Further, n_3 is well above zero. Thus, the pattern of missing values is monotone. To generate imputations for the missing values in $u_{i,2}$ and $u_{i,3}$, we need to randomly and independently draw values from the conditional distribution (4.8) for all i which can be written as the product of two conditional distributions, the distribution of $u_{i,2}$ given $u_{i,1}$ and $\boldsymbol{\theta}_2$, times the distribution of $u_{i,3} \mid u_{i,2}, u_{i,1}, \boldsymbol{\theta}_3$ (cf. (4.10)). For the continuous variable $u_{i,2}$ we could assume $u_{i,2} \mid u_{i,1} \sim N(\beta_{2,0} + u_{i,1}\beta_{2,1}, \sigma_2^2)$ for all i, and $\boldsymbol{\theta}_2 = (\beta_{2,0}, \beta_{2,1}, \log \sigma_2)^T$. For the binary variable a logistic model may be adequate, where

$$\Pr(u_{i,3} = 1 \mid u_{i,1}, u_{i,2}, \boldsymbol{\theta}_3) = \frac{\exp(\eta_i)}{1 + \exp(\eta_i)} = \frac{1}{1 + \exp(-\eta_i)},$$

$\eta_i = \beta_{3,0} + u_{i,1}\beta_{3,1} + u_{i,2}\beta_{3,2}$ and $\boldsymbol{\theta}_3 = (\beta_{3,0}, \beta_{3,1}, \beta_{3,2})^T$. To generate imputations we could then proceed as follows:

1. Assuming that the two conditional models are not of applied-scientific interest, no prior knowledge about the parameters is available. Hence given that there are no contradictory arguments, we could assume $\boldsymbol{\theta}_2$ and $\boldsymbol{\theta}_3$ to be distinct and choose flat priors for both, i.e., prior distributions that are proportional to constants.
2. Derive the observed-data posterior distributions.
   (a) Derive the observed-data posterior distribution of $\boldsymbol{\theta}_2$: Given the likelihood function for $u_{i,2} \mid u_{i,1}, \boldsymbol{\theta}_2$ and the prior distribution for $\boldsymbol{\theta}_2$, the posterior distribution of $\boldsymbol{\theta}_2$ is the product of the posterior distribution of $\boldsymbol{\beta}_2 = (\beta_{2,0}, \beta_{2,1})^T$ conditional on some σ_2^{*2} generated from the posterior distribution of σ_2^2 times the posterior distribution of σ_2^2. The former is the normal distribution with mean $\hat{\boldsymbol{\beta}}_2$ and variance $\text{Var}(\hat{\boldsymbol{\beta}}_2) = \sigma_2^{*2}\mathbf{V}$, where $\hat{\boldsymbol{\beta}}_2$ is the ML estimator of this linear normal regression and $\text{Var}(\hat{\boldsymbol{\beta}}_2)$ is its variance (see Appendix A.3.2). The posterior distribution of σ_2^2 can be derived from the result that $\hat{\sigma}_2^2(n_2 - 2)/\sigma_2^2$ follows a $\chi^2_{n_2-2}$ distribution (see Rubin, 1987, pp. 166–167). Estimate the linear model for $u_{i,2} \mid u_{i,1}$ by the maximum likelihood method to get ML estimates $\hat{\boldsymbol{\beta}}_2$ and $\hat{\sigma}_2^2$ based on all units for which both $u_{i,1}$ and $u_{i,2}$ are observed.
   (b) Derive the observed-data posterior distribution of $\boldsymbol{\theta}_3$: Given the above logistic model for $u_{i,3} \mid u_{i,2}, u_{i,1}, \boldsymbol{\theta}_3$, the posterior distribution of $\boldsymbol{\theta}_3$ can in large samples be approximated by the normal distribution with mean equal to the ML regression estimate $\hat{\boldsymbol{\theta}}_3$ and variance equal to the estimated variance $\widehat{\text{Var}}(\hat{\boldsymbol{\theta}}_3)$. Although the posterior distribution of $\boldsymbol{\theta}_3$ may be very different from a normal distribution in small or even moderate samples, it is typically approximated by the normal distribution (cf. Rubin, 1987, pp. 169–170). Estimate the binary logistic model for $u_{i,3} \mid u_{i,2}, u_{i,1}$ by the maximum

likelihood method to get ML estimate $\hat{\boldsymbol{\theta}}_3$ and an estimate of its variance, which depends on $\boldsymbol{\theta}_3$ as the only unknown parameter, based on all units for which $u_{i,1}$, $u_{i,2}$ and $u_{i,3}$ are observed (see Appendix A.3.2).

3. (a) Randomly draw values for $\boldsymbol{\theta}_2$ from the observed-data posterior distribution: Randomly select a value, say w from the $\chi^2_{n_2-2}$ distribution and calculate $\tilde{\sigma}_2^2 = \hat{\sigma}_2^2(n_2-2)/w$. Randomly draw a value $\tilde{\boldsymbol{\beta}}_2$ from the normal distribution $N(\hat{\boldsymbol{\beta}}_2, \tilde{\sigma}_2^2\mathbf{V})$, where $\mathbf{V} = (\mathbf{U}_{(1)}^T\mathbf{U}_{(1)})^{-1}$ and $\mathbf{U}_{(1)}$ is a $(n_2 \times 2)$-matrix of ones (for the constant, $\beta_{2,0}$) in the first column and observed $u_{i,1}$-values in the second column.
   (b) Generate imputations for unobserved $u_{i,2}$'s: For each unit with missing $u_{i,2}$ randomly draw a value from the $N(0, 1)$ distribution, say $\tilde{z}$ and generate an imputation $\tilde{u}_{i,2}$ as $\tilde{u}_{i,2} = (1\ u_{i,1})\,\tilde{\boldsymbol{\beta}}_2 + \tilde{z}\tilde{\sigma}_2$ independently for all units with missing $u_{i,2}$.
4. (a) Randomly draw values for $\boldsymbol{\theta}_3$ from the observed-data posterior distribution: Randomly draw a value $\tilde{\boldsymbol{\theta}}_3$ from the normal distribution with expectation $\hat{\boldsymbol{\theta}}_3$ and variance $\widehat{\text{Var}}(\hat{\boldsymbol{\theta}}_3)$.
   (b) Generate imputations for unobserved $u_{i,3}$'s: For each unit with missing $u_{i,3}$ predict the probability of observing $u_{i,3} = 1$ given the ML estimate $\hat{\boldsymbol{\theta}}_3$ and the observed or imputed values of $u_{1,i}$ and $u_{2,i}$. Then randomly draw a value for $u_{i,3}$ from the Bernoulli distribution with these predicted probabilities independently for all i with missing value $u_{i,3}$.

Performing steps 3–4 M times generates M imputations for each missing value in the data set. □

Note that within the process of generating imputations, all incompletely observed variables enter a regression model as the dependent variable. Often models need to be estimated that are not of applied-scientific interest and about which no empirical results are available. For example, if in a data set the variable 'age' is incompletely observed, a regression model of 'age' on, e.g., 'wage' needs to be specified and estimated. Since there may neither be theoretical nor empirical results to justify a specific model, the decision for one or another model is somehow arbitrary and the usually implicitly adopted model may not coincide with the true data generating process. For example, the true data generating process for the binary variable in the example above could involve an interaction of $u_{i,1}$ and $u_{i,2}$, which we missed in the imputation model. If the model is not severely misspecified, however, this may still allow (confidence) valid inferences (see Sect. 4.3.1) because for frequentist inferences not the correct observed-data posterior distribution of $\boldsymbol{\theta}$ (4.1) but only its mean and variance (and large sample arguments) are necessary (see Sect. 4.3.4).

On the other hand, there may be cases in which a better option is to ignore imputed values and use only the completely observed units for a regression analysis, for example, if only the dependent variable in the model of applied-scientific interest is affected by missing values (see Sect. 2.5).

Imputation under ignorability and a monotone-distinct structure of the missing data mechanism is well justified. This also applies to other specific structures, for example in combination with missing data patterns arising from matrix sampling or file matching (see Sect. 1.4) which allow, under some additional assumptions, the application of simple imputation techniques similar to the one described above. In general, however, real data sets will rarely show a corresponding benign pattern of missing and observed data.

4.4.3 Beyond Monotone-Distinct Structures

Justification of an imputation procedure is much harder in case of an arbitrary pattern of observed and missing values. At the centre of the observed-data posterior distribution (4.9) is—if the standard assumption of independent observations is justified—the distribution $f(\mathbf{u}_{i,(1)} \mid \boldsymbol{\theta})$ which can be written as a sequence of conditional distributions. However, if the missing data pattern is arbitrary, it is unclear how to specify the individual conditional models: Depending on the pattern of observed and missing values, group specific models for each observed pattern would have to be specified and estimated. It would not be easy to justify prior distinctness of the corresponding parameters. The imputation models would also be difficult to justify and would in general not coincide with the models specified in (4.9). Claiming ignorability would also be daring: Let us suppose a data set with a pattern as in the first two columns (variables $\mathbf{u}_1$ and $\mathbf{u}_2$) of the right graphic of Fig. 1.2 in Chap. 1 and assume that $(u_{i,1}, u_{i,2})$ are iid but that $u_{i,1}$ and $u_{i,2}$ are not independent. To justify ignorability of the missing data mechanism, one could assume three response groups: One group for which the missing values of both variables are MCAR, a second group with missing values in $\mathbf{u}_1$ which may be MAR, depending on the observed values in $\mathbf{u}_2$ but not in addition on the missing values in $\mathbf{u}_1$ and a third group of units for which the missing values in $\mathbf{u}_2$ are possibly MAR, depending on observed values in $\mathbf{u}_1$ but not in addition on the missing values in $\mathbf{u}_2$. Without additional variables that define these groups, however, the justification for this classification would be very weak and inferences may be invalid.

One strategy in case of an arbitrary pattern of missing values could be to delete just enough data values to create a monotone pattern (see Rubin, 1987). This is not a trivial task and may lead to ignoring a large amount of information because the crucial point is that not only the number of values to be deleted is relevant, but the amount of information deleted with these values. As a strategy to roughly assess the amount of missing information to be deleted, descriptive techniques, like means, variances or correlations can be applied to the incomplete data set before and after deleting the values in question. If changes are large, then one should probably not adopt the strategy of deleting values. Otherwise, after deleting values and given a monotone missing data pattern, techniques as described in Sect. 4.4.2 can be applied. Of course, the deleted values have to be imputed again. This strategy can be a feasible way if only a small number of values are affected. However, it seems to be rarely realized in applications.

Another strategy described in Rubin (1987) is to fill in as few as possible imputations, generated by a simple method which is possibly not well justified, to just create a monotone missing data pattern and then apply techniques as described in Sect. 4.4.2. Adopting this strategy is associated with the hope that these somehow created imputations are dominated by the imputations generated based on the theoretically justified method for monotone-distinct structures in the sense that inferences based on the imputed data set are still approximately valid. This strategy is adopted by a popular imputation strategy described in Sect. 4.4.6 and illustrated in Chaps. 5 and 6.

4.4.4 Arbitrary Missing Data Patterns: A General Procedure

As described at the beginning of the last section, given an arbitrary missing pattern, it is difficult to specify the distributions (4.8) and (4.9) and hence to derive (4.6) analytically so that values for $\mathbf{u}_{(0)}$ can be generated. Numerical techniques that considerably simplify this task are subsumed under the topic Markov-Chain-Monte-Carlo methods (MCMC methods).

These techniques are designed to approximate integrals like (4.6) by simulation. The idea is, as in the case of the EM-algorithm (see Sect. 3.3.2), to replace a difficult task by a sequence of simpler tasks whose solution converges to the solution of the difficult task. At the heart of these algorithms are sampling steps where variable values are successively drawn over steps $t = 0, 1, 2, \ldots$ from simple conditional distributions, the transition kernel (Roberts, 1996). A transition kernel is the conditional distribution of the variable of interest at step $t \geq 1$ given the values generated in previous step $t - 1$ of the chain. However, the variables whose values are realized in some step $t > 1$ of this chain are not independent from the variables realized in step zero. Under some regularity conditions (e.g., Roberts, 1996; Tierney, 1996), however, which according to Schafer (1997) are met in most situations of practical interest, this dependence declines for an increasing t and the distribution from which the values are selected converges to an invariant (or stationary) distribution. For an appropriately chosen kernel this is the distribution of interest, also called the target distribution.

A particularly interesting technique in the context of generating imputations is the Gibbs sampler (Geman & Geman, 1984; for an introduction, see, e.g., Casella & George, 1992). In case of a complicated multivariate distribution, this algorithm draws successively $k = 1, \ldots, K$ parts of the vector variable from appropriate conditional distributions instead of drawing the complete vector at once. At a given step t of the MCMC chain, these components are realized from conditional distributions of the corresponding component conditional on, in step t, already updated components, say $1, \ldots, k - 1$, and not yet updated components from step $t - 1$, say $k + 1, \ldots, K$. That is, each MCMC step t is further split into simpler sub-steps $k = 1, \ldots, K$. Because each of these K conditional distributions are conditional on all other components of the variable vector, they are also called fully conditionals (cf. Schafer, 1997). Conditions for convergence of the distributions to the target distribution are, among others, that the target distribution is a genuine probability distribution and that the conditional probability distributions at each step t must correspond to this target distribution (cf. Schafer, 1997).

A special case of this technique is given by alternating, in step t of the chain, between drawing from distribution (4.8), $f(\mathbf{u}_{(0)}^{(t)} \mid \mathbf{u}_{(1)}, \boldsymbol{\theta}^{(t-1)})$, and the complete-data posterior distribution $p(\boldsymbol{\theta}^{(t)} \mid \mathbf{u}_{(1)}, \mathbf{u}_{(0)}^{(t)})$, where the superscripts (t) and $(t-1)$ denote variables selected in the tth and $(t-1)$th step, respectively. Note that this technique uses the complete-data posterior distribution instead of the observed-data posterior distribution, because it is generally easier to simulate data from the former than from the observed-data posterior (4.9). Because the observed-data posterior is 'augmented' by the imputations to get the complete-data posterior distribution, Schafer (1997) uses the label 'data augmentation' algorithm (cf. Li, 1988; Tanner, 1996; Tanner & Wong, 1987).

One strategy to generate imputations is to first specify the target distribution, i.e., the posterior predictive distribution of the variables to be imputed, and then, after choosing appropriate conditional distributions, run the data augmentation algorithm until the distribution of the generated values converged and corresponding draws do not depend on values selected at $t = 0$. Assume that this happens after J steps. The M imputations to be generated should be M independent draws from the posterior predictive distribution. The first set of imputations may be generated by drawing values for $\mathbf{u}_{(0)}$ in the Jth step of the Markov chain. To generate M imputations one can either start a new chain for each m and run the algorithm until convergence or continue the first chain for additional J steps until a second set of independent draws can be made and repeat this procedure until M imputations are generated.

Before imputations can be drawn from the posterior predictive distribution, the joint posterior distribution of $\mathbf{u}_{(0)}$ and $\boldsymbol{\theta}$ must have converged. However, monitoring whether the joint posterior distribution of $\mathbf{u}_{(0)}$ and $\boldsymbol{\theta}$ converged is inconvenient in most applications due to the high dimensionality of the problem. It can be simplified, however, by noting that convergence of the posterior distribution of $\boldsymbol{\theta}$ is sufficient for convergence of the posterior distribution of $\boldsymbol{\theta}$ and $\mathbf{u}_{(0)}$, as the former depends on the posterior distribution of $\mathbf{u}_{(0)}$ (Schafer, 1997).

One condition for convergence is that the target distribution exists and is a genuine probability distribution. However, it is not easy to specify the posterior distribution (4.6), for example, in a data set with several continuous, truncated and categorical variables, where the continuous variables may follow different distributions. In this case, it may be hazardous to specify even (4.8).

The target distribution exists in general if appropriate conditional distributions and a proper prior distribution are chosen for $\boldsymbol{\theta}$. However, even then it may happen for specific data sets that, for example, relevant subgroups are only sparsely populated such that not all parameters are identified, which is more likely if a data set is not completely observed. In addition, although proper prior distributions lead to proper posterior distributions, this may not be the case if improper prior distributions are chosen, even if they lead to proper posterior distributions in complete-data situations (Schafer, 1997, p. 81). Hence, if in doubt a proper prior should be chosen in these situations (cf. Sect. 1.5.2).

To avoid these problems, Schafer (1997, 2001), Schafer and Yucel (2002) propose using specific fixed multivariate posterior predictive distributions for the variables with missing values, like a (conditional) multivariate normal distribution (Schafer, 1997) as implemented in the software `NORM` (Schafer, 1999b). Alternatively, one may assume that a multivariate posterior predictive distribution exists given univariate conditional distributions for variables with missing values. Such an approach that can be interpreted as an approximation to an MCMC method, also denoted as imputation by fully conditional specification, is realized, e.g., in packages `IVEware` (Raghunathan, Lepkowski, Van Hoewyk, & Solenberger, 2001; Raghunathan et al., 2016) and `mice` (van Buuren & Groothuis-Oudshoorn, 2011).

It is, however, not easy to decide whether values generated in step t of a Markov chain can be interpreted as being realizations from a stationary distribution. To support the decision, several tools are available and one may either monitor the behaviour of parameters (Schafer, 1997) over t or directly of the potential imputations (van Buuren & Groothuis-Oudshoorn, 2011). To assess convergence, either parameter values or statistics of the potential imputations like means, quantiles, variances or autocorrelations may be plotted against t. If generated parameter values or distributions of variable values converged, then means, quantiles and variances should be stable. If generated parameter values or distributions of variable values are independent, then autocorrelations should be close to zero. Unfortunately, it is not easy to decide whether values or distributions actually converged, even if parameter values or statistics do not change substantially over t for several iterations, because this may change after some additional iterations. Similarly, from correlations close to zero, one cannot infer (almost) independence and hence parameter or variable values may still be non-linear dependent. Irregular or erratic behaviour of one or more statistics should give rise to think about the models and whether they might be too flexible or overidentified, i.e., if too many parameters are included. On the other hand, behaviour that implies fast and stable convergence in several statistics usually suggests that the problem is well defined if the models are not too parsimonious. In general, monitoring convergence of different aspects of several parameter or variable values at the same time usually gives a good impression whether underlying models are well identified. For a more detailed treatment see, e.g., (Schafer, 1997, Section 4.4).

4.4.5 Generating Imputations by Joint Modeling

The advantage of a method that generates multiple imputations assuming a specific multivariate posterior predictive distribution $f(\mathbf{u}_{(0)} \mid \mathbf{u}_{(1)}, \boldsymbol{\theta})$ is that if the algorithm has converged and the M imputations are values selected sufficiently far apart from each other from the chain of generated values, then the imputations can be interpreted as independent random draws from the target posterior distribution. If the models for the imputations approximate the true data generating process sufficiently well, then the multiple imputation-based inferences tend to be valid.

The downside of this approach is that it is not very flexible: The number of manageable joint posterior predictive distributions is restricted. For example, Schafer (1999b) assumes a multivariate normal distribution. In applications, however, variables may be far from being normally distributed and data sets may be made up from continuous and discrete variables. To allow imputation also under non-normal distributions Schafer (1999b) proposes to transform variables, impute and then transform back. To impute categorical variables, for example binary or ordered categorical variables, e.g. Schafer (1997, 1999b) suggests to impute values using the normal assumption and then round to the nearest possible value. We will deal with this ad-hoc technique, which is not exclusively used in the context of generating imputations based on joint modeling, in Sect. 4.5. Application of the joint modeling approach is illustrated in Sect. 5.5.1.

4.4.6 Generating Imputations by Fully Conditional Specification

Fully conditional specification is a very flexible way of generating imputations which does not require specification of the multivariate posterior predictive distribution. Instead, for each variable with missing values a univariate regression model is specified, a strategy which enables the use of a great variety of different models. In a first round, the procedure to generate imputations could proceed as described in Sect. 4.4.2 and the last paragraph of Sect. 4.4.3. Once the data set is completed, new imputations are generated for each incompletely observed variable using all the other variables with observed or already imputed values. These new imputations overwrite the imputations generated in the preceding round.

The costs of the flexibility of this approach are that it is often unclear whether a common multivariate posterior predictive distribution exists. On the other hand, it is not yet well understood what happens if a genuine multivariate posterior distribution does not exist.

With respect to the first problem, encouraging results are presented by Liu, Gelman, Hill, Su, and Kropko (2014) who show that, besides some technical conditions, if all the conditional distributions implied by the adopted regression models are compatible then the common distribution of those variables affected by missing values converges to a Bayesian posterior distribution. Hence, multiple imputation-based inferences tend to be valid if this distribution is sufficiently close to the true data generating process and the complete-data set analysis is valid. Conditional models are compatible if there exists a joint model such that all the conditional models can be written as sub-models of this joint model. For example, if (and only if) $y \mid x$ is a linear regression model with homoscedastic errors and $x \mid y$ is a linear regression model then the common distribution of y and x is normal (Spanos, 1995). Therefore, in this example the regression of y on x and the reverse regression from x on y are compatible (for more examples, see Liu et al. 2014). Furthermore, van Buuren, Brands, Groothuis-Oudshoorn, and Rubin (2006) confirm these results and further find in a simulation study that—concerning the second problem—at least in the linear models and for the specific situations considered, valid inferences are possible even if the imputation models are incompatible.

4.5 Further Topics and Open Problems

In this section we address several specific topics relevant for generating multiple imputations in different situations. Some refer to challenges for which solutions are available, others address issues that are still awaiting to be solved.

4.5.1 Transforming, Rounding and Trimming

The distribution of a variable to be imputed is often not normal. For example, the distribution may be skewed, flat, truncated or even discrete. On the other hand, the normal linear regression imputation model is fast and computationally robust even in medium to small data sets. Hence it is tempting to handle as many missing data situations as possible with this imputation method. And in fact, several strategies have been proposed to adopt this imputation technique even in situations where it is obvious or is least suspected that the normality assumption is violated.

If continuous variables are assumed to be not normal, a strategy that has been proposed is to transform the observed values to normality, impute and then transform back (e.g. Raghunathan et al. 2016, van Buuren 2012, Schafer, 1997, 1999b; Schafer & Graham 2002). At the same time Schafer and Graham (2002) or He and Raghunathan (2009) are cautious with respect to suggesting the use of transformations and von Hippel (2013) recommends this strategy only in specific cases. To understand the different conclusions let us consider various possible situations and the relevant components of the imputation and estimation procedure for a simple linear regression setting with y being the dependent and x the independent variable.

Let us first ignore x and let y be MCAR for some units i ($i = 1, \ldots, n$). Assume we are interested in the marginal distribution of y. If y is normally distributed, then the distribution of the observed values will only randomly deviate from a normal distribution. Imputations can then easily be generated from a normal linear model where only a constant is included, i.e., no transformation is required but may introduce bias if not carefully chosen.

If the normality assumption of y is questionable, generating imputations based on the normal model may still allow valid inferences if the mean is of interest as implied by the 'self-correcting' property of multiple imputation (see Sect. 4.5.2) and a simulation study of He and Raghunathan (2009). However, if inferences about probabilities in the tails of non-normal distributions are of interest, then the same simulation study implies that inferences based on the normal imputation model must be expected to be invalid. In these cases transforming the data seems obvious. Then, a first step might be to choose an appropriate transformation from a large family of possible techniques. Examples are the exponential, log, logit, power or Box-Cox transformation (von Hippel 2013; for an overview and critical discussion of the Box-Cox transformation, see Sakia 1992). Another strategy, considered by He and Raghunathan (2009), is to generate imputations from a standard normal distribution and then transform these values such that their distribution approximates the estimated distribution of the target variable. This can be done with the help of the gh distribution where two parameters, g and h, which need to be estimated, govern the skewness and kurtosis of the distribution (see He & Raghunathan, 2009). The simulation results presented in He and Raghunathan (2009) imply that the latter strategy may allow valid inferences about probabilities in the tails of strongly heavy tailed distributions whereas the strategy of generating imputations from a normal model tends to lead to undercoverage in these cases. On the other hand, for values whose distribution in the sample is skewed von Hippel (2013) considers transformations like the log, the square root and the fourth-root transformation and concludes that these transformations allow valid inferences with respect to mean and variance of the imputed variable if the distribution of the transformed values is close to a normal distribution. If not, then at least the variance tends to be biased.

In a more relevant scenario, beside y there are additional completely observed or already imputed variables. For simplicity, however, we will assume that only one completely observed variable, x, is available. When x is included into the imputation model, the relevant distribution for generating imputations is the distribution of y conditional on x. If y and x are bivariate normally distributed, then the conditional distribution of y given x is also normal (see Appendix A.2.5) and hence including x into the normal linear imputation model allows valid and, if missing y-values are MCAR, more precise inferences than ignoring x if y and x are not independent. Note that from the normality of y it does neither follow that x is normal nor that the conditional distribution of y depending on x is normal even if x is normally distributed (see Appendix A.2.4). In applications the conditional distribution of $y \mid x$ cannot easily be derived from the distribution of observed y-values if y depends on x. Then a flexible strategy, like adopting the gh distribution in generating imputations, that does not require the relevant distribution to be precisely known may be advantageous. However, results from a simulation study reported in He and Raghunathan (2009) imply that imputation based on the normal linear model or a gh distribution conditional on x with missing values being MCAR in y may lead to valid inferences over a wide range of situations even if the normality assumption is violated. In situations with distributions deviating markedly from the normal, the actual rates with which confidence intervals cover true regression coefficients is moderately too small under the normal linear but also under the gh imputation. Thus, in these cases, imputation under a gh distribution seems to be superfluous.

In a different setting, the probability of observing y may depend on x, i.e., missings in y are MAR. As is shown in Sect. 2.5 of Chap. 2, imputation or any other method to compensate for missing values is not required because inferences based on a regression of y on x will be valid as long as the assumed regression model would allow valid inferences without missing values. If the model of applied-scientific interest is a linear regression model with a normally distributed error term and this assumption is approximately correct, then imputations generated under a Bayesian normal linear imputation model will allow valid inferences in sufficiently large samples. Hence, given the model for the complete-data set is not misspecified a transformation of the observed y-values would not only be superfluous but could even introduce bias if the transformation is not appropriate. Note that y will very likely follow a non-normal distribution if x follows a non-normal distribution or when the missing values in y are MAR. In both cases the distribution of $y \mid x$ may be normal. Hence transforming the observed values of y to be approximately normal as proposed in the literature may make things worse as compared to ignoring the missing data problem in this case (cf. von Hippel, 2013).

Note that situations in which missing values are MCAR or missing values in y, the dependent variable in a regression model of scientific interest, are MAR are not only rare but it is often superfluous to consider transformations in these cases because the observed part of the data set is a simple random sample from the complete-data set conditional—in the latter case—on the completely observed variable x. It may even be misleading if an inappropriate transformation is chosen. However, the above results give an idea about whether the transformation strategy can help to generate imputations such that final inferences are valid. In fact, the above results imply that in many cases, if interest is in functions of means of (conditional) distributions, the normal linear imputation model is rather robust and may allow valid inferences in many situations even if the normality assumption is violated. Adopting a transformation strategy can be an option when the tails of a (conditional) distribution that deviates markedly from the normal are of interest. Instead of a rigid transformation, like the log or square-root transformation, that requires rather precise knowledge about the (conditional) distribution of the variable to be imputed, it is probably less risky to adopt a flexible approach, like adopting the gh distribution to generate imputations. However, from this strategy it is a small step towards a strategy that generates imputations from more flexible models, as described in Chap. 6.

Summing up, the strategy of transforming observed values so that their distribution looks sufficiently normal may not only be superfluous but should generally be avoided. If it has to be assumed that the distribution in question deviates markedly from the normal distribution, then imputations should be generated based on the generalized additive model of location scale and shape (GAMLSS) or quantile regression (see Chap. 6). In small data sets where these flexible methods may not be appropriate, probably adopting the gh distribution as proposed by He and

Raghunathan (2009) might be a solution. However, more research is needed to evaluate this strategy for a large variety of situations.

To impute categorical, for example binary or ordered categorical variables, e.g. Schafer (1997, 1999b) proposes to impute values using the normal assumption and then round to the nearest possible value. Unfortunately, Horton, Lipsitz, and Parzen (2003) have shown that this may lead to biased estimators. On the other hand, imputing under the normality assumption without rounding even binary or discrete metric variables may allow (approximately) valid inferences although the imputed values are not values that could be observed (cf. de Jong et al., 2016; Horton et al., 2003). However, there are occasions where continuous imputed variables may not be an option. For example, if the corresponding imputed variable enters a model of applied-scientific interest as the dependent variable. In those cases, imputations should be generated using appropriate models that respect the level of measurement adequately. For example, to generate imputations for binary, ordered or unordered variables, corresponding logit models may be appropriate and for a count variable, e.g., Poisson or negative binomial models may be appropriate (see Chap. 6).

Variables in a data set may have restricted domains. For example, reaction time cannot be negative or the number of correct answers in a test can only vary between zero and thirty. To generate imputations which are plausible in the sense that they can take on values only in the restricted domain of such a variable, von Hippel (2013) distinguishes two situations: censoring and truncation. Censoring refers to the technique of generating imputations from an appropriate unrestricted distribution, e.g. the normal distribution, and then round out-of-range values to the nearest bound of the restricted domain. Truncating denotes the technique where imputations are generated from an unrestricted model until they fall within the desired interval. A more efficient version that generates imputations from a truncated predictive distribution is based on the Sampling-Importance-Resampling algorithm (e.g., Raghunathan et al. 2001, 2016).

In the best but presumably rare cases, censoring or truncating, like rounding or applying some inflexible transformation to an incompletely observed variable, seems not to be preferable over generating imputations based on an unrestricted but misspecified normal linear imputation model. In fact, these naive techniques may lead to invalid inferences in most cases (e.g., von Hippel 2013; Rodwell, Lee, Romaniuk, and Carlin 2014). A more sophisticated approach is to generate imputations from the corresponding truncated normal predictive distribution. However, von Hippel (2013) reports technical problems with available algorithms, like non-convergence, to generate imputations following this strategy and hence does not recommend it. Based on his results, von Hippel (2013) concludes that the normal linear imputation model generates imputations such that (approximately) valid inferences are possible for means, variances and regression parameters even if the assumption of normally distributed errors is wrong, but inferences are invalid for parameters depending on the shape of the distribution, like percentiles. Based on similar results using naive techniques, Rodwell et al. (2014) recommend to generate imputations using an unrestricted imputation model.

Clearly, simple solutions to generate plausible values as imputations do not allow valid inferences in general. Like the simple ad-hoc methods discussed in Chap. 3, these techniques are not theoretically justified but are rather adopted based on a desired distributional shape of imputed values or the wish to get only possible values for the imputations. These methods may not be proper. Proper imputation methods usually require careful modeling of the predictive distribution and thus of the imputation model. More research is needed to develop and systematically evaluate flexible imputation methods, like the quantile regression imputation for bounded variables proposed in Geraci and McLain (2018), for general non-normal, discrete and truncated variables.

4.5.2 *Imputation of Functions of Variables*

Another problem arises from higher-order polynomial and interaction terms or, more generally, transformed variables. For example, if x is an incompletely observed continuous variable and it is assumed that in a model estimated in downstream analyses x^2 or the interaction with another variable z is of interest, then the question is how to generate imputations for x.

One idea underlying the strategy 'passive imputation' or 'impute-then-transform' is to ignore, in a first step, the transformed variable in question and impute only the untransformed variable. After imputations have been generated, the imputed values are transformed so that, e.g., x and x^2 are both available for the imputation of other variables. The advantage of this idea, besides its simplicity, is that the transformed variable can take on only possible values. However, see Sects. 4.3.1 and 4.3.4.1 for a discussion of this criterion.

Unfortunately, passive imputation makes an imputation method improper, because the imputation model simply ignores the transformed variable when generating imputations for the untransformed variable. Thus, if the transformed variable, e.g., x^2, has an effect on the dependent variable y in the model of applied-scientific interest, this strategy implies a misspecified imputation model and thus invalid inferences, which has been demonstrated not only for continuous but also for binary variables y, e.g., by von Hippel (2009) (see also Seaman, Bartlett, & White, 2012).

A theoretical explanation is illustrative as it does not only explain this result but also highlights a general problem with some available imputation methods and their uninformed application, a topic we will pick up later in this chapter. For the explanation, a result repeatedly used in this book (cf. Sects. 3.3.2, 3.5.2, 4.4.6 and Example 4.2) proved in Spanos (1995) is needed: The regression of a continuous variable y on a variable x is characterized by

$$E(y \mid x) = \beta_0 + x\,\beta_1 \qquad \text{with} \qquad \text{var}(y \mid x) = \sigma^2$$

and the regression of x and y is characterized by

$$E(x \mid y) = \zeta_0 + y\,\zeta_1$$

if and only if

$$(y\ x)^T \sim N(\boldsymbol{\mu}, \boldsymbol{\Sigma}) \ .$$

This result can be extended to multidimensional variables **y** and **x**.

If x^2 has an effect on y, i.e., $E(y \mid x) = \beta_0 + x\beta_1 + x^2\beta_2$, where $\beta_2 \neq 0$, then the regression relationship of x on y is

$$E(x \mid y) = -\left(\beta_1 \pm \sqrt{\beta_1^2 - 4\beta_0\beta_2 + 4\beta_2 y}\right)/(2\beta_2) \ , \quad \beta_1^2 \geq 4\beta_2(\beta_0 - y) \ ,$$

obviously not linear in y. A linear imputation model for $x \mid y$ would be a misspecified model and the imputation method would be improper.

To solve this problem, von Hippel (2009) proposes a 'transform then impute'-strategy, also denoted as 'just another variable'-technique (JAV, e.g., Bartlett, Seaman, White, & Carpenter, 2015). The idea is to treat a transformed variable, say x^2 as a new variable, $z = x^2$, and impute this variable like any other variable. The apparent disadvantage of this technique is that imputed values z_* might not be equal to the transformed (imputed) values of the untransformed variable, $z_* \neq x_*^2$. However, given the discussion in Sects. 4.3.1 and 4.3.4.1 this is not a criterion related to proper imputation methods.

Following this imputation strategy, the assumed model of interest is given by

$$E(y \mid x) = \beta_0 + x\,\beta_1 + z\,\beta_2 \ , \quad \mathrm{var}(y \mid x) = \sigma^2 \ ,$$

where $z = x^2$. To generate imputations, von Hippel (2009) proposes either to follow the joint modeling approach or the fully conditional specification strategy, both under the normality assumption and assuming that the missing data mechanism is ignorable. Under the fully conditional specification strategy, imputation could proceed as under a monotone-distinct structure. In a first step impute x given y using

$$E(x \mid y) = \zeta_{x,0} + y\,\zeta_{x,1}$$

and, in a second step, impute z given y and x,

$$E(z \mid y, x) = \zeta_{z,0} + y\,\zeta_{z,1} + x\,\zeta_{z,3}$$

assuming normality of the errors in the imputation models. Generating imputations according to the common model would use

$$E((x \;\; z)^T \mid y) = \boldsymbol{\zeta}_0 + y\,\boldsymbol{\zeta}_1$$

with errors being (bivariate) normally distributed. The imputation models are estimated based on the completely observed cases and then, based on the estimated model parameters, adopted to generate imputations.

However, given the result in Spanos (1995) and the assumed model of applied-scientific interest, these imputation models are only correctly specified if (and only if) $(y \;\; x \;\; z)^T$ follows a common normal distribution $N(\boldsymbol{\mu}, \boldsymbol{\Sigma})$. This, however, is not possible as z is a squared variable. Hence, the imputation model is misspecified and the imputation method is not proper. If the relationship is almost linear, in the example if β_2 is close to zero, or the missing data mechanism thins out an area where the linear imputation model is not severely misspecified then a misspecification of the imputation model may not have serious consequences, even more so in small samples given the 'self-correcting' property of multiple imputation.

Self-correcting property means that a misspecified imputation model tends to lead to exaggerated within and between variances and thereby 'mask' a possible bias in the estimator of scientific interest (Rubin, 1996, 2003). The within variance will tend to be larger than if the 'correct' model would have been chosen due to a lower goodness of fit. The between variance will be larger because the variation of the estimated imputation models over the M imputation steps will be increased. Therefore, biases in the estimators of scientific interest tend to be masked by larger variances as if a 'correct' imputation model would have been chosen as long as the imputation model is not severely misspecified. This effect, however, depends on the selectivity of the missing data mechanism and the true data generating process. If missing values are MAR then the missing data mechanism may be selectively thinning out certain regions of the sample space. If this occurs systematically in a region where the true relationship deviates considerably from the relationship assumed in the imputation model, then a possible bias may not be masked by an overestimated variance and inferences cannot be expected to be valid anymore. This may be even more pronounced in large samples than in small samples because usually the standard deviation of estimators converges to zero with increasing sample size (cf. Rubin, 1996, 2003).

The dependence of inferences on the distribution of the variables using the JAV strategy and whether the missing values are MCAR or MAR are illustrated in a simulation study by Seaman et al. (2012). They consider imputation of squared terms, interactions in linear and binary models and show that adopting the JAV strategy may lead to invalid inferences if the missing values are MAR.

Another approach proposed by Vink and van Buuren (2013), denoted as 'polynomial combination' approach, deals with the specific problem of imputing squared continuous variables in linear regression models. They propose, in the above example, to multiply impute x and x^2 by a technique called 'predictive mean matching' (PMM; see Sect. 4.5.7) following the JAV strategy and (multiply) estimate β_1 and β_2

from the regression of y on x and x^2 based on the imputed data sets. They then define $z = x\,\beta_1 + x^2\,\beta_2$, again based on observed and imputed x-values, and generate imputations z^* for those z for which x was not observed using PMM. Imputations for x are generated using

$$x^*_{1/2} = -\left(\hat{\beta}_1 \pm \sqrt{\hat{\beta}_1^2 + 4\hat{\beta}_2\, z^*}\right)/(2\hat{\beta}_2)\,, \quad \hat{\beta}_2 \neq 0\,, \quad \hat{\beta}_1^2 \geq -4\hat{\beta}_2\, z^*\,.$$

If $\hat{\beta}_1^2 = -4\hat{\beta}_2\, z^*$ there is one solution to this equation. To decide which of the two possible solutions, x_1^* or x_2^*, should be chosen if $\hat{\beta}_1^2 > -4\hat{\beta}_2\, z^*$, Vink and van Buuren (2013) propose to estimate a logistic regression with dependent variable indicating whether the observed $x \leq -\hat{\beta}_1/(2\hat{\beta}_2)$ or not. This model is estimated for the completely observed part of the data set and then applied to the incomplete part to predict whether to use x_1^* or x_2^* as an imputation for x.

Simulation results in Bartlett et al. (2015) imply that this imputation method may allow valid inferences with respect to coverage rates in specific situations if the missing values are MCAR, but tends to coverage rates being too low if the missing values are MAR. The reason for these results could be the use of PMM, which is not without problems (see Sect. 4.5.7; cf. Schenker and Taylor 1996). A serious limitation of this imputation method is that it is restricted to the imputation of squared continuous variables. If other functions of a variable with missing values has to be assumed then other, but always very specific procedures need to be applied.

A possibly promising approach to impute interactions, non-linear functions of predictor variables or non-linear relationships in regression models is proposed by Bartlett et al. (2015). The basic idea is to generate imputations from models which are compatible with the model of applied-scientific interest. However, this approach requires that the model of applied-scientific interest is known at the imputation stage, because this (parametric) model is necessary to decide whether a generated value can be accepted as an imputation. Hence this strategy is not a solution for situations in which the model or models of scientific interest is or are unknown. The results of a limited simulation study suggest that this strategy may lead to valid inferences in settings where these restrictions are met and even in situations in which the above discussed strategies fail.

4.5.3 Imputing Subgroups

In data sets based on questionnaires it might be important to differentiate between groups of units during the imputation process for which variables should be imputed and other groups for which certain variables should not be imputed. Consider the variables ‘gender’ with possible answers ‘female’ and ‘not female’ and ‘number of pregnancies’ with missing values for some units. If the value of variable ‘gender’ is observed or imputed as ‘not female’, then the variable ‘number of pregnancies’ does not apply. The question then is: Should this variable be imputed to simplify the imputation process or not?

A simple solution would be to set the variable 'number of pregnancies' to zero if the first variable is imputed as 'not female' and then go on to impute other variables. Another strategy could be to impute the variable 'number of pregnancies' for both groups, impute other variables and set the values of 'number of pregnancies' to missing for 'not female' after finishing the imputation step. Alternatively, only the 'female' group could be imputed and the values for the 'number of pregnancies' variable could be left missing for the 'not female' group.

Let us consider the three strategies in more detail. The first strategy implies an improper imputation method in most situations, because the 'non-female' group would be assigned values for a variable that does not exist and these arbitrary but invariant values would then be used to impute the values of other (existing) variables of both groups. Put differently, a conditional imputation approach—conditional on non-existing variable values 'number of pregnancies'—would be adopted to impute values of other variables for the 'not female' group where a marginal approach with respect to the variable 'number of pregnancies' would be needed. Thus, this strategy leads in general to systematically misspecified imputation models.

Example 4.4 (To Impute or Not to Impute: Strategy 1) Suppose a data set with three continuous variables of interest, y, x and z where x is completely observed, y and z are incomplete with z more observed than y, so that the pattern of missing values is monotone. However, assume that there are two groups of units such that for group A the variable z exists and is observed for all units and, for group B, z does not exist and is not observed. The missing data mechanisms of z and y are ignorable.

In a first scenario for group A, $(y\ x\ z)^T \sim N(\boldsymbol{\mu}_A, \boldsymbol{\Sigma}_A)$, where

$$\boldsymbol{\mu}_A = \mathbf{0}_{3\times 1} \quad \text{and} \quad \boldsymbol{\Sigma}_A = \begin{pmatrix} 1 & 0.7 & 0.4 \\ 0.7 & 1 & 0.3 \\ 0.4 & 0.3 & 1 \end{pmatrix}$$

and for group B $(y\ x)^T \sim N(\boldsymbol{\mu}_B, \boldsymbol{\Sigma}_B)$, where

$$\boldsymbol{\mu}_B = \mathbf{0}_{2\times 1} \quad \text{and} \quad \boldsymbol{\Sigma}_B = \begin{pmatrix} 1 & 0.7 \\ 0.7 & 1 \end{pmatrix} .$$

The following steps can easily be derived from results given in Appendix A.2.5.

This scenario implies that the marginal effect of x on y is the same in both groups:

$$y = 0.7\, x + \epsilon\ , \quad \epsilon \sim N(0, 0.51)\ . \tag{4.11}$$

However, assume that the database producer who generates imputations does not know which models are of applied-scientific interest and will be estimated later by the analyst. Following strategy one, zeros would be imputed for all unobserved values in z and then y would be imputed. Assuming that the missing data mechanism is ignorable and since the missing data pattern is monotone, the imputation model for y would then be estimated based on the observed values of $(y\ x\ z)$ in group A. The true data generating process and thus the imputation model from the observed part that mimics this process (rounded to three decimal places)[3] is

$$y = 0 + 0.637\, x + 0.209\, z + \epsilon_A\,, \qquad \epsilon_A \sim N(0, 0.470) \qquad \text{for group A}\,.$$

In the next step, the observed values in x and z would be inserted into the imputation model to generate imputations for y in group A based on values for the parameters randomly selected from their posterior distribution and error terms randomly selected from a normal distribution. Repeating this procedure would allow the generation of imputations such that inferences are valid for group A. However, to generate imputations for group B the same model and parameter values would be adopted but with z values set to zero. This leads to an assumed imputation model

$$y = 0 + 0.637\, x + \epsilon_B\,, \qquad \epsilon_B \sim N(0, 0.470) \qquad \text{for group B}\,, \tag{4.12}$$

with implied $\text{var}(y) \approx 0.877$ and correlation between y and x of 0.681 (rounded to three decimal places). Comparing (4.12) with (4.11) shows that the imputation model for group B would be misspecified. Clearly, if z had no effect on y conditional on x in group A, then this imputation strategy would allow valid inferences. □

Following the second strategy, imputations would be generated for the variable 'number of pregnancies' in the 'not female' group based on relationships in the 'female' group. Imputing further variables using these imputed values as predictor variables assumes that the variable 'number of pregnancies' has the same effect for the 'female' and the 'not female' group on the variables to be imputed. Whether or not the resulting imputation model is correctly specified and allows valid inferences, depends on the true data generating process and the model of applied-scientific interest estimated in downstream analyses. For example, if the variable 'number of pregnancies' has no effect on the variable to be imputed conditional on fully observed or already imputed variables, then this second strategy may allow valid inferences. Otherwise this imputation method will be proper only in very specific situations, like the one considered in Example 4.4.

Example 4.5 (To Impute or Not to Impute: Strategy 2) Suppose the same situation as in Example 4.4, but let now

$$\boldsymbol{\mu}_B = \mathbf{0}_{2\times 1} \quad \text{and} \quad \boldsymbol{\Sigma}_B = \begin{pmatrix} 0.877 & 0.637 \\ 0.637 & 1 \end{pmatrix}\,,$$

[3]More precisely, the parameter values are $\beta_x = 0.6373626$ for the parameter that weights x, $\beta_z = 0.2087912$ for the parameter weighting z and $\sigma^2_{\upsilon_A} = 0.4703297$.

which implies

$$y = 0.637\,x + \epsilon_B, \quad \epsilon_B \sim N(0, 0.470)\;,$$

again rounded to three decimal places.[4] Adopting the second strategy, z would be imputed based on a model for $z \mid x$ and then y would be imputed based on $y \mid x, z$ in group A. The imputation model for z with known parameters would be

$$z = 0.3\,x + \nu_A\;, \qquad \nu_A \sim N(0, 0.91) \qquad \text{for group A}\;. \tag{4.13}$$

Generating values z^* for z according to this model and imputing these values into the imputation model for y would lead to

$$y = 0.637\,x + 0.209\,z^* + \epsilon_A\;, \qquad \epsilon_A \sim N(0, 0.47) \qquad \text{for group A}\;,$$

with true rounded parameter values. Note that (4.13) implies—again true parameter values are rounded to three decimal points—imputations for y in group B generated from model

$$y = 0.637\,x + 0.209\,(0.3\,x + \nu_A) + \epsilon_A\;, \quad \nu_A \sim N(0, 0.91), \quad \epsilon_A \sim N(0, 0.47)$$

which is equivalent to

$$y = 0.7\,x + \epsilon\;, \qquad \epsilon \sim N(0, 0.51) \quad \text{cf. (4.11)}\;,$$

which, again, would be a misspecified imputation model in the current context. □

The third strategy seems to be obvious but implies that groups of units are imputed separately which in turn requires that a sufficient number of observed values are available for the imputation tasks within each group. Of course, smaller samples sizes will lead to an increased amount of noise in the imputations. Furthermore, if several variables that do not apply to all units divide the sample into several (disjunct) subsamples then these groups may be too small to be imputed separately. The advantage over the above described strategies is that no hard to justify (often implicit) assumptions about non-existing variables need to be made.

As a consequence, if subgroups are large enough, the imputation method of choice would generate imputations separately for each group. If this is not feasible then strong assumptions about underlying relationships and imputation models may be necessary and should transparently be communicated.

[4]The exact values are $\text{var}(y) = 0.8765608$ and $\text{cov}(y, x) = \beta_x = 0.6373626$, where β_x is the parameter weighting x, and $\sigma_\nu^2 = 0.4703297$.

4.5.4 The Imputation Models: (Non-)ignorability

For most implementations of multiple imputation methods, the underlying assumption is that the missing data mechanism is ignorable. Although the method of multiple imputation could also be adopted if the missing data mechanism is non-ignorable, all-purpose software written for these situations is not available at the time of writing this book. The problem is that rich and precise information from outside the data set must be available and it is hardly predictable—and therefore not easy to write a program for general use—how exactly this information should affect the imputations.

There is a way to make the assumption of ignorability more plausible, by including as many variables as possible into the imputation step (e.g., Rubin 1996, Collins, Schafer, & Kam 2001). This includes not only variables that might be included in models estimated in downstream analyses, but also variables which might be relevant for selecting the sample, like indicators that define strata, or variables thought to be important for the response mechanism, like group indicators, age or occupation. Furthermore, all these variables could enter the imputation step as a polynomial of degree two or three or even higher. In addition, interactions of two or three or more variables may be taken into account.

This strategy is not without problems, however. One problem is that it is usually not known how this information should be considered in the imputation step. Another challenge is that including many variables and functions thereof may lead to exact linear dependencies or multicollinearity. In the former case, estimation of the imputation model will stop with a warning in many software packages. In the latter case, typically the computing time to generate the imputations will be long and variances of the imputed values tend to be large. Thus, these problems can be identified either by errors or warnings from the imputation algorithm or by inspection of descriptive statistics, like the variance, for the imputed part of the data set. If one of these problems occur, variables deemed to be less important may be ignored in the corresponding imputation model.

4.5.5 Reproducible Results

Within the last years it has become increasingly important to publish, together with research results, supplementary material like data sets and code used to analyse the data. If a public use data set is analysed that provides weights and multiple data sets, this is technically easy to realize given enough server space. If weights and multiple imputations are generated only for the analysis at hand, then weights might be added to the data set just as additional variables. Since the number of imputations may be larger, it might be favourable to publish only the code that generated the imputations. To be able to reproduce the results, however, and since the method of multiple imputation is a method based on simulations, it would be important to control the random seed, i.e., the starting value for the pseudo-random number generators. In R this is the `set.seed()` command, or if e.g. the package `mice` is used, the `seed` option. If this—or similar functions in other software packages—is not set to a specific value, then the starting value will be generated from the internal computer time and/or the process identifier (usually a number) and therefore will be different for every run.

Another kind of reproducibility is to check whether the results remain stable even if different starting values are used. For serious inferences they should of course not vary substantially. One aspect to note when this stability is checked, is to choose a sufficient number of imputations. In Sect. 4.3.5 we already discussed the criteria to choose the number of imputations. Varying the starting values for the random number generators, increasing the number of imputations step by step and comparing the results gives an impression on the stability of the inferences. Assuming that the complete-data set analysis is well specified, very slow convergence or, for a decided-to-be-sufficient M, substantially different results for different starting values may indicate an ill-posed imputation problem. In that case, the imputation models should possibly be reformulated.

The above described procedures are appropriate if the imputations are generated at the analysis stage. Usually this is not the case if imputation and analysis stages are separate steps, for example, if the imputed data set is a public use data set provided by an institution. In that case the procedure described in the last paragraph could be realized at least approximately if the number of imputations are very large, like hundreds or more imputations, and by randomly sampling the imputed data sets. If the number of imputations is small, they could simply be added to the data set to be published.

4.5.6 Some Additional Notes

Imputing real data sets is not straightforward even with current software solutions. General requirements on software solutions and the process of generating imputations will be discussed in the following subsections.

Specific requirements that received not much attention in the literature have been discussed in Sects. 4.5.2, 4.5.3, and 4.5.5, and it turned out that solutions are often not easy to find. As in the case of ad-hoc methods (see Sect. 3.2) simple solutions may lead astray even if they are embedded into multiple imputation methods.

Imputing real data sets may call for solutions not considered in this book. For example, if some components of an observed sum, e.g., household income, are missing or if the distribution of a variable to be imputed seems to deviate markedly from the desired posterior predictive distribution. In the latter case, it is often proposed to apply some transformation. However, when applying this technique it should be kept in mind that to generate imputations the theoretical distribution of the variable to be imputed conditional on all predictors is relevant, but what is observed in a data set is the unconditional distribution of the observed and possibly very selective subsample. Thus the latter may not be very informative with respect to the former.

Some imputation software provide options to solve these problems. However, care should be taken that the proposed techniques are justified by theoretical arguments or at least backed up by systematic simulation studies. Otherwise, they are questionable like the ad-hoc methods considered in Sect. 3.2 and may allow valid inferences only in very specific situations.

4.5.7 Choosing from a Large Number of Imputation Techniques

Most software for statistical analyses provide functions to generate multiple imputations. Often the same function makes several methods available. For example, the function `mice` provides around 20 different techniques to generate imputations. Thus it is not easy to decide which technique to choose in a certain application. In this section, we will discuss imputation in some specific situations and provide some general guidelines to select an imputation method.

4.5.7.1 Basic Requirements and General Comments

For valid inferences of scientific interest using the combining rules presented in Sect. 4.3.3 imputations should approximate independent draws from the posterior predictive distribution (4.5). Assuming that the complete-data set estimator is valid, it is not necessary for valid inferences that the posterior distribution of the MI based estimator of scientific interest is correctly specified. For valid inferences only its mean conditional on the observed values should be approximately unbiased for the estimate in the complete-data set or the statistic or parameter of scientific interest and its variance estimator should not underestimate its true variance over repeated sampling. Therefore, in applications not only imputations from the 'true' posterior predictive distribution may allow valid inferences, but also imputations generated from a model that approximates this posterior distribution.

The method of multiple imputation has been shown to work in general by theoretical arguments (Rubin, 1987, 1996; Meng 1994; Tsiatis 2006) and many simulation studies if the imputation method is proper or confidence proper. If different entities impute and analyse the imputed data set then different information might be used at the imputation and the analysis stage. In a first scenario, variables ignored for generating imputations are used to analyse the multiply imputed data set. According to Rubin (1996) even ignoring mildly important predictor variables in the imputation model may allow confidence valid inferences due to the 'self-correcting' property of MI. If the variable ignored at the imputation stage is in fact irrelevant but is included in the model of applied-scientific interest, then more information is used at the imputation as compared to the analysis stage. In this case the estimator of the model of applied-scientific interest is called 'superefficient' because extra information is used at the imputation stage that leads to a smaller variance of this estimator. At the same time the variance is overestimated and thus inferences are conservative. This is the situation illustrated in Example 4.2 (see Tables 4.1 and 4.2). A MI based estimator is 'strongly superefficient' if its variance is even smaller than the variance of the complete-data estimator (cf. Table 4.2). On the other hand, more information may be used at the analysis stage than in the imputation step (cf. Meng, 1994). For example, at the analysis stage it could be known that a variable is independent from all other variables in a model of applied-scientific interest. In the imputation step, however, this variable is used to impute a variable that enters the regression model at the analysis stage as a predictor. In this case, if the analysis model is valid and the imputations are generated from an appropriate model, the final inferences will still be valid.

In applications a data set often includes variables whose relationships are not of scientific interest and therefore are unknown. As an example consider a data set which, amongst others, includes variables wage, tenure, schooling, occupation and body height. Suppose that only body height is not completely observed and needs to be imputed. Thus an imputation model has to be specified and estimated. Without additional information and given that height can be treated as a continuous variable, a linear regression model of height on wage, tenure, schooling and occupation could be chosen. However, since this relationship is not of general scientific interest, it is not easy to justify this imputation model. Does wage have a (statistical) effect on height? If yes and given the research on effects of various variables on wage (cf. Sect. 2.5), should the logarithm of wage be included instead of wage? Should tenure be included as a second-order polynomial? In fact, empirical results suggest that there might be a non-linear relationship between the logarithm of wage and body height, different for males and females, which would not justify a linear imputation model for height (e.g., Hübler, 2009). If the logarithm of wage is ignored at the imputation stage, then the relationship between wage and body height would be underestimated in downstream analyses. Due to the self-correcting property, inferences about the effect of height on wage could still be confidence valid as long as the sample size is not too large but an estimator of the relationship would be biased.

Hence, imputation models should be carefully chosen and expert knowledge can be helpful to select predictor variables and appropriate imputation models. Available imputation techniques range from restrictive Bayesian models, like the Bayesian linear or logistic regression model (cf. Example 4.3) to semi- or nonparametric and robust imputation models.

4.5.7.2 Imputation Techniques

A sensible Bayesian imputation model that includes all relevant (functions of) variables tends to allow confidence valid inferences if it is not severely misspecified.

Hence, if there is no evidence for strong non-linear relationships or these relationships are known and can be modeled, if the missing data mechanism is ignorable and not highly selective, then choosing a parametric Bayesian imputation model may be an appropriate choice.

Less restrictive imputation techniques are based on the class of 'hot-deck' techniques (Rubin, 1987). The idea is to find for each unit with a missing value in x, say, several units in the same data set for which x has been observed and choose, usually randomly, one unit out of this set to 'donate' its value to the unit with missing x. Usually the set of possible donors is a set of neighbours, i.e., units which are close in the observed variables to the unit with x missing. These methods are called k-nearest neighbour techniques (k-NN techniques) and the specific version depends on the distance function. A common technique is called 'predictive mean matching' (PMM; e.g., van Buuren et al., 2006), where a regression is estimated for the completely observed part of the data set and then, based on the estimated linear relationship between the incompletely observed variable in question and the observed variables, the distance of each completely observed unit and the incompletely observed unit is estimated by the squared difference of the predicted values, i.e., the squared Euclidean distance.

Advantages of these techniques are that they do not require restrictive assumptions about the relationship between the variable to be imputed and the corresponding predictors, that they are easy to implement and are computationally fast. However, there is an unpleasant bias/variance trade-off: If the number of neighbours is too small, then imputations for the same unit and variable will not be independent. On the other hand, if the number of possible donors is too large, then the estimator of applied-scientific interest may be biased because this imputation method implicitly assumes that within a given cell, implicitly defined by the neighbours, missing values are MCAR (cf. de Jong et al., 2016; Schenker & Taylor, 1996). A drawback closely related to the latter point is that if the missing data mechanism is selective and thins out data points, for example, in an extreme region, then the observed values of neighbours may be far away and/or may systematically be different from the unobserved values which may lead to biased estimation. In fact, simulation results suggest (e.g., de Jong et al., 2016; He & Raghunathan, 2009) that predictive mean matching imputation may lead to invalid inferences in these cases.

A promising version of hot-deck imputation is proposed by Siddique and Belin (2008) and implemented in slightly extended version by Gaffert, Meinfelder, and Bosch (2016) as package `midastouch` in `R`. In this hot-deck version all completely observed cases have a positive probability of becoming a donor, the probability being a function of the distance to the incompletely observed unit. A small simulation study in Gaffert et al. (2016) implies that this version may overcome some of the problems of k-NN methods and may thus be adopted to generate imputations if the distributional assumptions and the assumed relationship in parametric Bayesian imputation models are hardly justified. Note that the problem due to imputing only observed values in the presence of a selective missing data mechanism that deletes values in border regions is not solved by this method. For an application, see Sect. 5.4.3.

To overcome the problem of non-linear relationships but at the same time generate model-based imputations de Jong et al. (2016) proposed an imputation method based on a flexible class of generalized additive models for location scale and shape (GAMLSS; Rigby & Stasinopoulos, 2005; Stasinopoulos & Rigby, 2007). Within this model class non-linear relationships along with additional aspects of the conditional distributions can be estimated, which makes this imputation method very flexible. It is implemented in an R-package `ImputeRobust` (Salfrán & Spiess, 2017, 2018; R Core Team 2018) that can be interpreted as approximating Bayesian imputation. Results of a simulation study suggest that this imputation method may allow valid inferences even when the relationship between the variable to impute and predictors is non-linear and parametric Bayesian and PMM methods fail (de Jong et al., 2016). The price to be paid for this additional flexibility are wider confidence intervals and, for computational stability, a need for larger samples. Hence this imputation method may allow valid inferences in large samples when the assumptions of parametric models may be violated, which is the case if, e.g., quadratic or higher-order terms need to be included into the imputation model and/or the missing data mechanism is selective.

Function `ImputeRobust` can also be adopted to generate non-continuous imputations, e.g., binary, polytomous or count variables. To generate imputations for a count variable within the framework of parametric models usually a Poisson regression model is adopted. However this is a very restrictive model. A more flexible approach to generate imputations for zero-inflated and overdispersed count variables has been proposed by Kleinke and Reinecke (2013). Again, a simulation study reported in Kleinke and Reinecke (2013) implies that this imputation method may lead to valid inferences when standard Poisson models to generate imputations fail. `ImputeRobust` and `countimp` can both be used together with R-package `mice` (van Buuren & Groothuis-Oudshoorn, 2011). See Sects. 6.3 and 6.2 for an application of these packages.

Several other imputation methods have been proposed and are available, some as options within widely used packages. Not all of these imputation methods are justified based on the multiple imputation theory of Rubin and thus allow confidence valid inferences based on the combining rules given in Sect. 4.3.3 (see Rubin, 1987). In the case of more complex data sets, like clustered data, imputation models should take the corresponding structure into account. The theory is the same as for simpler data structures, but most imputation methods are available only for simpler cases, like non-clustered cross-sectional data. This is due to the fact that flexible non-restrictive statistical models to generate imputations and stable algorithms to estimate them are not yet readily available. Those that are available to generate imputations in mixed models are based on strong assumptions and may be used only in very specific situations. Thus, there is still room for developing imputation functions that allow to generate imputations such that valid inferences are possible in more general situations. However, available imputation methods are considered and discussed in Chaps. 5 and 6.

Since a theoretical justification is often difficult or the underlying assumptions cannot be assumed to hold and it may therefore not be obvious if imputations are generated respecting the relevant aspects of the posterior predictive distribution (4.6), it is important to check whether simulation results are available. If yes, simulation studies should cover a wide range of possible situations including non-normally distributed variables and non-linear relationships, at least varying the sample sizes, fraction of missing values (or better missing information), the selectivity of the missing data mechanism and the true relationship of variables. It would further be informative to simulate problems that arise when real data sets are to be imputed, like multicollinearities, outliers or different missing data mechanisms even for the same incompletely observed variable. To evaluate the methods, simulation studies should report the bias of the estimators, the width of confidence intervals (or the estimated variances) and, very important, the rates with which true values are covered by confidence intervals.

Based on this information—and after thorough inspection of the data set at hand—one may make an informed decision about which imputation technique may be used for the specific data set at hand. In many cases this might not be the default option provided by the software package used to generate imputations. If imputation and analyses are carried out by different entities then as much information as possible about the imputation procedure should be provided with the imputations.

4.6 Summary

In this chapter the method of multiple imputation to compensate for missing values was discussed. The theory of multiple imputation has been proposed by Rubin (1987) and was further generalized and justified by Rubin (1996), Meng (1994), Tsiatis (2006) and others. The theory justifies the use of multiple imputation as long as the assumptions underlying the models adopted to generate imputations are approximately met. Today the method is available via many software packages and functions.

However, not all of the imputation functions realize proper imputation methods that allow valid statistical inferences. On the other hand, available software solutions do not allow the treatment of all situations of practical interest. Therefore, applying an imputation method requires knowledge of the underlying assumptions and restrictions. If the imputer and the analyst are different entities, then the imputation model should be as general and flexible as possible, possibly sacrificing efficiency. If both, imputer and analyst, are the same entity and if enough information is available, then the imputation models may be tailored towards the analyses of interest. But in any case, generating imputations should not be an automated process. To allow valid scientific inferences, imputation methods and models have to be chosen carefully, which also requires expert knowledge about the field in which the data set will be used.

References

Barnard, J., & Rubin, D. B. (1999). Small-sample degrees of freedom with multiple imputation. *Biometrika, 86*(4), 948–955.

Bartlett, J. W., Seaman, S. R., White, I. R., & Carpenter, J. R. (2015). Multiple imputation of covariates by fully conditional specification: Accommodating the substantive model. *Statistical Methods in Medical Research, 24*(4), 462–487.

Casella, G., & George, E. I. (1992). Explaining the Gibbs sampler. *The American Statistician, 46*(3), 167–174.

Collins, L. M., Schafer, J. L., & Kam, C. M. (2001). A comparison of inclusive and restrictive strategies in modern missing data procedures. *Psychological Methods, 6*(4), 330–351.

de Jong, R., van Buuren, S., & Spiess, M. (2016). Multiple imputation of predictor variables using generalized additive models. *Communications in Statistics – Simulation and Computation, 45*(3), 968–985.

Gaffert, P., Meinfelder, F., & Bosch, V. (2016). *Towards an MI-proper predictive mean matching* (Discussion Paper). https://www.uni-bamberg.de/fileadmin/uni/fakultaeten/sowi_lehrstuehle/statistik/Personen/Dateien_Florian/properPMM.pdf.

Geman, S., & Geman, D. (1984). Stochastic relaxation, Gibbs distributions, and the Bayesian restoration of images. *IEEE Transactions on Pattern Analysis and Machine Intelligence, 6*(6), 721–741.

Geraci, M., & McLain, A. (2018). Multiple imputation for bounded variables. *Psychometrika, 83*(4), 919–940.

Graham, J. W., Olchowski, A. E., & Gilreath, T. D. (2007). How many imputations are really needed? Some practical clarifications of multiple imputation theory. *Prevention Science, 8*(3), 206–213.

He, Y., & Raghunathan, T. E. (2009). On the performance of sequential regression multiple imputation methods with non normal error distributions. *Communications in Statistics – Simulation and Computation, 38*(4), 856–883.

Horton, N. J., Lipsitz, S. R., & Parzen, M. (2003). A potential for bias when rounding in multiple imputation. *The American Statistician, 57*(4), 229–232.

Hübler, O. (2009). The nonlinear link between height and wages in Germany, 1985–2004. *Economics and Human Biology, 7*(2), 191–199.

Kleinke, K., & Reinecke, J. (2013). Multiple imputation of incomplete zero-inflated count data. *Statistica Neerlandica, 67*(3), 311–336.

Kuchler, C., & Spiess, M. (2009). The data quality concept of accuracy in the context of public use data sets. *AStA Wirtschafts- und Sozialstatistisches Archiv, 3*(1), 67–80.

Li, K. H. (1988). Imputation using Markov chains. *Journal of Statistical Computation and Simulation, 30*(1), 57–79.

Li, K. H., Raghunathan, T. E., & Rubin, D. B. (1991). Large-sample significance levels from multiply imputed data using moment-based statistics and an F-reference distribution. *Journal of the American Statistical Association, 86*(416), 1065–1073.

Liu, J., Gelman, A., Hill, J., Su, Y.-S., & Kropko, J. (2014). On the stationary distribution of iterative imputations. *Biometrika, 101*(1), 155–173.

Meng, X.-L. (1994). Multiple-imputation inferences with uncongenial sources of input. *Statistical Science, 9*(4), 538–558.

Nielsen, S. F. (2003). Proper and improper multiple imputation (with discussion). *International Statistical Review, 71*(3), 593–627.

R Core Team. (2018). *R: A language and environment for statistical computing*. Vienna: R Foundation for Statistical Computing. https://www.R-project.org.

Raghunathan, T. E., Lepkowski, J. M., Van Hoewyk, J., & Solenberger, P. (2001). A multivariate technique for multiply imputing missing values using a sequence of regression models. *Survey Methodology, 27*(1), 85–95.

Raghunathan, T. E., Solenberger, P., Berglund, P., & Van Hoewyk, J. (2016). *IVEware: Imputation and variance estimation software (Version 0.3)*. Ann Arbor, MI: Survey Methodology Program, Survey Research Center, Institute for Social Research, University of Michigan. http://www.src.isr.umich.edu/software/iveware-documentation/

Rigby, R. A., & Stasinopoulos, M. D. (2005). Generalized additive models for location, scale and shape. *Journal of the Royal Statistical Society: Series C (Applied Statistics), 54*(3), 507–554.

Roberts, G. O. (1996). Markov chain concepts related to sampling algorithms. In W. R. Gilks, S. Richardson, & D. J. Spiegelhalter (Eds.), *Markov chain Monte Carlo in practice* (pp. 35–57). London, UK: Chapman & Hall.

Robins, J. M., & Wang, N. (2000). Inference for imputation estimators. *Biometrika, 87*(1), 113–124.

Rodwell, L., Lee, K. J., Romaniuk, H., & Carlin, J. B. (2014). Comparison of methods for imputing limited-range variables: A simulation study. *BMC Medical Research Methodology, 14*(1), 57.

Rubin, D. B. (1987). *Multiple imputation for nonresponse in surveys*. New York, NY: Wiley.

Rubin, D. B. (1996). Multiple imputation after 18+ years. *Journal of the American Statistical Association, 91*(434), 473–489.

Rubin, D. B. (2003). Discussion on multiple imputation. *International Statistical Review, 71*(3), 619–625.

Sakia, R. M. (1992). The Box-Cox transformation technique: A review. *The Statistician, 41*(2), 169–178.

Salfrán, D., Jordan, P., & Spiess, M. (2016). *Missing values: On criteria to evaluate imputation methods* (Discussion Paper No. 4). Hamburg, Germany: University of Hamburg, Department of Psychology Methods and Statistics.

Salfrán, D., & Spiess, M. (2017). `ImputeRobust`: Robust multiple imputation with generalized additive models for location scale and shape [Computer software manual]. https://CRAN.R-project.org/package=ImputeRobust (R Package Version 1.2).

Salfrán, D., & Spiess, M. (2018). Generalized additive model multiple imputation by chained equations with package `imputerobust`. *The R Journal, 10*(1), 61–72.

Schafer, J. L. (1997). *Analysis of incomplete multivariate data*. London, UK: Chapman & Hall.

Schafer, J. L. (1999a). Multiple imputation: A primer. *Statistical Methods in Medical Research, 8*(1), 3–15.

Schafer, J. L. (1999b). NORM users guide (version 2) [Computer software manual]. University Park, PA: The Methodology Center, The Pennsylvania State University. https://www.methodology.psu.edu/training/missing-data/.

Schafer, J. L. (2001). Multiple imputation with PAN. In L. M. Collins & A. G. Sayer (Eds.), *New methods for the analysis of change* (pp. 357–377). Washington DC, WA: American Psychological Association.

Schafer, J. L., & Graham, J. W. (2002). Missing data: Our view of the state of the art. *Psychological Methods, 7*(2), 147–177.

Schafer, J. L., & Yucel, R. M. (2002). Computational strategies for multivariate linear mixed-effects models with missing values. *Journal of Computational and Graphical Statistics, 11*(2), 437–457.

Schenker, N., & Taylor, J. M. G. (1996). Partially parametric techniques for multiple imputation. *Computational Statistics & Data Analysis, 22*(4), 425–446.

Seaman, S., Bartlett, J. W., & White, I. R. (2012). Multiple imputation of missing covariates with non-linear effects and interactions: An evaluation of statistical methods. *BMC Medical Research Methodology, 12*(46), 1–13.

Siddique, J., & Belin, T. R. (2008). Multiple imputation using an iterative hot-deck with distance-based donor selection. *Statistics in Medicine, 27* (1), 83–102.

Spanos, A. (1995). On normality and the linear regression model. *Econometric Reviews, 14*(2), 195–203.

Stasinopoulos, M. D., & Rigby, R. A. (2007). Generalized additive models for location scale and shape (GAMLSS) in R. *Journal of Statistical Software, 23*(7), 1–46.

Tanner, M. A. (1996). *Tools for statistical inference*. New York, NY: Springer.

Tanner, M. A., & Wong, W. H. (1987). The calculation of posterior distributions by data augmentation. *Journal of the American Statistical Association, 82*(398), 528–540.
Templ, M., Kowarik, A., & Filzmoser, P. (2011). Iterative stepwise regression imputation using standard and robust methods. *Computational Statistics and Data Analysis, 55*(10), 2793–2806.
Tierney, L. (1996). Introduction to general state-space Markov chain theory. In W. R. Gilks, S. Richardson, & D. J. Spiegelhalter (Eds.), *Markov chain Monte Carlo in practice* (pp. 59–74). London, UK: Chapman & Hall.
Troyanskaya, O., Cantor, M., Sherlock, G., Brown, P., Hastie, T., Tibshirani, R., et al. (2001). Missing value estimation methods for DNA microarrays. *Bioinformatics, 17*(6), 520–525.
Tsiatis, A. A. (2006). *Semiparametric theory and missing data*. New York, NY: Springer.
van Buuren, S. (2012). *Flexible imputation of missing data*. Boca Raton, FL: Chapmann & Hall/CRC.
van Buuren, S., Brands, J. P. L., Groothuis-Oudshoorn, C. G. M., & Rubin, D. B. (2006). Fully conditional specification in multivariate imputation. *Journal of Statistical Computation and Simulation, 76*(12), 1049–1064.
van Buuren, S., & Groothuis-Oudshoorn, K. (2011). `mice`: Multivariate imputation by chained equations in R. *Journal of Statistical Software, 45*(3), 1–67.
Vink, G., & van Buuren, S. (2013). Multiple imputation of squared terms. *Sociological Methods & Research, 42*(4), 598–607.
von Hippel, P. T. (2009). How to impute interactions, squares and other transformed variables. *Sociological Methodology, 39*(1), 265–291.
von Hippel, P. T. (2013). Should a normal imputation model be modified to impute skewed variables? *Sociological Methods & Research, 42*(1), 105–138.
von Hippel, P. T. (2018). How many imputations do you need? A two-stage calculation using a quadratic rule. *Sociological Methods & Research, 2018*, doi:10.1177/0049124117747303.

Chapter 5
Multiple Imputation: Application

5.1 Overview

In this chapter, we discuss the most important and most commonly used multiple imputation tools in R[1] for both multivariate and clustered data sets, including packages `mice`, `norm2`, `Amelia`, `mi`, `pan`, as well as function `aregImpute()` from package `Hmisc`, and show practical applications. We give hands-on step by step tutorials regarding how to carry out MI in practice.

For the examples in Chaps. 5 and 6, we use data from four waves of an empirical (panel) data set, which we introduce in Sect. 5.2.1. The dependent variable here is a discrete count variable. Counts are defined as non-negative integer values, which may be modeled as continuous in an imputation process, for example, when it is used as a predictor in a regression model of applied scientific interest (see Sect. 4.5.1). If an incompletely observed count variable enters a model of interest for count variables as the dependent variable, however, then it should be treated as a count variable during the imputation process. In addition, the distribution of count variables conditional on predictors is often assumed to be skewed and both, imputation and subsequent analysis models, should allow for this possible skewness. While we demonstrate standard parametric and more robust (semi- and non-parametric) MI methods for both continuous and count variables, it is beyond the scope of this book to demonstrate all available procedures for all possible variable types. We, for example, do not demonstrate imputation of binary or (ordered) categorical variables. However, once the basic principles are clear, it will be very straightforward for readers to adjust imputation methods and models accordingly.

[1] Table 5.1 gives an overview of the download frequencies of various MI packages in R.

K. Kleinke et al., *Applied Multiple Imputation*,
Statistics for Social and Behavioral Sciences,
https://doi.org/10.1007/978-3-030-38164-6_5

Table 5.1 RStudio download frequencies of various MI packages

	Year					
Package	2013	2014	2015	2016	2017	2018
Amelia	8785	18,172	32,416	58,405	75,865	109,393
Hmisc	142,606	331,111	634,051	1,037,841	1,359,935	1,500,417
jomo	0	125	7150	9651	12,622	362,213
mi	6301	12,385	72,843	125,670	157,774	179,074
mice	18,547	37,739	63,498	132,188	268,856	487,282
norm	2728	4861	9773	10,805	9350	16,147
norm2	0	0	0	1023	1676	1209
pan	5748	9156	14,020	16,475	21,244	165,463

Note. The table shows the download frequencies of the respective R packages (timespan: 01 January 2013–31 December 2018). Package download counts were obtained from the Rstudio CRAN mirror using function `dlstats::cran_stats()`

An explicit objective of the following two chapters is to keep the practical examples relatively simple and easy to follow. We therefore use one data set and one motivating example throughout Chaps. 5 and 6. Here, we focus on the incomplete dependent variable in our model of applied scientific interest (see Sect. 5.2.2), a scenario which has gained the most attention so far in the literature. The predictors in our data set are completely observed. An advantage of this scenario is that when the MAR assumption holds (which we assume in our applications), we can use the model estimates based on the remaining observations as a benchmark to compare the various imputation methods against. We can thus discuss the strengths and weaknesses of the respective methods in comparison to the benchmark.

Note that as already mentioned, the predictor variables in our example data set are completely observed. Imputation of incomplete predictor variables is not the focus of this book. A main problem when incomplete predictors need to be imputed is that in general the imputation model differs from the model of applied scientific interest: If the model of interest from y on x is a normal linear homoscedastic regression model, then the reverse regression, i.e., the regression from x on y is usually not linear homoscedastic (see Sect. 3.3.2); if the model of interest is a specific multilevel model, then choosing the same model to generate imputations for a predictor will usually be a misspecified model. The problems that arise when incomplete predictors need to be imputed, especially, when these predictors are then used to form interaction terms or higher-order relationships (like quadratic or cubic terms), as well as what software solutions are currently available, is discussed extensively in Spiess, Kleinke, and Reinecke (in press).

5.2 Data and Substantive Model

5.2.1 The CrimoC data

For the practical examples throughout this chapter we use incomplete empirical panel data from the "Crime in the modern City" study (CrimoC, e.g., Boers, Reinecke, Seddig, & Mariotti, 2010; Reinecke & Weins, 2013), which examined the emergence and development of juvenile delinquency over time in adolescence. Data were collected in schools in two larger German cities: Münster with about 275,000 inhabitants and Duisburg with about 500,000 inhabitants. The study in Münster started in 2000 with around 2,000 7th-graders. The study in Duisburg started in 2002 with a sample of about 3,400 7th-graders. For our illustrations, we use data from four waves of the Münster study: Our example data set `crim4.dat`, which is available in the supplementary material of the book, consists of $N = 2,064$ students, who were interviewed annually from grade 7 to 10. The average age of participants at Wave 1 was 13 years (Weins & Reinecke, 2007). A detailed description of this data set is given in Reinecke and Weins (2013). The variables in the data file `crim4.dat` are:

`id`	the participant identifier
`FEMALE`	the gender indicator
`RE`	school type indicator "Realschule"
`GY`	school type indicator "Gymnasium"
`HA`	school type indicator "Hauptschule"
`ACRIM–DCRIM`	delinquency score at wave A–D (A = year 2000; D = year 2003)

Data were collected via self-administered classroom interviews. Delinquency was measured with 16 questions to get the prevalences of various offences like burglary or assault with or without a weapon (for details, see Table 8 in Reinecke & Weins, 2013). Students indicated for each offence, if they committed this delinquent behaviour in the 12 months prior to the interview (1 = yes; 0 = no). Variables `ACRIM–DCRIM` denote the sums of these different offences, where letters A–D denote the respective panel wave (A = year 2000; B = 2001; C = 2002; D = 2003). Indices `ACRIM–DCRIM` can range between 0 and 16, with higher values indicating a more versatile criminal activity. Reinecke and Weins (2013) expected to find the typical age-crime-curve, a curvilinear development of delinquency over time, i.e., the means of `ACRIM–DCRIM` were expected to increase until around the age of 15, and to decrease thereafter (see also Moffitt, 1993).

Furthermore, in our practical examples, we are not only interested in modeling the age-crime-relationship, but also to investigate the effects of gender and school type on the age-crime relationship (cf. Reinecke & Weins, 2013): The German secondary education system consists of different school types, three of which we distinguish here: 'Gymnasium' is the highest branch and prepares students for

Table 5.2 The CrimoC data—descriptive statistics

	Mean	Std. Dev.	Min	P25	P50	P75	Max	Sum	NAs
FEMALE	0.495							1022	0
RE	0.323							666	0
GY	0.432							892	0
HA	0.245							506	0
ACRIM	0.604	1.355	0	0	0	1	12		689
BCRIM	1.062	1.991	0	0	0	1	15		397
CCRIM	1.292	2.215	0	0	0	2	16		343
DCRIM	1.005	1.763	0	0	0	1	16		579

Note. ACRIM–DCRIM are the repeatedly measured delinquency scores, where letters A–D denote the respective measurement timepoint (A = 2000; D = 2003). FEMALE is the gender indicator, RE, GY and HA the school type indicators. The table displays means, standard deviations and percentiles for continuous variables and observed absolute and relative frequencies (columns Sum and Mean, respectively) for the categorical variables. NAs is the count of missing observations

higher education (e.g., university) and finishes usually after grade 12 (or 13). The intermediate branch 'Realschule' finishes after grade 10. The reference category in our example data set ('Hauptschule') denotes the lowest branch and prepares students for vocational education. Reinecke and Weins (2013) found that both gender and school type predicted individual differences in the development of delinquent behaviours over time. Their model results show a higher prevalence of delinquent behaviour of boys and of adolescents attending the lowest branch of school ('Hauptschule').

Descriptive statistics of the variables in `crim4.dat` are displayed in Table 5.2. The distribution of delinquency scores appears to be heavily skewed with a large percentage of zero counts. Most students did not report any punishable offence at any measurement time point. The assumed non-normal distribution of delinquency scores conditional on predictor variables needs to be taken into account, when choosing a suitable imputation and data analysis model. We will come back to that issue later on.

Missing data patterns are displayed in Table 5.3. The gender and school type indicators are completely observed and are not included in Table 5.3. Note that only 813 out of the 2064 cases (39.3%) are complete cases. Using listwise deletion in this case would discard a lot of valuable information. If the data are not MCAR, invalid inferences are to be expected. Reinecke and Weins (2013) argued that the MCAR assumption is not likely to hold: adolescents with missing data are overproportionally male, and the percentage of students attending the lowest branch, i.e., 'Hauptschule' is about twice as high among adolescents with missing data than among adolescents without missing data. Unlike complete case analysis, multiple imputation can make use of these partially observed cases to predict missing information: There are 1251 respondents with only one or two panel waves missing. Since these repeated measurements cannot be expected to be independent, it is plausible that missing information at one or two panel waves can be predicted by

Table 5.3 The CrimoC data—missing data patterns

	ACRIM	BCRIM	CCRIM	DCRIM
813	1	1	1	1
262	0	1	1	1
38	1	0	1	1
10	1	1	0	1
184	1	1	1	0
293	0	0	1	1
20	0	1	0	1
49	1	0	0	1
114	0	1	1	0
17	1	0	1	0
264	1	1	0	0

Note. ACRIM–DCRIM denote the repeatedly measured dependent variable—the delinquency index, where letters A–D denote the respective measurement timepoint (A = 2000; D = 2003). 1 = observed value; 0 = missing value; the first column gives the observed frequency of the respective missing data pattern

the observed delinquency at other time points. For pragmatic reasons, cases with three or more missing waves are excluded from the analysis. These are cases where either only cross-sectional information about their delinquent behaviour could be collected, and consequently no information about the development of this variable over time was present, or no information at all about delinquency could be collected (cf. Reinecke & Weins, 2013). Two main reasons that could be identified for these patterns are problems with the pseudonymization code from wave one to wave two (Pöge 2005, 2008). Some students were not able to reproduce their code at the second panel wave and therefore their records could not be matched from wave one to the subsequent waves. The other reason was that some families moved away during the course of the study. Note that if these kinds of drop out are selective somehow, excluding those cases could produce a selective sample and subsequent inferences could be biased. For a more in-depth discussion, see (Pöge 2005, 2008).

5.2.2 *Growth Curve Models*

To model the age-crime relationship, we specify a growth curve model. Furthermore, as the data are counts, it is usually more plausible to assume a Poisson or a negative binomial distribution for the delinquency scores rather than the usual normal model. As the distribution of the scores is highly skewed (with a large number of zero counts), a so-called zero-inflated Poisson (abbreviated ZIP) growth curve model is used to model the age-crime curve. For readers who are not familiar with growth models or zero-inflation models, we will provide a brief introduction in the following two paragraphs. The third paragraph summarizes results of our substantive application of a ZIP growth curve model. A brief introduction to growth curve models, as well as comparisons with similar model classes is furthermore given in Reinecke and Seddig (2011).

5.2.2.1 Growth Curve Modeling in a Nutshell

Growth models are typically used to model change in a variable of interest across time. In comparison to standard ordinary least squares regression, growth models do not assume a constant starting level and constant level of change for all individuals in the data set. Instead they estimate, how individuals vary in starting levels and change over time. They furthermore allow inclusion of predictors, why individuals differ in their starting levels and levels of change. A graphical representation of an unconditional growth model (i.e., a model without predictors) with four measurement time points is displayed in Fig. 5.1.

The general measurement model equation for the growth curve model for the ith unit is

$$\mathbf{y}_i = \boldsymbol{\Lambda}\boldsymbol{\eta}_i + \boldsymbol{\epsilon}_i, \quad E(\boldsymbol{\epsilon_i}) = E(\eta_{ji}\boldsymbol{\epsilon_i}) = \mathbf{0} \quad \text{for all } i = 1, \ldots, n,\ j = 1, \ldots, J,, \tag{5.1}$$

where $\mathbf{y}_i = (y_{1i} \cdots y_{Ti})^T$ are manifest (observed) indicators at time points $t = 1, \ldots, T$ (in our example variables ACRIM–DCRIM) and $\boldsymbol{\eta}_i = (\eta_{1i} \cdots \eta_{Ji})^T$ are the latent growth factors, here the latent intercept, slope and quadratic slope,

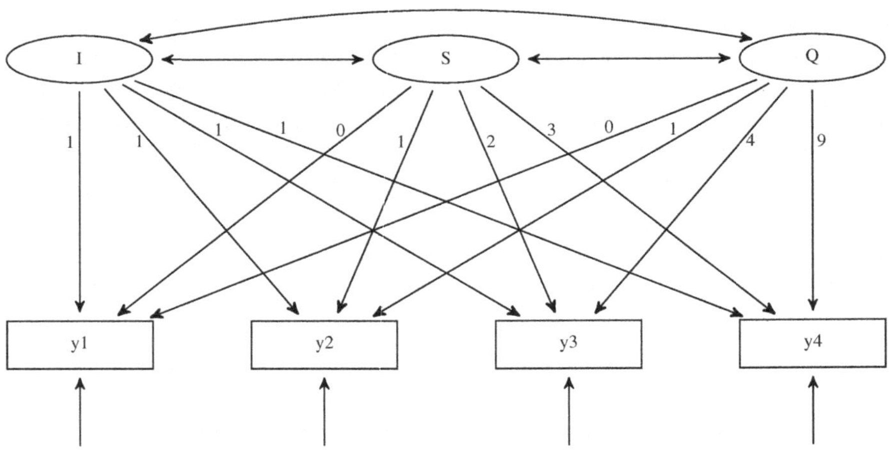

Fig. 5.1 Unconditional growth model. Delinquency at four time points ($y_1, \ldots, y_4$), I = intercept, S = slope, Q = quadratic slope. Factor loadings are constrained to represent the (constant) intercept, the linear and quadratic slope, respectively

respectively (i.e., I, S and Q in Fig. 5.1). $\boldsymbol{\epsilon}_i = (\epsilon_{1i} \cdots \epsilon_{Ti})^T$ are time-specific measurement errors that will be assumed to be iid, and

$$\Lambda = \begin{pmatrix} 1 & 0 & 0 \\ 1 & 1 & 1 \\ 1 & 2 & 4 \\ 1 & 3 & 9 \end{pmatrix}$$

is called the matrix of factor loadings in the context of growth curve models.

Latent growth factors $\boldsymbol{\eta}_i$ are random variables described as a function of their means $\boldsymbol{\alpha}$ (which show the average development across p panel waves within a homogeneous population) and random errors $\boldsymbol{\zeta}_i = (\zeta_{1,i} \cdots \zeta_{J,i})^T$, where the $\zeta_{j,i}$ will again be assumed to be iid for all j, i:

$$\begin{bmatrix} \eta_{1i} \\ \eta_{2i} \\ \eta_{3i} \end{bmatrix} = \begin{bmatrix} \alpha_1 \\ \alpha_2 \\ \alpha_3 \end{bmatrix} + \begin{bmatrix} \zeta_{1i} \\ \zeta_{2i} \\ \zeta_{3i} \end{bmatrix}, \quad E(\boldsymbol{\zeta}_i) = E(\eta_{ji}\boldsymbol{\zeta}_i) = \mathbf{0} \quad \text{for all } j, j', i. \tag{5.2}$$

In applications more general models may be specified. For example, a vector of predictors $\mathbf{x}_i$ can be included into the model to explain why individuals differ in growth factors η,

$$\boldsymbol{\eta}_i = \boldsymbol{\alpha} + \boldsymbol{\Gamma}\mathbf{x}_i + \boldsymbol{\zeta}_i \,, \tag{5.3}$$

with $\boldsymbol{\Gamma}$ being a $(J \times p)$-matrix of regression coefficients, where p is the number of predictors, or the above assumptions about the errors can be relaxed (see Bollen and Curran (2006) for a more detailed discussion).

In addition to the above assumptions it is often assumed that $\boldsymbol{y}_i$ is a continuous variable and (approximately) multivariate normally distributed for all i. Extensions to non-normal situations are available in various software packages. M*plus* (Muthén & Muthén, 2017), for example, allows to fit growth curve models assuming a Poisson or negative binomial distribution, or zero-inflation variants of these distributions (see below for details). In case of discrete Poisson distributed observed variables y_{ti}, with

$$f(y_{ti}) = \frac{\exp(-\mu_{ti})\mu_{ti}^{y_{ti}}}{y_{ti}!} \,,$$

where μ_{ti} denotes the mean parameter of the distribution, the growth model equation becomes

$$\log(\mathbf{y}_i) = \boldsymbol{\Lambda}\boldsymbol{\eta}_i + \boldsymbol{\epsilon}_i \,.$$

5.2.2.2 Zero-Inflation Modeling in a Nutshell

Zero-inflation models are usually fitted to data sets in which the dependent count variable has more zero values than would be predicted by typical standard count data models like the Poisson or the negative binomial model. Zero-inflation models (Lambert, 1992) are mixture models and assume two data generating processes: the count process and the zero-inflation process. Usually, the zero model is a logit model, which predicts, if a participant is in the so-called certain zero group or in the count group. Then, a count model, for example, a Poisson or negative binomial model predicts the respective count for each participant who is not in the zero group.[2] Typically different sets of predictors can be specified for the zero and the count part of the model. For a comprehensive discussion of count models, and guidelines regarding model selection, see Hilbe (2011).

5.2.2.3 The Zero-Inflated Poisson Growth Curve Model by Reinecke and Weins (2013)

As we have seen in Table 5.2, indices `ACRIM–DCRIM` are highly skewed and have a large percentage of zero counts—meaning that most participants did not report any criminal activity. Reinecke and Weins (2013) have therefore used a zero-inflated Poisson growth curve model to analyse the data.[3]

Their model included a latent intercept term, and additionally a latent linear slope and quadratic slope for both the zero part and the count part of the model. Furthermore, these quantities are regressed on gender and school type.[4] M*plus* input to get FIML estimates of the model parameters can be found in the supplementary material of the book (File: `FIML.inp`). Parts of the M*plus* output are listed in Table 5.4.

Let us point out and interpret some of the results: First of all, the positive linear slope (S) and negative quadratic slope (Q) reflect the typical age-crime-curve, meaning that delinquency—on average—first increases over time, and then decreases later on in adolescence. Furthermore, the estimated odds of not being delinquent at Wave 1 are about 50% higher for girls than for boys: The regression

---

[2]Note that classical zero-inflation models allow two sources of zeros. They can stem either from the zero-process or from the count process. A highly similar model class (so-called hurdle models) allows only one source of zeros. These models fit a zero-truncated Poisson or negative binomial model for the count process.

[3]From today's perspective, a more appropriate model would have been the zero-inflated negative binomial model, which allows to estimate a dispersion parameter (Hilbe, 2011). However, this model was not available in standard SEM software like M*plus* (Muthén & Muthén, 2017) at that time.

[4]To keep computation times of the examples in this book low, we only estimate and report the 'fixed' part of the model, i.e., we assume variances and covariances of the latent growth factors to be zero. Hence, $\eta_{ij} = \alpha_j$ for all i, j.

Table 5.4 Results of the growth curve ZIP model (FIML estimates)

	Est.	S.E.	Est./S.E.	p
Intercepts				
I	0.957	0.120	7.981	0.000
S	0.419	0.142	2.957	0.003
Q	−0.119	0.040	−2.986	0.003
II	0.000	0.000	–	–
SI	−0.885	0.199	−4.458	0.000
QI	0.222	0.060	3.707	0.000
Regressions				
I ON FEMALE	−0.415	0.146	−2.837	0.005
I ON RE	−0.314	0.152	−2.057	0.040
I ON GY	−0.356	0.154	−2.318	0.020
S ON FEMALE	−0.168	0.166	−1.008	0.314
S ON RE	0.189	0.182	1.039	0.299
S ON GY	0.090	0.182	0.493	0.622
Q ON FEMALE	0.061	0.046	1.323	0.186
Q ON RE	−0.052	0.051	−1.013	0.311
Q ON GY	−0.067	0.053	−1.262	0.207
II ON FEMALE	0.399	0.161	2.477	0.013
II ON RE	0.056	0.195	0.288	0.773
II ON GY	0.372	0.182	2.044	0.041
SI ON FEMALE	0.149	0.201	0.739	0.460
SI ON RE	0.391	0.247	1.584	0.113
SI ON GY	0.540	0.239	2.255	0.024
QI ON FEMALE	−0.016	0.060	−0.261	0.794
QI ON RE	−0.154	0.073	−2.118	0.034
QI ON GY	−0.212	0.074	−2.883	0.004

Note. I is the intercept, S and Q the linear and quadratic slopes in the count part of the model. II, SI and QI are the respective counterparts in the zero-inflation part of the model. These quantities are regressed on FEMALE (the gender indicator), RE, and GY (the school type indicators). Est. is the parameter estimate, S.E. the corresponding standard error. Est./S.E. is the test statistic to test the null hypothesis that the respective parameter is zero. p is the two-tailed p-value. The intercept of the zero model has been fixed to zero (cf. Muthén & Muthén, 2017, Example 6.7)

coefficient `FEMALE` predicting the intercept of the logit (i.e., zero vs. non-zero) part of the model is 0.399. Computing exp(0.399) = 1.49 gives the odds. Furthermore, the odds for not being delinquent are also higher for students attending Gymnasium in comparison to students from Hauptschule (exp(0.372) = 1.45). Thirdly, in the count (i.e., Poisson) part of the model, gender and school type predicted the intercept, i.e., the average delinquency rate at Wave 1. At the beginning of the study, girls on average showed a lower versatility of delinquent behaviours than boys (−0.415), and students attending the intermediate branch (Realschule, −0.314) or top level branch (Gymnasium, −0.356) exhibited a lower versatility in comparison to students attending Hauptschule. Gender and school type furthermore had no significant impact on the linear and quadratic slope, i.e., on the shape of the age-crime curve.

In addition, Reinecke and Weins (2013) compared results based on full information maximum likelihood estimation with results obtained by normal model multiple imputation. To be able to compare results obtained by the various imputation procedures discussed in this chapter with results from Reinecke and Weins (2013), we will fit the conditional ZIP growth curve model, which is presented in Table 7 in Reinecke and Weins (2013) to our imputed data sets. Comparisons and discussions of a large variety of different models (e.g., 'normal', Poisson and ZIP growth curve and growth mixture models) that are fitted to the CrimoC data may be found in Mariotti and Reinecke (2010).

5.3 Multiple Imputation of Missing Data

In this section, we revisit some of the points from Chaps. 1 to 4 and demonstrate their practical application in R:

1. missing data inspection,
2. creating the multiple imputations,
3. repeated data analysis, and
4. pooling of results.

5.3.1 Reading in the CrimoC data

The data file `crim4.dat` can be found in the supplementary material of the book. We load the data set into our R workspace using the flexible `read.table()` function. It is advisable to open the data file in a simple text editor first to see in what format the data are stored (e.g., comma separated, tab separated, etc.)—so that the arguments of `read.table()` can be set accordingly. In our case, the data are tab separated, and there are no variable names in the first row of the data file. Furthermore, the missing data indicator is '−999'.

With this information in mind, we can set the arguments of `read.table()`:

```
> dat <- read.table("./data/crim4.dat", col.names=c("id",
+         "FEMALE", "RE", "GY","HA", "ACRIM", "BCRIM", "CCRIM",
+         "DCRIM"), na.strings="-999", colClasses = c("numeric",
+         "factor", "factor", "factor", "factor", "numeric",
+         "numeric","numeric", "numeric"))
```

The first argument specifies the file name.[5] The second argument `col.names` provides the variable names: As already outlined in Sect. 5.2.1, `id` is the participant identifier, `FEMALE` is the gender indicator, `HA`, `RE`, and `GY` are the school type dummy variables, denoting the basic, intermediate and top level branch of the German secondary educational system, respectively, and `ACRIM`–`DCRIM` denote the repeatedly measured delinquency scores, where letters A–D indicate the respective panel wave. The argument `na.strings = "-999"` defines the missing data code that is used in the data file. The `colClasses` argument sets the classes of the variables in the data file, where `"factor"` defines a categorical variable and `"numeric"` indicates a numeric vector.

Note that we did not have to tell R, what field separator is used in `crim4.dat`. The default setting of the `read.table()` function is `sep = ""`. This works for data files where the field separator is any kind of 'white space', including one or more spaces or tabs. Furthermore, a default setting of `read.table()` is `header = FALSE`, which means that the variable names are not included in the first row of the data file. Finally, we store the data in a `data.frame` object called `dat`.

To quickly check that the data are read in correctly, we use the `head()` function. This function displays the first six rows of the data frame.

```
> head(dat)
  id FEMALE RE GY HA ACRIM BCRIM CCRIM DCRIM
1 1       0  0  0  1     2     0    NA    NA
2 2       0  0  0  1     1     4    NA    NA
3 3       1  0  0  1     0     0    NA    NA
4 4       1  0  0  1     0     1    NA    NA
5 5       1  0  0  1     0     0    NA    NA
6 6       1  0  0  1     0     1    NA    NA
```

It appears that the data are read in correctly. We can now have a closer look at the missing data processes in this data set.

5.3.2 Missing Data Inspection

Missing data inspection gives an idea of the quantitative extent of the missing data problem in the data set and of the selectivity of the missing data mechanism. At this stage, data analysts should also think about possible MNAR processes and what actions should be taken, if MNAR mechanisms are likely (e.g., doing a MNAR sensitivity analysis, for details see, e.g., van Buuren and Groothuis-Oudshoorn (2011) or choosing appropriate models like selection models, see Sect. 3.3.3). Also, a thorough missing data analysis is the basis for choosing a proper imputation method. Finally, missing data inspection can also help to find possible solutions,

[5]File `crim4.dat` can be found in subdirectory 'data' in the supplementary material of the book. To be able to reproduce the examples in the book, we ask readers to set the pathname of the supplementary material as working directory using the `setwd()` function.

when there are problems with the convergence of the MI procedure (see Sect. 4.4 and the discussions in the present section).

5.3.2.1 The Quantitative Extent of the Missing Data Problem

A good starting point to get an idea of the quantitative extent of the missing data problem is to look at the absolute and relative missing data frequencies.

```
> colSums(is.na(dat))
    id FEMALE      RE      GY      HA   ACRIM   BCRIM   CCRIM   DCRIM
     0      0       0       0       0     689     397     343     579
```

The `is.na()` function in R returns `TRUE` vs. `FALSE` statements, if a value in an R object like a vector, matrix or data frame is missing or observed. The `colSums` function treats a `TRUE` statement as '1' and `FALSE` as '0'. Consequently, the R code above gives the column wise sums of missing data, i.e., the missing data frequency per variable.

Dividing these sums by sample size multiplied by 100% gives the missing data percentages:

```
> round(colSums(is.na(dat))/nrow(dat) * 100, 2)
    id FEMALE      RE      GY      HA   ACRIM   BCRIM   CCRIM   DCRIM
  0.00   0.00    0.00    0.00    0.00   33.38   19.23   16.62   28.05
```

The `round()` function rounds the output to the specified decimal places—here 2. As already mentioned in Sect. 5.2.1, gender and school type indicators are completely observed. Missingness in the dependent variable ranges between 16.62% (Wave 3) and 33.38% (wave1). This is actually not too bad and quite typical for longitudinal studies (see, for example, Lally, Mangione, & Honig, 1988; McCord, 1978).

The missing data percentage is a rough indicator for the amount of missing information (see Sect. 4.3). However, it is only one factor that influences the quality of statistical inferences (e.g., Schafer, 1997). The quality of multiple imputation procedures also depends to a great extent upon how well missing information can be predicted by observed information in the data set. It is therefore essential to establish, if there are variables in the data set that are related to (a) the incomplete variables in the data set, and (b) related to missingness, so that these variables can be included in the imputation model later on (cf. Collins et al., 2001). Additionally, enough 'usable cases' of these variables need to be present.

5.3.2.2 Missing Data Pattern

The missing data pattern can be obtained, for example, by using the `md.pattern()` function from package `mice` (see also Sect. 2.6):

```
> library(mice)
> md.pattern(dat)
```

```
    id FEMALE RE GY HA CCRIM BCRIM DCRIM ACRIM
813  1      1  1  1  1     1     1     1     1    0
262  1      1  1  1  1     1     1     1     0    1
 38  1      1  1  1  1     1     0     1     1    1
 10  1      1  1  1  1     0     1     1     1    1
184  1      1  1  1  1     1     1     0     1    1
293  1      1  1  1  1     1     0     1     0    2
 20  1      1  1  1  1     0     1     1     0    2
 49  1      1  1  1  1     0     0     1     1    2
114  1      1  1  1  1     1     1     0     0    2
 17  1      1  1  1  1     1     0     0     1    2
264  1      1  1  1  1     0     1     0     1    2
     0      0  0  0  0   343   397   579   689 2008
```

The output of this function is a matrix containing the missing data pattern and some additional information. The value 1 denotes an observed value, 0 a missing value. The first column (more precisely the `row.names`) gives the observed frequency of the respective pattern. The last column gives the number of missing variables in each pattern. Variables and patterns are sorted by increasing numbers of missing data. The last row gives the sum of missing values in each variable. The last value in this row represents the total sum of missing values in this data set. The output tells us that there are 813 complete cases and that there are another $262 + 38 + 10 + 184 = 494$ cases with only one variable missing. The remaining cases have two missing variables.

Note that in the output above, the repeated delinquency measures `ACRIM`–`DCRIM` are not printed in chronological order. If this is desired, one could sort the function output manually:

```
> md.pattern(dat)[, c(1:5, 9, 7, 6, 8, 10)]
    id FEMALE RE GY HA ACRIM BCRIM CCRIM DCRIM
813  1      1  1  1  1     1     1     1     1    0
262  1      1  1  1  1     0     1     1     1    1
 38  1      1  1  1  1     1     0     1     1    1
 10  1      1  1  1  1     1     1     0     1    1
184  1      1  1  1  1     1     1     1     0    1
293  1      1  1  1  1     0     0     1     1    2
 20  1      1  1  1  1     0     1     0     1    2
 49  1      1  1  1  1     1     0     0     1    2
114  1      1  1  1  1     0     1     1     0    2
 17  1      1  1  1  1     1     0     1     0    2
264  1      1  1  1  1     1     1     0     0    2
     0      0  0  0  0   689   397   343   579 2008
```

5.3.2.3 Proportion of Usable Cases

The `md.pairs()` function in `mice` gives a more detailed picture of the number of 'usable cases' for missing data imputation. Of special interest is the slot[6] `$mr` of the function output. `$mr` gives the number of observed cases (columns) for each incompletely observed variable (rows):

```
> md.pairs(dat)$mr
        id FEMALE  RE  GY  HA ACRIM BCRIM CCRIM DCRIM
id       0      0   0   0   0     0     0     0     0
FEMALE   0      0   0   0   0     0     0     0     0
RE       0      0   0   0   0     0     0     0     0
GY       0      0   0   0   0     0     0     0     0
HA       0      0   0   0   0     0     0     0     0
ACRIM  689    689 689 689 689     0   396   669   575
BCRIM  397    397 397 397 397   104     0   348   380
CCRIM  343    343 343 343 343   323   294     0    79
DCRIM  579    579 579 579 579   465   562   315     0
```

We can ignore the first five rows since these variables are completely observed. Recall, for example, that there are 689 missing values in variable `ACRIM`. To get predictions for these 689 missing cases, 396 observations from Wave 2, 669 observations from Wave 3, and 575 observations from Wave 4, as well as the 689 completely observed gender and school type indicators could be used.

Dividing the numbers in `$mr` by the total number of missing values in the respective variable gives the proportion of usable cases—the fraction of cases with missing data on the target variable that has observed values on the respective predictor (van Buuren & Groothuis-Oudshoorn, 2011).

```
> delinq = dat[, c("ACRIM", "BCRIM", "CCRIM", "DCRIM")]
> mdp = md.pairs(delinq)$mr/colSums(is.na(delinq))
> round(mdp, 2)
      ACRIM BCRIM CCRIM DCRIM
ACRIM  0.00  0.57  0.97  0.83
BCRIM  0.26  0.00  0.88  0.96
CCRIM  0.94  0.86  0.00  0.23
DCRIM  0.80  0.97  0.54  0.00
```

Obviously, one would want these fractions to be rather large. If the proportion of usable cases is close to zero, the observed part of the predictor may provide only little information to generate imputations for the target variable and its inclusion into the imputation model may lead to large variation in the imputed values and thus to large standard errors for the estimator of applied scientific interest. If the proportion of usable cases is zero then, obviously, the corresponding variable cannot be used to generate imputations for the data set at hand.

[6]The output of the `md.pairs()` function is a list of four components named `rr`, `rm`, `mr`, and `mm`. These components can be accessed using the `$` operator. See `help("md.pairs")` for details.

5.3.2.4 Auxiliary Variables

Multiple imputation theory suggests to build rich imputation models. These are models that (in addition to containing all variables and higher-order relationships and interactions that are of interest to the data analyst) also include further variables—the so-called auxiliary variables, that are (a) highly related to missingness, and (b) highly related to the outcome variable(s). Including these variables into the imputation model may reduce bias and may also help to shift a potentially MNAR mechanism more in the direction of a MAR mechanism.

Applied researchers thus need to establish, if there are variables in the data set that are either (a) highly correlated with the incomplete variables, or (b) correlated with the missing data indicators.

A correlation matrix of the variables in the data set can be obtained in R by using the `cor()` function:

```
> round(cor(data.matrix(dat[, 2:9]), use =
+         "pairwise.complete.obs"), 2)
       FEMALE    RE    GY    HA ACRIM BCRIM CCRIM DCRIM
FEMALE   1.00  0.00  0.04 -0.04 -0.15 -0.21 -0.23 -0.19
RE       0.00  1.00 -0.60 -0.39  0.02  0.00  0.06  0.08
GY       0.04 -0.60  1.00 -0.50 -0.10 -0.14 -0.17 -0.17
HA      -0.04 -0.39 -0.50  1.00  0.10  0.17  0.13  0.12
ACRIM   -0.15  0.02 -0.10  0.10  1.00  0.53  0.36  0.31
BCRIM   -0.21  0.00 -0.14  0.17  0.53  1.00  0.61  0.47
CCRIM   -0.23  0.06 -0.17  0.13  0.36  0.61  1.00  0.63
DCRIM   -0.19  0.08 -0.17  0.12  0.31  0.47  0.63  1.00
```

The argument `use` determines, how to treat missing data. Here, we use the pairwise complete observed method, which is also referred to as ACA (see Sect. 3.2.1). Furthermore, note that we have excluded correlations with the subject identifier (the first variable in the data set), since these have no practical relevance.

When we look at the output above we observe a small negative relationship between gender and delinquency: Girls tend to exhibit a less versatile pattern of reported delinquent behaviours than boys. Furthermore there is a small negative relationship between school type and delinquency: Additionally, there are moderate to high intercorrelations between the repeatedly measured delinquency scores. This means that missing information regarding self-reported delinquency can be explained (at least to some extent) by observed delinquency from other panel waves.

The following R code gives the correlations between the variables in the data set and the missing data indicators of the repeatedly measured delinquency scores:

```
> R <- is.na(dat)
> colnames(R) <- paste("R.", colnames(dat), sep = "")
> dat2 <- data.frame(R, dat)
> round(cor(dat2[, 6:9], data.matrix(dat2[, 11:18]), use =
+         "pairwise.complete.obs"), 2)
        FEMALE    RE    GY   HA ACRIM BCRIM CCRIM DCRIM
R.ACRIM  -0.07  0.08 -0.19 0.14    NA  0.13  0.17  0.11
R.BCRIM  -0.07  0.05 -0.07 0.02  0.05    NA  0.13  0.13
R.CCRIM  -0.02 -0.02 -0.01 0.04  0.12  0.09    NA  0.02
R.DCRIM  -0.07 -0.02 -0.06 0.09  0.12  0.15  0.12    NA
```

`is.na(dat)` gives the missing data indicator matrix `R`. `R` has the same dimensions as `dat`. To be better able to distinguish the variables in `R` and `dat`, we use prefix `R.` to refer to variable names in `R`. We then correlate the missing data indicators of the repeatedly measured delinquency scores (`R.ACRIM`–`R.DCRIM`) with the following variables in `dat`: `FEMALE`, `RE`, `GY`, `HA`, and `ACRIM`–`DCRIM`. We observe some rather small correlations between missingness in the dependent variable and gender and school type, respectively. Girls are slightly more likely to complete the delinquency questions than boys and initially, students from 'Gymnasium' are more likely to complete the delinquency questionnaire than students from 'Hauptschule'. Note that non-zero correlations with the missing data indicators imply a deviation from MCAR.

Furthermore, an interesting finding is the small positive relationship between missing delinquency at one time point and observed delinquency at other time points. Ignoring this fact (i.e., failing to include the information from other panel waves in the imputation model) could shift the missing data mechanism towards MNAR.

5.3.2.5 Missing Data Process: MCAR, MAR or MNAR?

In the previous section we have tried to get an idea about missing data processes by inspecting the correlations of the variables in the data set with missing data indicators of the variables of interest. Descriptions of further simple tools for missing data diagnostics are given in Hill (1997). Furthermore, see Sect. 2.6 and the discussion in van Buuren and Groothuis-Oudshoorn (2011) about diagnostic plots to distinguish MCAR and MAR.

Usually, however, the far more interesting question is, whether MNAR processes have to be assumed. As there is no way to formally test for MNAR, there is also no way to rule out these processes. Based on the literature and based on theoretical considerations, it has to be thoroughly discussed if these processes are likely to have caused the missing data patterns in the present data set. For example, if some of the participants of the CrimoC study would fear that their anonymity could be compromised and they would expect legal prosecution, refusing to answer the questions about their delinquent behaviours would be the consequence. Thus, missing data in the delinquency scores would depend on the unobserved delinquency score and are thus MNAR. MNAR processes would require special MNAR modeling as we have seen in Sect. 3.3.3.

However, as MNAR modeling is often complex and hardly feasible for applied researchers (e.g., due to a lack of available 'general purpose' software), the most common procedure is to use MI under the MAR assumption with a rich imputation model (cf. Collins et al., 2001). The hope of building a rich model containing many variables and relationships between those variables is to push the missing data mechanism more in the direction of a MAR mechanism. Also note that, as MI model misspecifications and violated assumptions (e.g., the MAR assumption) affect mainly the missing part, MNAR processes can do more damage, the more missing data have to be filled-in. With only very few missing data and thus presumably a small amount of missing information, one may not be too worried about a slight violation of the MAR assumption. When more data are missing, MNAR processes could distort the results severely. In practice, MNAR sensitivity analyses could be conducted (cf. van Buuren & Groothuis-Oudshoorn, 2011) to assess, how and to what extent MNAR patterns of different strengths could distort one's parameter estimates.

5.3.3 *Choosing the Multiple Imputation Framework*

Now that we have a notion about the process underlying the missing data in this data set, the next step would be to decide on the framework for creating the multiple imputations: joint modeling (e.g., R packages `norm2`, `Amelia`, `pan`, `jomo`) or conditional modeling (e.g., R package `mice`), see Sect. 4.4. Recall, that the main difference between these two approaches is that in joint modeling—as the name suggests—a joint imputation model has to be specified for the variables to be imputed, whereas in conditional modeling, a separate imputation model is built for each incompletely observed variable. Our recommendation is that joint modeling may be used when it is feasible to specify a joint model, and when the usually restrictive distributional assumptions of the respective approach are likely to hold (e.g., multivariate normality). Conditional modeling on the other hand is a good and flexible alternative, when this is not the case. In this chapter, we will demonstrate the application of both joint modeling and conditional modeling MI techniques and discuss the advantages and disadvantages of the respective approaches with regard to our example data set.

5.3.4 *Building the Imputation Model*

The basic rule for the specification of imputation models is that it has to be at least as detailed as the subsequent analysis model, i.e., all variables that are of interest to the data analyst, as well as higher-order relationships (e.g., quadratic or cubic terms) and interaction terms must also be included in the imputation model (cf. Schafer, 1997; Schafer & Graham, 2002). Failing to include these terms would bias their estimates towards zero (if they have an effect), as during imputation, a zero-relationship between these variables would be assumed (Schafer, 1997). This bias tends to get larger with an increasing number of missing values in the variable to be imputed.

Also, information about cluster membership should be used adequately. In the remainder of the chapter, we will discuss the so-called wide format and long format imputation strategies. Wide format means that the repeatedly measured variables are stored as separate variables in the data file, whereas in long format data sets, the repeated measurements are stacked upon another and stored in a single variable.

In our examples, we include the repeatedly measured delinquency scores as well as information about school type and gender into the imputation models. In our example data set there are no further auxiliary variables. Further advice regarding the identification and inclusion of auxiliary variables is given in van Buuren and Groothuis-Oudshoorn (2011). We now demonstrate, how to set up the imputation models and impute the data using `mice` and other MI packages in R.

5.4 Multiple Imputation with `mice`

Recall from Chap. 4 that MI is a three-step process: In the first step, *m* complete-data sets are generated. Secondly, these completed data sets are then analysed separately using any standard complete-data technique (like a growth curve ZIP model, for example) and *m* sets of parameter estimates and standard errors are obtained. Thirdly, these *m* sets of model estimation results are integrated into an overall set of results using combination rules like Rubin's (1987) formulae. The `mice` package contains functions for each of the three steps (for an overview, see Table 5.5). The `mice()` function creates the *m* multiple imputations. The resulting object is of class `mids`, a multiply imputed data set.

The generic `with()` function (which calls `mice` function `with.mids()`) facilitates repeated data analysis and supports many commonly used statistical models like linear models, generalized linear models or analysis of variance, just to name a few. The resulting object of *m* model results is of class `mira`—a multiply imputed repeated analysis . The `pool()` function can then be applied to the `mira` object to obtain an overall combined MI estimate. This object is of class `mipo` – a multiply imputed pooled outcome. Applying the generic `summary()` function to this object produces typical MI output.

For some model types (like structural equation models, for example) that are not yet supported by `with.mids()`, we also show solutions to facilitate repeated data analysis and pooling of results (Sect. 5.7).

Very comprehensive descriptions of the conditional modeling `mice` package and its functionalities may also be found in van Buuren (2012) and van Buuren and Groothuis-Oudshoorn (2011). In this chapter, we focus only on the essentials to get novice `mice` users started.

Table 5.5 `mice`—multiple imputation by chained equations

Step	Function	`mice` object class
1. Multiple imputation	`mice()`	mids (multiply imputed data set)
2. Repeated data analysis	`with()`	mira (multiply imputed repeated analysis)
3. Pooling of results	`pool()`	mipo (multiply imputed pooled outcome)

Creating multiple imputations of missing data in mice is really straightforward and the default settings usually work fine. Imputations are created by the mice() function, which takes two important arguments: method and predictorMatrix.

5.4.1 Argument method

The argument method specifies the imputation procedure for each incompletely observed variable, and has to be a character vector of length equal to the number of variables in the data set. The first entry in method specifies the imputation procedure for the first variable in the data set, the second entry the method for the second variable, and so on. Variables that need not be imputed (e.g., because they contain no missing data) have method "". mice already comes with a variety of imputation functions and the number is ever growing. Currently, the default methods are "pmm", predictive mean matching for continuous data, "logreg", Bayesian logistic regression for binary variables and "polyreg", Bayesian polytomous regression for categorical variables with more than two levels. The information stored in method tells mice to call the corresponding imputation sub-function. These functions are called mice.impute.name, where name is the function identifier. For instance, a "pmm" entry in method would call the imputation function mice.impute.pmm() to fill in missing values in this variable.

mice also allows to call user-written imputation functions, which also have to follow the mice.impute.name-structure. The imputation functions from package countimp (for incomplete count data) or from package ImputeRobust (based on semiparametric generalized additive models), for example, work as add-ons to the mice package (see Chap. 6 for details).

5.4.2 Argument predictorMatrix

The imputation model for each incomplete variable is specified via the predictorMatrix argument. predictorMatrix must be a rectangular matrix of dimensions equal to the number of variables in the data set. Each row j in that matrix defines the imputation model of variable u_j. Zeros and ones indicate (0 = no; 1 = yes), if the respective variable u_k is used to predict missing data in u_j. By default, every other variable from the data set is used to predict missing information in a certain variable.

5.4.3 *Multiple Imputation by Predictive Mean Matching*

From Table 5.2 we know that the delinquency scores are not normally distributed. To the contrary, they are highly skewed. Consequently, an imputation procedure based on the normal model would not be appropriate for these data.[7] The `"norm"` method in `mice` (i.e., Bayesian linear regression) would impute normally distributed values, thus distorting the original distribution of the variable quite noticeably. Yu, Burton, and Rivero-Arias (2007) or Kleinke (2017), for example, have shown that normal model MI yields biased estimates, when empirical data depart too heavily from normality.

Predictive mean matching (method `"pmm"` in `mice`) on the other hand is believed to be more robust against violations of the normality assumption. However, see Yu et al. (2007) and Kleinke (2017) for the limits of PMM's robustness, when data are heavily skewed. An introduction to that method and further (critical) discussions of PMM can be found in Sect. 4.5.7, as well as in Dahl (2007); de Jong et al. (2016); He and Raghunathan (2009); Kleinke (2018); Schenker and Taylor (1996).

The implementation of classical predictive mean matching in `mice` is described in detail in van Buuren (2012, Algorithm 3.3). PMM can be enumerated among the hot-deck imputation procedures or the k nearest neighbour procedures. Current versions of `mice` by default sample from a pool of $k = 5$ donor cases. A newer donor selection alternative in R, which is based on the SAS macro MIDAS by Siddique and Belin (2008) (i.e., multiple imputation using distance-aided selection of donors) is discussed in Gaffert et al. (2016).

5.4.3.1 Application

The following application demonstrates, how to impute the CrimoC data by classical predictive mean matching, how to adjust the size of the donor pool and how to use the adaptive donor selection strategy `midastouch`, (Gaffert et al. 2016; Siddique & Belin 2008), which selects one donor from all available observations with probability inversely proportional to their distance from the recipient.

In Sect. 5.3.1, we have described, how to load the data file `crim4.dat` into the R workspace. The data are stored in a `data.frame` object called `dat`.

In this example, we do not need the participant identifier, nor the redundant dummy variable `HA` in our imputation model (since `HA` is the reference category). We therefore select a subset of `dat`, which we call `dat2` that includes the variables we want to use in our imputation models. This step is not essential. We could also have worked with the original data frame `dat`. However, when data sets are very

[7] Reinecke and Weins (2013) have split the zero-inflated count variables into zero vs. non-zero indicators and zero-truncated count variables. They imputed both variables jointly under the multivariate normal model.

large, it makes sense to use a subset of the original data that only contains the variables to be used for data imputation and subsequent data analysis. Otherwise, setting up method and predictorMatrix could become very cumbersome.

```
> dat2 <- dat[, c("ACRIM", "BCRIM", "CCRIM", "DCRIM", "FEMALE",
+          "RE", "GY")]
```

A good starting point is to do an initial run of mice(), so that mice can automatically set up method and predictorMatrix using its default settings:

```
> ini <- mice(dat2, maxit = 0)
```

The argument maxit = 0 tells mice not to run any iterations of the Gibbs sampler. method and predictorMatrix can now be easily extracted from the mids object ini. Recall that the default settings are to impute numeric vectors by predictive mean matching and to include all other variables in the respective imputation models:

```
> ini$method
 ACRIM   BCRIM   CCRIM   DCRIM  FEMALE      RE      GY
 "pmm"   "pmm"   "pmm"   "pmm"      ""      ""      ""

> ini$predictorMatrix
          ACRIM BCRIM CCRIM DCRIM FEMALE RE GY
ACRIM         0     1     1     1      1  1  1
BCRIM         1     0     1     1      1  1  1
CCRIM         1     1     0     1      1  1  1
DCRIM         1     1     1     0      1  1  1
FEMALE        0     0     0     0      0  0  0
RE            0     0     0     0      0  0  0
GY            0     0     0     0      0  0  0
```

Note that FEMALE, RE, and GY are completely observed. These variables thus have method "", and zero entries in the respective rows of the predictorMatrix.

In our first example, we are satisfied with the default settings and we do not make any adjustments to method or predictorMatrix.

Next, we proceed with a test run, i.e., we create a set of $m = 5$ imputations and assess convergence of mice's Gibbs sampler by visually inspecting the so-called Spaghetti plots.

```
> test.mice.pmm <- mice(dat2, m = 5, maxit = 20, printFlag =
+          FALSE, seed = 123456)
```

We have set the number of iterations to 20 (maxit = 20). This is usually enough to reach convergence (van Buuren & Groothuis-Oudshoorn, 2011).

By default, mice prints the iteration history to the console. This is especially useful for complex models that take a while to compute. Users then get visual feedback about the progress of the computations. By setting printFlag = FALSE in the function call, users can turn this off. Finally, as outlined in Chap. 4, we have defined a seed so that results of our examples are reproducible.

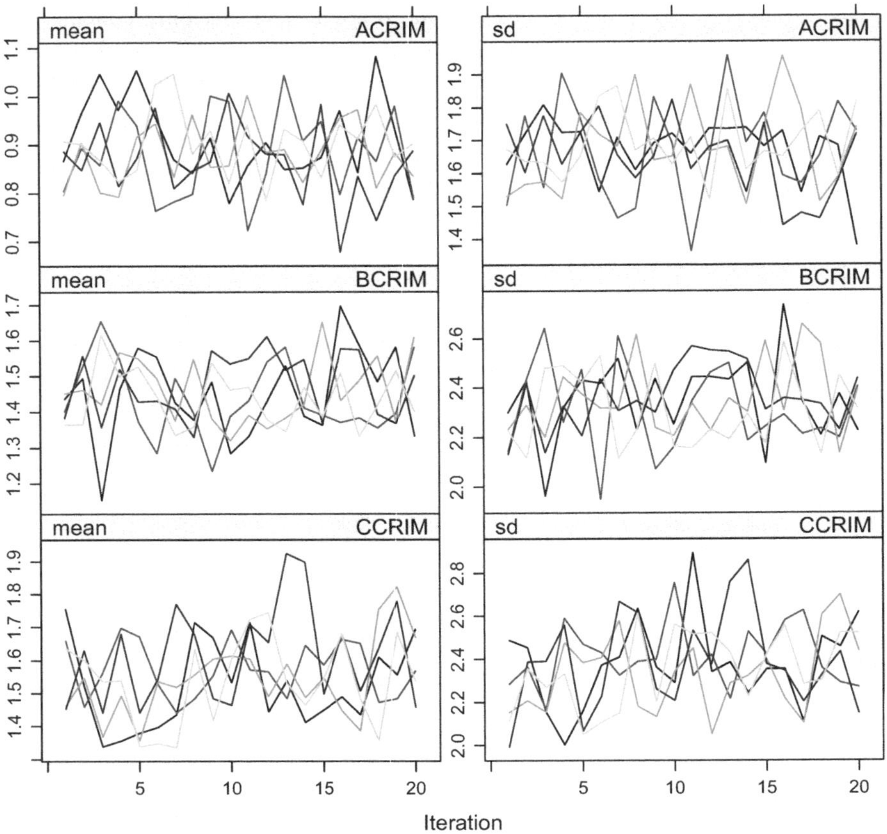

Fig. 5.2 Multivariate imputation by `mice.impute.pmm()`—Spaghetti plots for variables `ACRIM–CCRIM`

The output of the `mice` call is stored in object `test.mice.pmm`. By default, i.e., when argument `diagnostics = TRUE`, the object also contains diagnostic information that can be used to assess convergence. Applying the generic `plot()` function to an object of class `mids` produces the Spaghetti plot.

```
> plot(test.mice.pmm)
```

The plot is displayed in Fig. 5.2. It shows how the values of the means and standard deviations (vertical axes) of the incomplete variables change with each iteration (horizontal axes) for the $m = 5$ streams of imputations. The Gibbs sampler can be assumed to have converged when the streams are well intermingled like a heap of spaghetti on a plate (for details, see van Buuren & Groothuis-Oudshoorn, 2011). Parallel lines or any systematic pattern on the other hand would indicate that the algorithm got stuck. Figure 5.2 shows healthy convergence: We cannot see any clear trends and the streams are well intermingled. This means, we can proceed and create a full set of $m = 100$ imputations.[8]

```
> imp.mice.pmm1 <- mice(dat2, m = 100, maxit = 20, donors = 1,
+         print = FALSE, seed = 123456)
> imp.mice.pmm5 <- mice(dat2, m = 100, maxit = 20, print =
+         FALSE, seed = 123456)
> imp.mice.pmm20 <- mice(dat2, m = 100, maxit = 20, donors = 20,
+         print = FALSE, seed = 123456)
```

Adjustments to the default settings of `mice.impute.pmm()` can be made by simply entering the arguments to be altered into the main `mice()` call. They will be automatically passed down to `mice.impute.pmm()`. The number of donors to be sampled from can be set via the `donors` argument (default is $k = 5$) . To draw from a pool of $k = 1$ or $k = 20$ donors, we set `donors = 1` or `donors = 20`, respectively.

Selecting the adaptive pmm variant `midastouch` instead requires changing `mice`'s `method` entries. To this end, we extract `method` from any of our `mids` objects, for example, from `ini` and overwrite the pmm entries with `"midastouch"`.

```
> method <- ini$method
> method[1:4] <- "midastouch"
```

The altered `method` argument then has to be supplied to the `mice()` function.

```
> imp.mice.mt <- mice(dat2, method = method, m = 100, maxit =
+         20, printFlag = FALSE, seed = 123456)
```

Again, it is advisable to assess convergence by inspecting Spaghetti plots (not shown here).

Now, we have four sets of imputations (based on a fixed set of $k \in \{1, 5, 20\}$ donors and based on the flexible `midastouch` variant). The next step would be to do the repeated data analysis and pooling of results. In Sect. 5.7, we give various examples how to achieve this in R.

Additionally, since special software packages like M*plus* for example, support models that are currently not yet available in R, we also want to demonstrate, how to export the imputed data from R to be analysed by other statistical packages.

In our example, we want to fit the growth curve ZIP model from Reinecke and Weins (2013, see Section 5.2.2) to the imputed data. This model is currently not supported by any R function we are aware of. M*plus* on the other hand can fit this model and can also handle multiply imputed data sets.

---

[8]To reduce simulation error due to small numbers of imputations, we will create $m = 100$ sets of imputations in all applications throughout this book (see, for example, the recommendations by Graham et al., 2007 or Bodner, 2008). Even with modern computers, this can take a considerable amount of time, especially when imputation models are more complex. To reproduce the examples within a reasonable amount of time, readers could set the number of imputations to 5. Additionally, all sets of imputations are available from the supplementary material of the book.

Our function `prepare.mplus()`, which is available from the supplementary material of the book, extracts the completed data sets from the `mids` object, writes them to disk in ASCII format (here: `imp1.dat`–`imp100.dat`) and also creates a file containing the list of names of the completed data sets (called `implist.dat`), which is needed by M*plus* to automate the repeated data analysis and pooling of results (see the M*plus* user's guide for details, Muthén & Muthén, 2017):

```
> source("./functions/prepare.mplus.R")
> dir.create("./imputations/pmm/midastouch", recursive = TRUE)
> prepare.mplus(imp.mice.mt, dir =
+         "./imputations/pmm/midastouch")
```

Model results are summarized in Table 5.6. M*plus* input files are available from the supplementary material of the book.

The table also contains the FIML estimates from Reinecke and Weins (2013). Note that the sizes of coefficients and standard errors obtained by PMM differ somewhat from the FIML estimates. The latter are based on the (more appropriate) zero-inflated Poisson model (see Sect. 5.2.2). PMM on the other hand uses a normal linear regression model, but only for matching a potential donor to the incomplete case. It picks an observed case and uses its observed value to fill in the missing value. Quality of PMM's results thus depends (a) upon the availability of suitable donor cases and (b) on the appropriateness of the normal model used for data matching.

In Sect. 5.8, we discuss in greater detail, how to assess the plausibility of the generated imputations.[9] Actually, the descriptive techniques here and in the following sections mainly serve to detect unacceptable imputed values, like extreme outliers, and inappropriate distributions of the imputations. See also Sect. 4.3.1 about 'valid inferences'.

Table 5.7 contrasts the percentages of counts from 0 to 12 for the observed and imputed parts of the data, respectively, for the different PMM settings (see Sect. 5.8 for details). Compared to the observed data, PMM yielded fewer zeros. This result *could* stem from a misspecified imputation model. However, from a theoretical point of view, imputations are not implausible: As reported above, male students and students from Hauptschule are more likely to have missing delinquency scores (see Sect. 5.2.1). Furthermore, we know that boys show more versatile delinquent behaviours than girls and students from Hauptschule are also more delinquent than students from other school types, so we might expect less zeros and more non-zero imputations among the subgroup of participants with unobserved delinquency at wave one (Reinecke & Weins, 2013). In Chap. 6, we introduce imputation methods based on count data models and further semiparametric imputation methods. To further assess the plausibility of imputations obtained by PMM, we will compare model results with those obtained by the methods discussed in Chap. 6.

---

[9]Sometimes the term 'plausibility' refers to imputations that lead to valid statistical inferences. In our context, the true parameters are unknown. Here we regard imputations as plausible if they meet our expectations about these values and their distributions, based on what we know about the data

Table 5.6 Imputation by predictive mean matching

	FIML		$k = 1$		$k = 5$		$k = 20$		mt	
	Est.	S.E.	Est.	S.E.	Est.	S.E.	Est.	S.E.	Est.	S.E.
Intercepts										
I	0.96	0.12	0.95	0.08	0.94	0.09	0.94	0.08	0.93	0.09
S	0.42	0.14	0.42	0.10	0.43	0.12	0.44	0.10	0.43	0.11
Q	−0.12	0.04	−0.12	0.03	−0.13	0.04	−0.13	0.03	−0.12	0.03
II	0.00	0.00	0.00	0.00	0.00	0.00	0.00	0.00	0.00	0.00
SI	−0.88	0.20	−0.74	0.21	−0.69	0.29	−0.70	0.24	−0.80	0.21
QI	0.22	0.06	0.16	0.07	0.15	0.09	0.15	0.08	0.19	0.07
Regressions										
I ON FEMALE	−0.42	0.15	−0.42	0.10	−0.41	0.11	−0.41	0.10	−0.43	0.11
I ON RE	−0.31	0.15	−0.18	0.11	−0.17	0.11	−0.17	0.11	−0.14	0.11
I ON GY	−0.36	0.15	−0.31	0.11	−0.31	0.12	−0.30	0.11	−0.31	0.11
S ON FEMALE	−0.17	0.17	−0.10	0.12	−0.11	0.15	−0.12	0.13	−0.11	0.15
S ON RE	0.19	0.18	0.07	0.14	0.07	0.14	0.07	0.14	0.04	0.14
S ON GY	0.09	0.18	0.03	0.14	0.03	0.16	0.02	0.14	0.02	0.14
Q ON FEMALE	0.06	0.05	0.04	0.04	0.04	0.04	0.04	0.04	0.04	0.04
Q ON RE	−0.05	0.05	−0.02	0.04	−0.02	0.04	−0.02	0.04	−0.02	0.04
Q ON GY	−0.07	0.05	−0.03	0.04	−0.03	0.05	−0.03	0.04	−0.03	0.04
II ON FEMALE	0.40	0.16	0.46	0.14	0.49	0.20	0.47	0.17	0.39	0.16
II ON RE	0.06	0.20	0.07	0.17	0.09	0.24	0.10	0.19	0.04	0.18
II ON GY	0.37	0.18	0.40	0.17	0.42	0.23	0.43	0.18	0.38	0.16
SI ON FEMALE	0.15	0.20	0.14	0.21	0.12	0.26	0.14	0.23	0.14	0.22
SI ON RE	0.39	0.25	0.29	0.25	0.30	0.34	0.26	0.28	0.34	0.26
SI ON GY	0.54	0.24	0.43	0.24	0.41	0.33	0.39	0.28	0.47	0.25
QI ON FEMALE	−0.02	0.06	−0.02	0.06	−0.01	0.08	−0.02	0.07	−0.01	0.07
QI ON RE	−0.15	0.07	−0.11	0.08	−0.12	0.10	−0.11	0.09	−0.13	0.08
QI ON GY	−0.21	0.07	−0.16	0.08	−0.16	0.10	−0.15	0.09	−0.19	0.08

Note. I is the intercept, S and Q the linear and quadratic slopes in the count part of the model. II, SI and QI are the respective counterparts in the zero-inflation part of the model. These quantities are regressed on FEMALE (the gender indicator), RE, and GY (the school type indicators). Est. is the parameter estimate, S.E. the corresponding standard error. k denotes the size of the donor pool in classical predictive mean matching. mt (function `mice.impute.midastouch()`) is the distance-aided donor selection procedure implemented by Gaffert et al. (2016)

5.4.4 Summary

We have given a brief introduction to the `mice` package in R and have demonstrated, how to apply different imputation methods in `mice`, namely classical predictive

set and based on the underlying theory. For the CrimoC data, for example, we can expect boys and students from Hauptschule to receive higher delinquency scores on average.

Table 5.7 Comparison of average percentages of counts obtained by predictive mean matching—variable ACRIM

	0	1	2	3	4	5	6	7	8	9	10	11	12
Observed													
	72.00	14.62	5.67	3.27	1.82	1.02	0.51	0.51	0.22	0.07	0.07	0.15	0.07
Imputed													
$k = 1$	62.33	16.74	8.46	5.13	2.53	2.02	0.85	0.78	0.38	0.06	0.13	0.40	0.18
$k = 5$	63.55	16.47	7.81	4.91	2.81	1.73	0.76	0.80	0.37	0.05	0.15	0.43	0.15
$k = 20$	63.65	16.57	7.40	4.82	3.11	1.81	0.82	0.76	0.39	0.07	0.17	0.27	0.17
`midastouch`	64.96	16.48	6.86	5.03	2.74	1.55	0.57	0.66	0.36	0.09	0.14	0.38	0.18

Note. k denotes the size of the donor pool in classical predictive mean matching. `midastouch` is the distance-aided donor selection procedure proposed by Gaffert et al. (2016)

mean matching and the more flexible PMM variant `midastouch`. Van Buuren (2012) summarizes the caveats of predictive mean matching as follows: 'The method works best with large samples [. . .]. Predictive mean matching cannot be used to extrapolate beyond the range of the data, or to interpolate within the range of the data if the data at the interior are sparse. Also, it may not perform well with small data sets. Bearing these points in mind, predictive mean matching is a great all-around method [. . .]' (p. 74). However, as we have argued previously, PMM has a built-in problem due to the unknown number of nearest neighbours to choose the donors from and due to its limited robustness when data are heavily skewed and contain an excess number of zeros. We once again refer readers to Sect. 4.5.7.2, for a critical discussion of predictive mean matching, as well as Schenker and Taylor (1996) and de Jong et al. (2016). In Chap. 6, we will discuss imputation methods (e.g., based on zero-inflation models) that are more appropriate for skewed count data.

5.5 Other R Packages and Functions for Multivariate Data Imputation

To give a comprehensive overview of all available packages and to demonstrate how imputations are generated with each package is beyond the scope of this book. However, we want to draw attention to some packages and functions that are frequently used in applied research (see Table 5.1): packages `norm2`, `Amelia`, `mi` and function `aregimpute()` from package `Hmisc`.

5.5.1 `norm2`

`norm2` creates multiple imputations based on the joint multivariate normal model. A description of the routines used in `norm2` can be found in Schafer (1997) and

Schafer (2016). For a description of the general approach assuming a specific joint distribution of all variables with missing values given the observed values based on the MCMC method, see Sect. 4.4.3. The MCMC algorithm adopted in `norm2` is implemented in function `mcmcNorm()`. Maximum likelihood estimates of the model parameters obtained by an EM algorithm (function `emNorm()`) can be used as starting values for the MCMC algorithm. See Schafer (2016) for further details.

Note that currently there are two R packages available that have implemented Schafer's (1997) algorithms: `norm` and `norm2`. Schafer originally provided his `norm` software only as a Windows standalone programme and for S-PLUS. `norm` was later ported to R. However, it seems that the first package is no longer maintained[10] and it misses important functionality, for example, the possibility to assess convergence of the MCMC algorithm. In 2016, Schafer published a new refurbished version of `norm` under the name `norm2` (for a list of improvements, see the R-package manual).

5.5.1.1 Application

For the CrimoC data, normal model MI is not the optimal strategy. However in this section, we adopt this imputation approach together with a transformation and rounding strategy so that the distribution of the transformed observed values is closer to a normal distribution and continuous imputations are rounded to non-negative integer values. Note that we discussed rounding and transforming of observed data to fit a prespecified distribution assumed for the complete variable at several places, see Sects. 2.6, 4.4.5, and 4.5.1. Hence, we do not advocate the strategy of transforming observed values, but adopt this approach to demonstrate the use of the `norm2` package, as suggested by Schafer (2016). Rounding in the case of count variables may be an acceptable strategy if a count model needs to be fit later on (cf. Sect. 4.4.5). In Chap. 6 we will discuss better strategies to generate imputations for skewed discrete variables. Another caveat is that the clustered structure of the data cannot explicitly be modeled with this package, which may also introduce bias.[11]

Since the delinquency scores in our example data set are not normally distributed, we follow the approach used in Reinecke and Weins (2013) to make the normality assumption of the variables with observed values somewhat more plausible: We split the zero-inflated count variable into two variables: (a) a variable that indicates if the observation for case i is zero or non-zero, and (b) in case of a non-zero observation, the second variable gives the respective count. Both indicators and count variables are then imputed under the joint multivariate normal model. After the m imputations

[10] At the time of writing, the most recent version 1.0-9.5 of the `norm` package was published in February 2013.

[11] Panel data however could be imputed in wide format, which would implicitly consider the longitudinal information (for a discussion, see Sect. 5.6.3.1).

are generated, imputations of the indicator variables are rounded to 0 and 1, and 1's are replaced by the respective count (which is also rounded to the nearest integer value). This strategy is chosen because to analyse the data using the ZIP model from Reinecke and Weins (2013), we need the imputations of the repeatedly measured delinquency scores to be counts, i.e., non-negative integer values. R code and a detailed documentation, how to use `norm2` is available from the supplementary material of the book.[12]

For the examples in this section, we have created a `matrix` object `dat3`, which contains the zero indicators and count variables, and information about gender and school type. A numeric `matrix` is the required input of the `norm2` functions, since `norm2` was originally meant to be used on multivariate normal data only. `data.frame` objects are automatically transformed into `matrix` objects. Here, the `norm2` functions do not handle categorical variables in a sensible way, for example, by replacing a factor by a set of dummy variables. This has to be done manually by the user beforehand.

```
> head(dat3[, 1:8])
  acrim.z acrim.c bcrim.z bcrim.c ccrim.z ccrim.c dcrim.z dcrim.c
1       1       2       0      NA      NA      NA      NA      NA
2       1       1       1       4      NA      NA      NA      NA
3       0      NA       0      NA      NA      NA      NA      NA
4       0      NA       1       1      NA      NA      NA      NA
5       0      NA       0      NA      NA      NA      NA      NA
6       0      NA       1       1      NA      NA      NA      NA
```

In `dat3`, the '`z`'-variables denote the binary count indicators, the "`c`"-variables give the respective counts: For example, `acrim.z` is the binary count indicator for Wave 1. This variable has the value 0, if the corresponding value in `ACRIM` is 0, and 1 otherwise. `acrim.c` gives the corresponding number of delinquent behaviours. If `acrim.z` is 0, `acrim.c` is `NA`, i.e., missing.

The next step is to obtain starting values for the MCMC algorithm using `emNorm()`[13]:

```
> emResult <- emNorm(cbind(acrim.z, acrim.c, bcrim.z, bcrim.c,
+         ccrim.z, ccrim.c, dcrim.z, dcrim.c) ~ FEMALE + GY + RE,
+         data = dat3)
```

In the `norm2`-syntax, the incomplete response variables appear before the ~ sign. Multiple incomplete response variables have to be combined using the `cbind()` function. Completely observed predictors can be placed on the right-hand side of the ~ sign. These variables do not have to be normally distributed.

[12]We once again would like to caution applied researchers to use normal model MI after transformation on highly non-normal data. Transformations and roundings were applied in the past, when more appropriate strategies and models were not yet available.

[13]Note that `emNorm()` produces maximum likelihood estimates of the mean vector and covariance matrix of the variables in the model, which can also be directly used as input for further statistical analyses (e.g., structural equation models).

The generic `summary()` function displays the EM output, a part of which is listed below:

```
Method:                               EM
Prior:                                "uniform"
Convergence criterion:                1e-05
Iterations:                           263
Converged:                            TRUE
Max. rel. difference:                 9.5012e-06
-2 Loglikelihood:                     1543.875
-2 Log-posterior density:             1543.875
Worst fraction missing information: 0.9452
```

Our main interest at this stage is if and after how many iterations the EM algorithm has converged. Usually, EM's convergence is a good indicator that subsequently the MCMC algorithm will also converge: According to Schafer and Olsen (1998) the MCMC algorithm tends to converge faster than the EM algorithm. Thus, if EM reports convergence after c cycles, it is very likely that the MCMC algorithm will also converge and that it will probably have converged after c number of cycles. On the other hand, if EM does not converge, MCMC will most likely run into convergence problems, as well. Schafer (2016) discusses some situations, where EM produced estimation problems.

In our application, using the default settings, i.e., a noninformative uniform prior, EM has converged after 263 iterations. Applied researchers however need to be aware that, a "`Converged: TRUE`" statement in the output of the `summary` function does not necessarily mean that EM has converged to the global unique maximum of the loglikelihood function. EM could also have reached a local maximum or saddle point. Schafer (1997) recommends to run EM multiple times using different sets of starting values. If EM has indeed reached the global maximum of the likelihood function, then both the likelihood value and the parameter estimates are the same regardless of the starting values. An example is given in Schafer (2016).

Furthermore, we need to point out another important value of the function output: the estimate of the worst fraction of missing information $\hat{\lambda}$, which is 0.9452. Fraction of missing information ranges between 0 and 1 and expresses, how much information about the parameters is contained in the missing part of the data relative to the observed part (Schafer, 1999b). An estimate for the worst fraction of very close to 1 indicates that at least one parameter in the model is not identified or that the model is weakly identified.

Weakly identified models are often a consequence of an unfortunate missing data pattern: Suppose, for example, you are interested in the relationship between variables y, x_1 and x_2. If there are only very few cases, for which y and x_2 have been jointly observed, the partial correlation of y and x_2 given x_1 cannot be estimated well. If there are no joint observations, the partial correlation cannot be estimated at all and the model is not identified in that regard (Schafer, 1999b). Inspecting missing data patterns and missing data patterns by variable pairs (see Sect. 5.3.2) might help to identify such problems.

In our case, however, the not identified parameters are a result of our recoding scheme: Splitting a zero-inflated count variable into a binary indicator and a partially missing count variable leads to a not identified normal model. The conditional distribution of the count variable given that the binary indicator has a value of zero and the relationship between the count and the binary variable is not identified. To illustrate what happens here, let us take a look at the zero-indicator and the count variable of the first time point.

```
> table(dat3$acrim.z)

  0   1
990 385
```

There are 990 cases, where `acrim.z = 0`, and 385 cases where `acrim.z = 1`.

When we build a contingency table of counts of `acrim.c` given that `acrim.z = 0`, `acrim.z = 1`, and `acrim.z = NA`, we see, that `acrim.c` is always missing, when `acrim.z = 0`.

```
> table(dat3$acrim.z, acrim.c, useNA="ifany")

      acrim.c
         1   2   3   4   5   6   7   8   9  10  11  12 <NA>
  0      0   0   0   0   0   0   0   0   0   0   0   0  990
  1    201  78  45  25  14   7   7   3   1   1   2   1    0
  <NA>   0   0   0   0   0   0   0   0   0   0   0   0  689
```

This means that by design, the data contain no information about the relationship between `acrim.z` and `acrim.c`, and the correlation between `acrim.z` and `acrim.c` cannot be estimated. After removing the 990 missing cases, where `acrim.c = NA`, `acrim.z` is a constant and thus the standard deviation is zero.

When the model is weakly identified or not identified, MCMC may fail to converge, because a proper posterior distribution may not exist (Schafer & Olsen, 1999): Across the iterations the time series for unidentified (and closely related parameters) may drift aimlessly. However, as Schafer and Olsen (1999) argue, an MCMC algorithm 'might fail to converge in a global sense, yet behave well with respect to the parameters of interest' (p. 30).

To see if this is the case, we run 1000 iterations of the MCMC algorithm and inspect plots of the time series (TS) and autocorrelation functions (ACF) of the model parameters.

```
> set.seed(123456)
> mcmcResult <- mcmcNorm(emResult, iter = 1000)
```

By default, the `mcmcNorm` function stores three time series objects: `series.worst`, which contains the simulated values of the worst linear function of the parameters from all iterations (for details, see Schafer, 1997, 2016), `series.beta`, the simulated values of the β coefficients, and `series.sigma`, the simulated values of the variances and covariances. The generic `plot` function

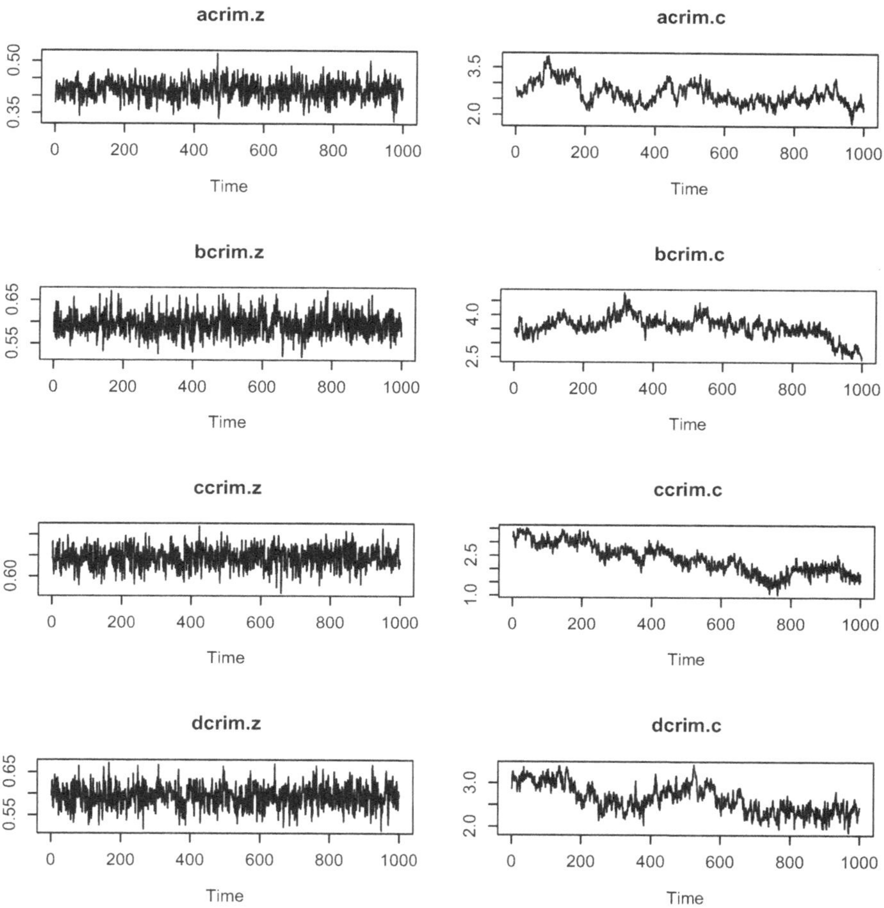

Fig. 5.3 MCMC under a uniform prior—TS plots of the β-coefficients of the zero and count indicators

can be used to display TS and ACF plots of the respective parameter. Plots of the 8 intercept terms are shown in Figs. 5.3 and 5.4.

Convergence can be assumed, when TS plots show an unsystematic up and down zigzag pattern without any clear, longer lasting trends, and when autocorrelations die down rapidly—as is the case for the zero indicators. However, TS plots of the count indicator intercepts show trends that last over several hundreds of iterations. Also, the corresponding autocorrelations do not die down, even after several hundreds of iterations. They even oscillate, which would not occur under proper conditions (Schafer, 1999b).

With this example, we wanted to stress the need to always assess convergence of the MI algorithm: If non-convergence is not recognized and parameters drift to

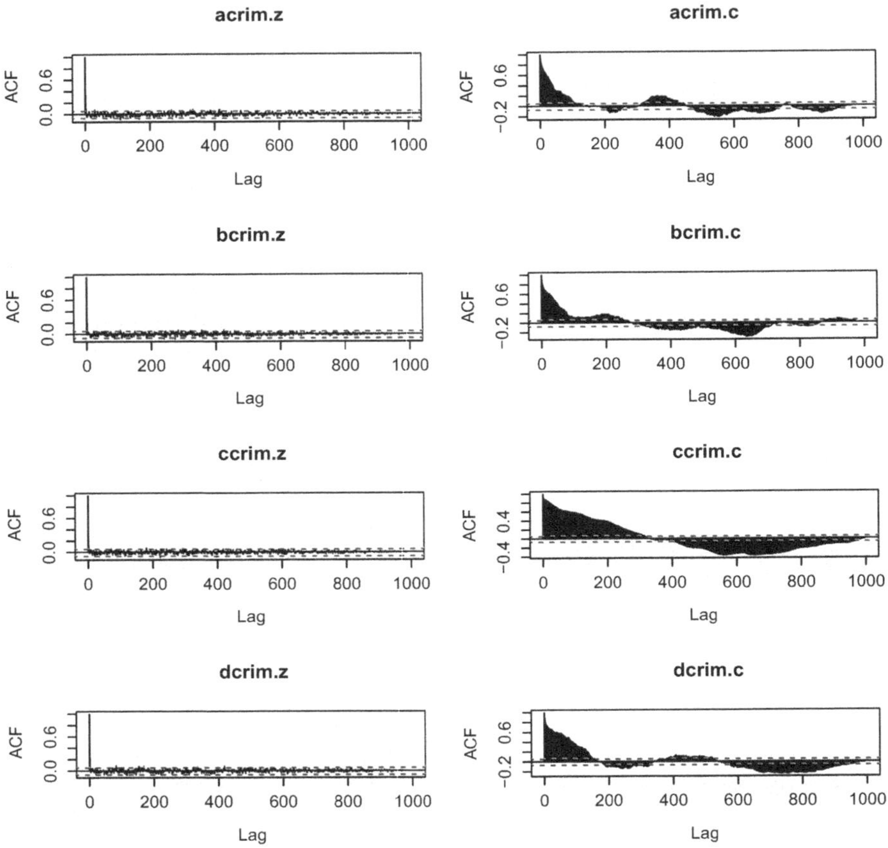

Fig. 5.4 MCMC under a uniform prior—ACF plots of the β-coefficients of the zero and count indicators

implausible values, the resulting imputations might be implausible and statistical inferences might be invalid (Schafer, 1999b, see also Section 5.8 for methods to assess the plausibility of imputed values).

When the model is weakly identified, using a ridge prior rather than the standard noninformative prior can help to stabilize the estimation of these parameters (Schafer, 1997, Chap. 5). It smooths the estimated correlations toward zero (see Schafer, 1997, pp. 155–156). The hyperparameter ξ, a positive real number, determines the amount of smoothing. In the user's guide of the `norm` for Windows software, Schafer (1999b) notes that there 'are no strict rules for selecting the hyperparameter. A small value is desirable, but if it is too small then the problem might not be solved. In practice, you should probably use a value no greater than 5% or 10% of the actual sample size or number of cases in your data set, to avoid introducing large biases in correlations that are well estimated' (p. 46).

In our example, 10% of the sample size would be about 200, so we could rerun emNorm, now specifying two additional arguments: prior = "ridge", and setting prior.df = 200, the hyperparameter.

```
> emResult2 <- emNorm(cbind(acrim.z, acrim.c, bcrim.z, bcrim.c,
+         ccrim.z, ccrim.c, dcrim.z, dcrim.c) ~ FEMALE + GY + RE,
+         data = dat3, prior = "ridge", prior.df = 200)
```

This time EM converged after 311 iterations. Next, we rerun mcmcNorm and check, if using the ridge prior with a hyperparameter of $\xi = 200$ has sufficiently stabilized the estimation.

```
> set.seed(123456)
> mcmcResult2 <- mcmcNorm(emResult2, iter = 1000)
```

This seems to be the case (see Figs. 5.5 and 5.6).

To generate $m = 100$ imputations, we run a total of $1000 * 100 = 100{,}000$ iterations and draw each imputation after 1000 iterations, respectively (impute.every = 1000).

```
> set.seed(123456)
> mcmcResult_m100 <- mcmcNorm(emResult2, iter = 1e+05,
+         impute.every = 1000)
```

The object mcmcResult$implist contains the list of $m = 100$ imputed data sets.

Note that the norm2 package does not contain functions to automate the repeated data analysis and pooling of results. In the supplementary material of the book, we provide tutorials, how to facilitate the process. In Sect. 5.5.5, we compare results of the growth curve ZIP model from Sect. 5.2.2 based on normal model MI with norm2 to results obtained by other packages.

5.5.2 Amelia

Similar to norm and norm2, MI with package Amelia is based on the multivariate normal model.[14] Imputations are created by the amelia() function.

```
> set.seed(123456)
> imp.amelia <- amelia(x = dat3, m = 100, noms = c("FEMALE",
+         "RE", "GY"))
```

Argument x specifies the data object to be imputed (here: matrix dat3 from Sect. 5.5.1). Like in mice, argument m sets the number of imputations.

amelia() furthermore can handle unordered and ordered categorical variables: argument noms defines nominal variables in the data file; ordinal variables can

[14] https://cran.r-project.org/package=Amelia. Descriptions of the algorithm, and detailed documentation of the software may be found at the project website https://gking.harvard.edu/amelia.

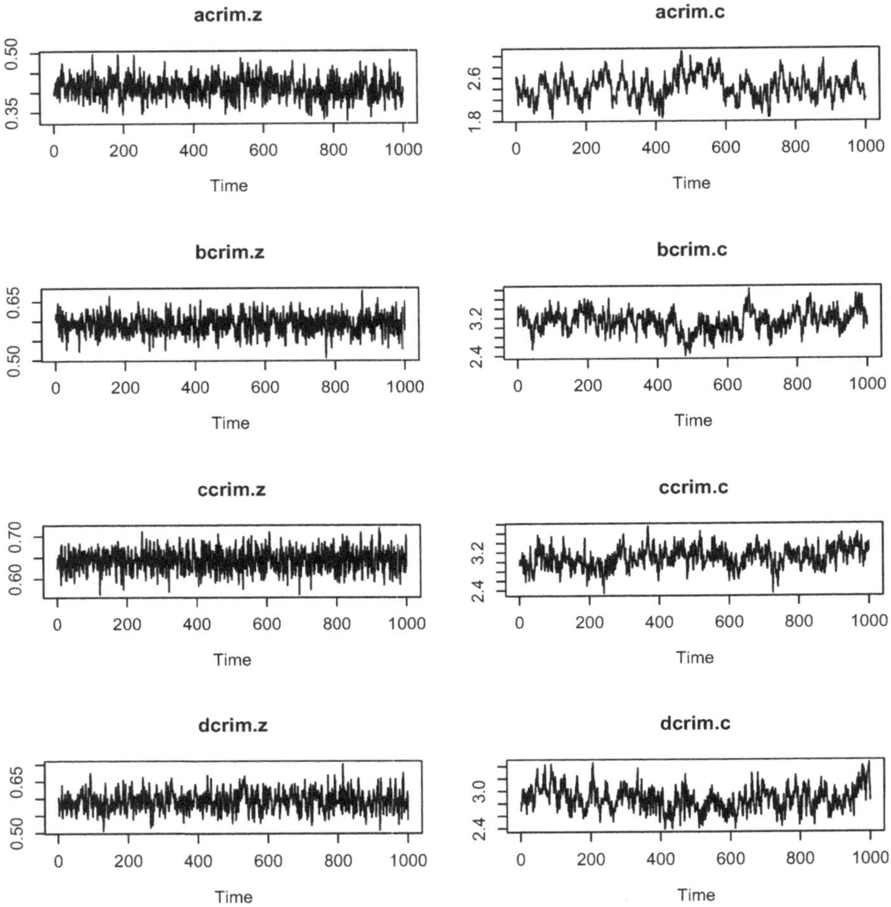

Fig. 5.5 MCMC under a ridge prior with hyper parameter $\xi = 200$—TS plots of the β-coefficients of the zero and count indicators

be listed under `ords` (for details, see the package documentation at https://gking.harvard.edu/amelia).

```
> set.seed(123456)
> imp.amelia.ords <- amelia(x = dat2, m = 100, ords = c("ACRIM",
+          "BCRIM", "CCRIM", "DCRIM"), noms = c("FEMALE", "RE",
+          "GY"))
```

These arguments ensure that imputations match the respective data measurement scale, for example, integer values for ordinal variables. The list of m imputed data sets is stored in slot `$imputations` of the resulting object. A useful tool is `write.amelia()`. As the name suggests, the function writes the m completed data sets to disk for further analysis with other statistical packages like M*plus*, for

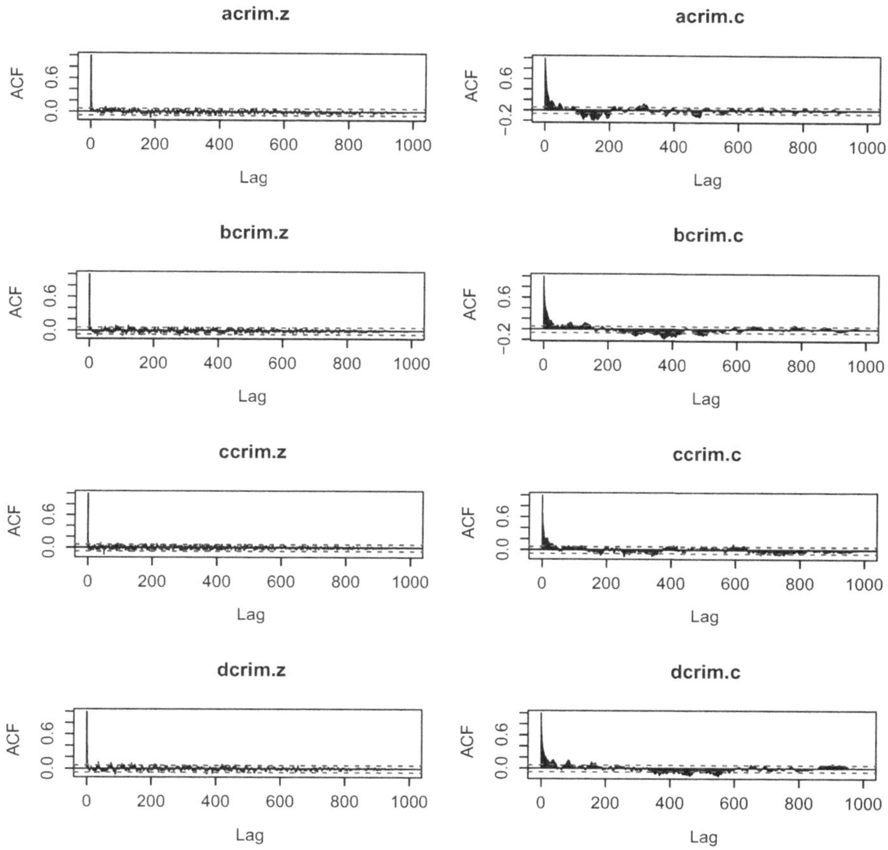

Fig. 5.6 `mcmcNorm()` under a ridge prior with hyper parameter $\xi = 200$—ACF plots of the β-coefficients of the zero and count indicators

example. The following code produces $m = 100$ data files, labelled `imp1.dat` – `imp100.dat`:

```
> write.amelia(imp.amelia.ords, file.stem =
+         "./imputations/other/Amelia/ords/imp", extension =
+         ".dat", format = "table", quote = FALSE, row.names =
+         FALSE, col.names = FALSE)
```

Arguments `row.names`, `col.names` and `quote` can be used as in R's `write.table()` function.

Furthermore, the generic `plot()` function produces graphs that help determine, if the distribution of the obtained imputations shows any peculiarities:

```
> plot(imp.amelia.ords, lwd = 2, col = c("black", "gray80"))
```

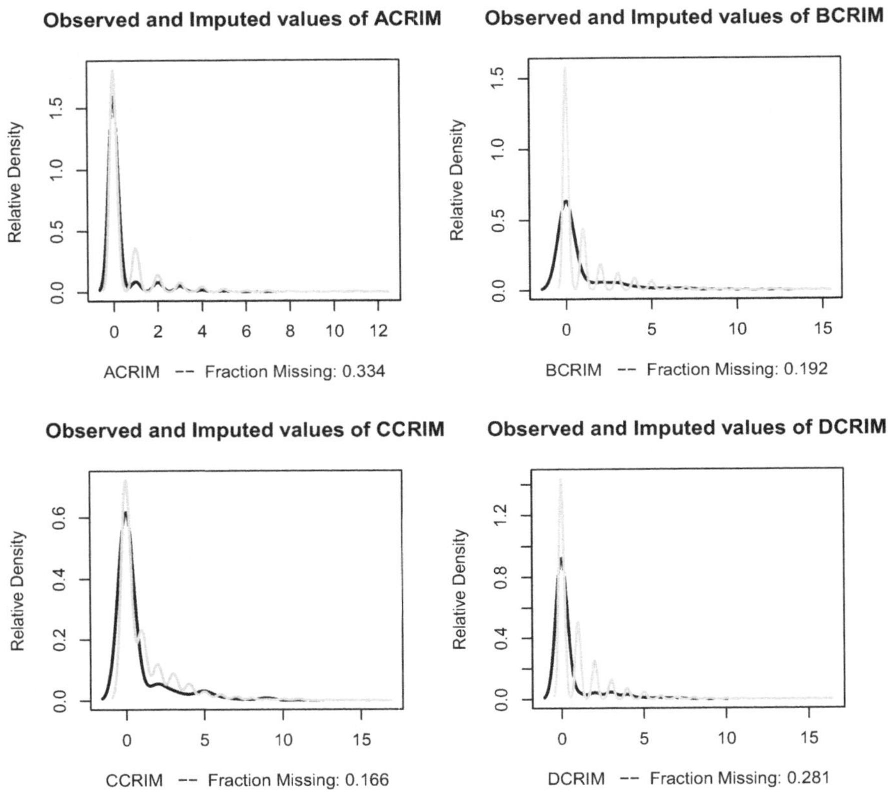

Fig. 5.7 Multivariate multiple imputation by the `amelia()` function—comparison of observed (light grey) and imputed values (black)

The generated plot is displayed in Fig. 5.7. It shows the distributions of the observed and imputed data (light grey and black, respectively). Noticeably differing distributions could indicate that the missing values are not MCAR. Extreme differences might reflect misspecified or weakly identified imputation models or extremely selective missing data mechanisms. The distributions of imputed values in Fig. 5.7 are inconspicuous, so that there are no indications for one of these extreme scenarios.

5.5.3 *mi*

Package mi[15] creates multiple imputations under the conditional modeling framework. Note that the commands of the current version of mi (1.0) are quite different from the structure described in Su, Gelman, Hill, and Yajima (2011), which is based on mi version 0.09-13. Some functions described in Su et al. (2011) no longer exist. Applied researchers should refer to the current package vignette[16] for guidance on how to use the package.

We want to give a very brief overview on how to create imputations with package mi: First, users need to convert their data file into a missing_data.frame object, which includes additional information used by the mi() imputation function.

```
> mdf <- missing_data.frame(dat2)
> show(mdf)
Object of class missing_data.frame with 2064 observations on 7
variables

There are 11 missing data patterns

Append '@patterns' to this missing_data.frame to access the
corresponding pattern for every observation or perhaps use
table()

             type missing method  model
FEMALE     binary       0   <NA>   <NA>
RE         binary       0   <NA>   <NA>
GY         binary       0   <NA>   <NA>
ACRIM  continuous     689    ppd linear
BCRIM  continuous     397    ppd linear
CCRIM  continuous     343    ppd linear
DCRIM  continuous     579    ppd linear

         family     link transformation
FEMALE     <NA>     <NA>           <NA>
RE         <NA>     <NA>           <NA>
GY         <NA>     <NA>           <NA>
ACRIM  gaussian identity    standardize
BCRIM  gaussian identity    standardize
CCRIM  gaussian identity    standardize
DCRIM  gaussian identity    standardize
```

Like mice() (see Sect. 5.4), missing_data.frame() tries to detect the variable type automatically and sets a default imputation method accordingly. In our example, ACRIM–DCRIM are identified as continuous. The default imputation method for continuous variables is a Bayesian linear model. Imputations are drawn from the posterior predictive distribution (method ppd in the output above).

[15]https://cran.r-project.org/package=mi.

[16]https://cran.r-project.org/web/packages/mi/vignettes/mi_vignette.pdf.

If users are not satisfied with the defaults, other methods could be selected. For example, we could change the `type` entries for variables `ACRIM`–`DCRIM` to `count`, using the `change()` function:

```
> mdf2 <- change(mdf, y = c("ACRIM", "BCRIM", "CCRIM", "DCRIM"),
+          what = "type", to = "count")
```

This would change the imputation model to a Bayesian quasipoisson model (see Chap. 6 for an overview on count data models).

In cases where none of the parametric imputation methods have an adequate fit to the data, predictive mean matching (PMM) is often chosen (see Sect. 4.5.7 and 4.5.2). Again, changing the imputation method correspondingly is quite straightforward:

```
> mdf3 <- change(mdf, y = c("ACRIM", "BCRIM", "CCRIM", "DCRIM"),
+          what = "method", to = "pmm")
```

Imputations are then created using the `mi()` function. Like in the previous sections, we set the seed of the random number generator to make the examples reproducible.

```
> set.seed(123456)
> imp.mi <- mi(mdf3, n.chains = 100, parallel = FALSE)
```

Argument `n.chains` defines the number of chains that are executed in parallel, and consequently the number of sets of imputed values to be generated. The default number of iterations each chain cycles through is `n.iter = 30`. By setting `n.chains` to 100, we obtain 100 completed data sets.

While the `plot()` function from package `Amelia` (Sect. 5.5.2) produces graphical output that allows to compare the distributions of observed and imputed values, `mi` can produce descriptive summary statistics for the observed and imputed parts of the data set using the generic `summary()` function:

```
> summary(imp.mi)$ACRIM
$is_missing
missing
FALSE  TRUE
 1375   689

$imputed
   Min. 1st Qu.  Median    Mean 3rd Qu.    Max.
-0.2228 -0.2228 -0.2228  0.1363  0.1463  4.2067

$observed
   Min. 1st Qu.  Median    Mean 3rd Qu.    Max.
-0.2228 -0.2228 -0.2228  0.0000  0.1463  4.2067
```

For repeated data analysis and MI pooling, the list of m imputed data sets can be extracted from the object of `mi-class` using the `complete()` function:

```
> imputed.data <- mi::complete(imp.mi, m = 100)
```

Note that `mice` also has a `complete()` function. By writing `mi::complete`, we tell R to use the `complete()` function from package `mi`.

5.5.4 aregImpute

A further useful function to create multiple imputations is `aregImpute()` from package `Hmisc`.[17] For a brief description of `aregImpute()`, see de Jong et al. (2016). By default, the function imputes missing data by a non-parametric PMM algorithm that is supposed to work for both continuous and categorical variables. The function also supports normal model PMM. The size of the donor pool (default in version 4.0-3 is $k = 3$) can be adjusted by the user. Also weighted probability sampling of donors is supported (see Sect. 5.4 for another distance-aided donor selection strategy—`midastouch` that is available in `mice`). Furthermore, various types of matching can be used, see Morris, White, and Royston (2014) for details, and van Buuren (2012, Section 3.4.2).

```
> set.seed(123456)
> imp.aregImpute <- aregImpute(~ACRIM + BCRIM + CCRIM + DCRIM +
+          FEMALE + RE + GY, data = dat2, type = "normpmm", nk =
+          0, n.impute = 100)
```

The imputation model is specified using typical R formula syntax. `aregImpute` automatically detects factors and handles them accordingly. Argument `type` defines the imputation method. Here, we use normal model predictive mean matching. `nk = 0` tells the program that the non-categorical variables (here: `ACRIM`–`DCRIM`) are treated as linear (see the documentation of package `Hmisc` for details). By default, donor matching is done by weighted probability sampling. If this is not desired, argument `match` could be set to `"closest"` for nearest neighbour PMM (i.e., $k = 1$) or to `"kclosest"`, where additional argument `"kclosest"` then defines the size of the donor pool (default is 3). Finally, argument `n.impute` sets the number of imputations to be drawn.

Unfortunately, extracting the imputed data sets from the function output is not so straightforward in comparison to `mice`, `Amelia`, or `mi`. The following code shows, how completed data sets can be obtained from the `aregImpute` output, and how the completed data sets could be written to disk for further analysis with other software packages:

```
> for (m in 1:100) {
+ com <- cbind.data.frame(impute.transcan(imp.aregImpute,
+          imputation = m, data = dat2, list.out = TRUE, pr =
+          FALSE, check = FALSE))
+ out <- cbind(1:nrow(com), com[, c("FEMALE", "RE", "GY",
+          "ACRIM", "BCRIM", "CCRIM", "DCRIM")])
+ write.table(out, paste("./imputations/other/aregImpute/imp",
+          m, ".dat", sep = ""), quote = FALSE, row.names = FALSE,
+          col.names = FALSE)
+ }
```

[17] https://cran.r-project.org/package=Hmisc.

Function `impute.transcan()` is used to create a complete-data set (similar to the `complete()` functions from packages `mice` or `mi`). For further information about the arguments of function `impute.transcan()`, see `help("impute.transcan")`. We use a `for` loop to cycle through all 100 imputations and write the 100 data files to disc in ASCII format for further analysis.

5.5.5 Comparison of Results

Table 5.8[18] displays maximum likelihood (FIML) results from Reinecke and Weins (2013) and contrasts them with MI results obtained by `norm2`, `Amelia`, `mi`, and `aregImpute`. Parameter estimates are obtained by the program M*plus* (Muthén & Muthén, 2017). Neither of the imputation methods applied in this section was originally meant to be used on highly skewed discrete data. One of the earliest MI solutions, Bayesian multiple imputation under the joint multivariate normal model creates imputed values that are normally distributed. In past times, where no other software packages were available, applied researchers used normal model MI in combination with rounding or various data transformations to handle non-normal data. In our demonstration of `norm2` package, we followed the approach by Reinecke and Weins (2013) to split the zero-inflated count variable into two variables to make the normality assumption of the imputation model somewhat more plausible. Splitting the variables during the imputation stage and putting the variables back together has to be done manually by the user. `Amelia` is more user-friendly in that regard. The `noms` and `ords` statements handle nominal and ordinal variables and produce output that follows the respective scale of measurement. However, in our case, negative integer values still had to be rounded manually before fitting the count model to the imputed data. A `count` argument is not yet available in `Amelia`. Using predictive mean matching as imputation method, for example, via the `mi` package or `aregImpute()` function makes rounding unnecessary, as PMM imputes actual observed values. However, most PMM implementations still are based on a normal regression model and are expected to produce biased model results, when the original empirical data are too heavily skewed. Additional problems of PMM are discussed in Sect. 4.5.7.2.

It is therefore not astounding that MI estimates differ somewhat from the original FIML results (Table 5.8). The main purpose of this section was to familiarize readers with popular MI packages and functions in R. Generally speaking, applied researchers should strive to use imputation methods and models of scientific interest that—at least approximately—meet all required assumptions for valid

[18] See Sect. 5.2.2 for details about the growth curve ZIP model. Note that the intercept of the zero model has been fixed to zero (cf. Muthén & Muthén, 2017, Example 6.7). See Sects. 5.5.1–5.5.4 for details about the respective imputation methods and models that are used to create the multiple imputations.

Table 5.8 Imputation by `Amelia`, `aregImpute()`, `mi`, and `norm2`

	FIML		Amelia		Amelia ords		aregImpute		mi		norm2	
	Est.	S.E.	Est.	S.E.	Est.	S.E.	Est.	S.E.	Est.	S.E.	Est.	S.E.
Intercepts												
I	0.96	0.12	1.02	0.08	0.62	0.09	0.94	0.08	0.96	0.10	0.99	0.07
S	0.42	0.14	0.34	0.11	0.74	0.14	0.44	0.10	0.45	0.13	0.38	0.09
Q	−0.12	0.04	−0.10	0.03	−0.37	0.04	−0.13	0.03	−0.13	0.04	−0.11	0.03
II	0.00	0.00	0.00	0.00	0.00	0.00	0.00	0.00	0.00	0.00	0.00	0.00
SI	−0.88	0.20	−0.83	0.20	0.71	0.34	−0.71	0.20	−0.69	0.26	−0.81	0.20
QI	0.22	0.06	0.20	0.06	−0.46	0.13	0.16	0.06	0.14	0.08	0.20	0.06
Regressions												
I ON FEMALE	−0.42	0.15	−0.36	0.08	−0.19	0.10	−0.41	0.10	−0.42	0.14	−0.36	0.09
I ON RE	−0.31	0.15	−0.21	0.10	−0.24	0.10	−0.16	0.10	−0.14	0.13	−0.24	0.10
I ON GY	−0.36	0.15	−0.35	0.10	0.23	0.02	−0.31	0.10	−0.31	0.12	−0.34	0.09
S ON FEMALE	−0.17	0.17	−0.15	0.12	0.14	0.16	−0.13	0.13	−0.08	0.19	−0.18	0.12
S ON RE	0.19	0.18	0.12	0.12	−0.31	0.17	0.06	0.13	0.01	0.16	0.13	0.13
S ON GY	0.09	0.18	0.09	0.13	−0.03	0.04	0.02	0.14	0.01	0.16	0.07	0.13
Q ON FEMALE	0.06	0.05	0.05	0.03	−0.04	0.05	0.05	0.04	0.04	0.06	0.06	0.04
Q ON RE	−0.05	0.05	−0.04	0.04	0.11	0.06	−0.02	0.04	0.00	0.05	−0.04	0.04
Q ON GY	−0.07	0.05	−0.05	0.04	−0.01	0.02	−0.03	0.04	−0.02	0.05	−0.05	0.04
II ON FEMALE	0.40	0.16	0.44	0.13	0.40	0.24	0.46	0.15	0.42	0.17	0.43	0.13
II ON RE	0.06	0.20	0.02	0.17	0.56	0.23	0.09	0.18	0.16	0.21	0.01	0.17
II ON GY	0.37	0.18	0.35	0.16	−0.69	0.12	0.42	0.17	0.50	0.22	0.35	0.16
SI ON FEMALE	0.15	0.20	0.12	0.19	0.06	0.43	0.11	0.21	0.08	0.26	0.13	0.19
SI ON RE	0.39	0.25	0.37	0.24	0.18	0.42	0.28	0.26	0.25	0.32	0.38	0.24
SI ON GY	0.54	0.24	0.51	0.23	−0.09	0.20	0.38	0.24	0.32	0.31	0.49	0.24
QI ON FEMALE	−0.02	0.06	−0.01	0.06	−0.10	0.17	0.00	0.06	0.03	0.08	−0.01	0.06
QI ON RE	−0.15	0.07	−0.15	0.08	−0.19	0.16	−0.11	0.08	−0.09	0.09	−0.14	0.08
QI ON GY	−0.21	0.07	−0.20	0.07	0.13	0.09	−0.14	0.08	−0.13	0.09	−0.19	0.08

Note. The table displays parameter estimates and standard errors of the zero-inflated Poisson growth curve model. Estimates are based on full information maximum likelihood estimation (FIML), normal model MI (package `norm2`), normal model MI (`amelia()` and `ords` statement), normal linear model predictive mean matching using `aregImpute`, and predictive mean matching using `mi`. I, S, and Q denote the intercept, slope and quadratic slope in the count part of the model, II, SI, QI the corresponding quantities in the zero-inflation part of the model. FEMALE is the gender indicator, RE (intermediate branch) and GY (top level branch) are school type indicators

inferences. This requires not only good statistical but also expert knowledge from the corresponding scientific field. If assumptions cannot be justified, then robust methods may be an avenue to proceed. In Chap. 6, we will discuss parametric count data imputation models as well as further semiparametric imputation procedures.

5.6 Multiple Imputation of Clustered or Panel Data Using Multilevel Models

In the previous sections, we have demonstrated the use of wide format multiple imputation strategies. Here, the repeated measurements are stored in separate variables and observed information from previous or later time points can be used to predict missing information at other time points. Imputation in wide format therefore implicitly considers longitudinal information and non-independence of observations. So far, however, we have not explicitly modeled the multilevel structure of the data using multilevel imputation models. In this section, we discuss imputation strategies that take information on cluster membership explicitly into account. These models require the data to be in long format meaning that the repeated measurements are stacked upon each other and stored in a single variable. Two other variables in the data set then indicate cluster membership and measurement time point. In this section we discuss advantages and disadvantages of long format over wide format imputation approaches for clustered or panel data.

Multiple imputation of clustered or panel data is a field that is currently of great interest to missing data researchers, as none of the currently existing multiple imputation solutions for complex data can be described as optimal. First of all, parametric procedures rely upon strong distributional assumptions like homoscedasticity or normality, which are often violated.[19] On the other hand, non- or semiparametric imputation methods often lack justification. Recent papers that contrast and review various strategies to impute complex clustered or panel data are, for example, Kleinke, Stemmler, Reinecke, and Lösel (2011), Andridge (2011), van Buuren (2011), Drechsler (2015), Enders, Mistler, and Keller (2016), Grund, Lüdtke, and Robitzsch (2016), Lüdtke, Robitzsch, and Grund (2017), Speidel, Drechsler, and Sakshaug (2018). So far, most evaluation studies of multilevel multiple imputation procedures used very simple models. For example, they investigated only missingness in the dependent variable, or evaluated scenarios where all model assumptions were fully met. Further research is needed before we can make sound recommendations regarding the robustness and general applicability of multilevel imputation procedures.

Before we elaborate on these points, we will give a brief introduction to multilevel models for those readers who are not yet familiar with statistical models for clustered or panel data.

[19]Shortcomings of some imputation techniques or consequences of misspecifications in simple data sets are discussed in de Jong et al. (2016) or He and Raghunathan (2009).

5.6.1 A Brief Introduction to Multilevel Regression Models

Usually, clustered or panel data violate the iid assumption of a standard (linear) regression model, as observations within the same cluster or panel are often more homogeneous than observations across different clusters. One solution to address this problem is to use a hierarchical linear model (also referred to as mixed-effects model, varying or random coefficient model, or multilevel regression model (Bryk & Raudenbush, 1992; Venables & Ripley, 2002). Linear mixed-effects models estimate the so-called fixed effects, i.e., parameters that are common to all elements in the population and that do not change across clusters or panel waves, as well as random effects, i.e., variances and covariances of intercepts and slopes across groups. Thus, in contrast to standard linear models, multilevel regression models do not assume that intercepts and slopes are constant across clusters. Predictors are usually added to the model which can explain individual or group differences of intercepts and slopes. A multilevel regression model can be written in the form

$$\begin{aligned} y_{ij} &= \beta_{0j} + \beta_{1j}x_{1ij} + \cdots + \epsilon_{ij} \\ \beta_{0j} &= \gamma_{00} + \gamma_{01}z_{1j} + \cdots + w_{0j} \\ \beta_{1j} &= \gamma_{10} + \gamma_{11}z_{1j} + \cdots + w_{1j} \\ &\ldots, \end{aligned} \tag{5.4}$$

where y_{ij} is the dependent variable of participant i in group j, and β are regression coefficients. ϵ_{ij} is the individual level error term, x_{ij} is an individual level predictor, z_j denote group level predictors, γ are the group-level regression coefficients, and w are the group-level errors or random effects. (5.4) can be collapsed into a single equation. With one individual and one group level predictor, (5.4) can be written as

$$\begin{aligned} y_{ij} &= \gamma_{00} + \gamma_{01}z_{1j} + w_{0j} + (\gamma_{10} + \gamma_{11}z_{1j} + w_{1j})x_{1ij} + \epsilon_{ij} \\ y_{ij} &= \gamma_{00} + \gamma_{01}z_{1j} + w_{0j} + \gamma_{10}x_{ij} + \gamma_{11}z_{1j}x_{1ij} + w_{1j}x_{1_ij} + \epsilon_{ij} \\ y_{ij} &= \underbrace{\gamma_{00} + \gamma_{01}z_{1j} + \gamma_{10}x_{ij} + \gamma_{11}z_{1j}x_{1ij}}_{\text{`fixed' part}} + \underbrace{w_{0j} + w_{1j}x_{1ij}}_{\text{`random' part}} + \epsilon_{ij}. \end{aligned} \tag{5.5}$$

With more predictors, (5.5) will become confusingly large. Therefore, matrix notation is recommended:

$$\mathbf{y}_j = \mathbf{X}_j\boldsymbol{\beta} + \mathbf{Z}_j\mathbf{w}_j + \boldsymbol{\epsilon}_j, \tag{5.6}$$

where $\mathbf{y}_j$ is a $n_j \times 1$ vector (the dependent variable with n_j representing the number of observations in the jth group), $\mathbf{X}_j$ is a design matrix with n_j rows and p columns containing the fixed effects predictors, $\mathbf{Z}_j$ is the design matrix with n_j rows and q columns containing the random effects predictors, $\boldsymbol{\beta}$ is a $p \times 1$ vector containing all parameters of the fixed part of the model, and $\mathbf{w}_j$ is a $q \times 1$ vector of random effects. Finally, $\boldsymbol{\epsilon}_j$ is a $n_j \times 1$ vector of individual level errors.

Linear mixed-effects models assume (a) a linear relationship between the dependent variable and the predictors, (b) normality of error terms at each level of the model, (c) homoscedasticity, (d) uncorrelated errors across the levels, and (e) uncorrelated errors at the highest level (for further information, see, for example, Hox, 2010).

5.6.2 *Strategies to Impute Clustered or Panel Data*

Graham (2009) discusses, how standard imputation solutions for multivariate data like imputation based on the multivariate normal model can be applied to impute clustered or panel data. The two strategies discussed in this paper are to either include indicator variables for cluster membership into the imputation model, or to impute data separately for each cluster.

In our experience, Bayesian normal model MI easily runs into estimation problems, when the imputation model contains more than about 100 variables.[20] Consequently, the first strategy might not be an option for larger data sets with many clusters or groups. Here, 100 variables are usually not enough. Graham (2009) remarks that he has 'seen this strategy work well with as many as 35 dummy variables, although a smaller number is desirable' (p. 564). Our CrimoC panel data set has 2064 cases (level 2 units). Including 2063 cluster dummy variables in the imputation model will not be feasible. A second drawback is that this strategy cannot account for slope variability. Thirdly, it is not possible to include level-2 predictors into the imputation model, since these would be perfectly collinear with the cluster dummies (Drechsler, 2015).

On the other hand, to impute each cluster or panel separately could also become very tedious and would involve some programming, since this strategy is currently not implemented in most standard MI packages.[21] Further problems occur, when cluster sizes become too small or clusters are completely unobserved (Drechsler, 2015).

An alternative solution would be imputation in long format using a standard multivariate model considering all clusters simultaneously. According to Allison (2001), this strategy works sufficiently well, when there are only a few observations in each cluster. In our example, we have only four repeated measurements, which is sufficiently small.

[20] Graham (2009) also recommends to keep the total number of variables in the imputation model below 100.

[21] An exception is the statistical package Stata. See the FAQ document 'How can I account for clustering when creating imputations with mi impute?', https://www.stata.com/support/faqs/statistics/clustering-and-mi-impute/.

Furthermore, imputation methods based on multilevel models are both available for the joint modeling MI framework (e.g., R packages `jomo` or `pan`), or for the conditional modeling framework (e.g., methods `2l.norm` or `2l.pan` in `mice`). Apart from R, multiple imputation routines are also implemented, for example, in SAS (macro `MMI IMPUTE`) and M*plus*. Furthermore there is the standalone (joint modeling) software `REALCOM-IMPUTE` by Carpenter, Goldstein, and Kenward (2011). Imputation here is typically based on a univariate or multivariate linear mixed-effects model.

5.6.2.1 Standard Versus Multilevel Multiple Imputation: A Discussion

Currently, van Buuren still recommends the use of standard imputation strategies like predictive mean matching MI for clustered or panel data, because according to van Buuren (2013) they often work sufficiently well (see also Vink, Lazendic, & van Buuren, 2015). However, there are scenarios where multilevel imputation models can yield better results (van Buuren, 2011). For a more in-depth discussion, see Drechsler (2015) and the references therein. On the other hand, the quality of currently available long format strategies like `pan` rely on distributional assumptions, which empirical data rarely meet. Simulations that systematically evaluated the available procedures in a variety of practically relevant scenarios are still scarce. Currently there is too little research to make a sound recommendation regarding which of the strategies is the best in a given scenario.

From a theoretical point of view, especially when following the congeniality discussion (Meng, 1994), multilevel data with missing values in the dependent variable should be imputed using a multilevel imputation model. However, robust two-level imputation procedures have yet to be developed (for new developments in this regard, see also Chap. 6). Thus, applied researchers often prefer a wide-format fixed effects imputation model, because these models are very easy to set up with standard MI software—as we have demonstrated in this chapter. Furthermore, imputation of incomplete predictor variables in multilevel models is a field where more research yet has to be done.

5.6.3 Application

In this section, we demonstrate the use of multilevel MI procedures in R: First, we show how multiple imputations are created by the two-level functions from package `mice`. Then, we illustrate the use of Schafer's `pan` package.

5.6.3.1 Multilevel Multiple Imputation in mice

Currently mice has two imputation methods for multilevel data, 2l.norm and 2l.pan.[22] As the function name suggests, these procedures only support two-level models. The imputation model of function mice.impute.2l.pan() is a special univariate case of the multivariate generalized linear mixed-effects model used by the pan software (for detailed information about the model, see Schafer & Yucel, 2002). Note that the pan model assumes homoscedasticity. mice.impute.2l.norm on the other hand allows for heterogeneous within-group variances. Both functions assume missing data to be MAR and the incomplete variable to be continuous.

Note that all multilevel imputation functions discussed in this section require long format data. So in the first step, we need to bring the data.frame object dat2, with which we have worked in the previous examples, into long format. We do this using R's reshape() function:

```
> dat.long <- reshape(data = dat2, varying = list(c("ACRIM",
+          "BCRIM", "CCRIM", "DCRIM")), direction = "long",
+          v.names = "DELINQ", times = 0:3, timevar = "TIME",
+          idvar = "ID")
> head(dat.long)
    FEMALE RE GY TIME DELINQ ID
1.0      0  0  0    0      2  1
2.0      0  0  0    0      1  2
3.0      1  0  0    0      0  3
4.0      1  0  0    0      0  4
5.0      1  0  0    0      0  5
6.0      1  0  0    0      0  6
```

The code above produces a data set containing the delinquency scores in long format (now labelled DELINQ) together with a newly created TIME variable (from 0–3), the subject identifier (ID), and the three complete predictors (FEMALE, RE, GY).

Analogous to Sect. 5.4, we proceed with an initial run of mice with maxit = 0 to set up method and predictorMatrix. Secondly, we change the imputation method of the dependent variable DELINQ to "2l.pan" (or alternatively, "2l.norm"). Finally, we set the imputation model for DELINQ to c(1,1,2,0,-2): As multilevel imputation models require the specification of both fixed and random factors, predictorMatrix here allows further entries in addition to '0' and '1'. As always, a '0' means that the variable is not included in the imputation model. '1' denotes a fixed effect, '2' a fixed *and* random effect and '−2' identifies the class variable. Currently only one class variable is allowed. In our example, ID is the class variable and TIME is entered as a fixed and random factor.

[22] Additional R packages like miceadds or countimp provide further two-level imputation functions for the mice framework.

This imputation model only assumes a linear relationship of the TIME variable. Inclusion of a quadratic term will be demonstrated later on.

```
> library(mice)
> ini <- mice(dat.long, maxit = 0)
> method <- ini$method
> method["DELINQ"] <- "2l.pan"
> pred <- ini$pred
> pred["DELINQ", ] <- c(1, 1, 1, 2, 0, -2)
```

Analogous to Sect. 5.4, we proceed with a test run to assess convergence:

```
> test.imp.2l.pan <- mice(dat.long, method = method, pred =
+        pred, m = 5, printFlag = FALSE)
> plot(test.imp.2l.pan)
```

The diagnostic plot (not shown here) shows proper convergence, and we can create a full set of $m = 100$ imputations:

```
> set.seed(123456)
> imp.2l.pan <- mice(dat.long, method = method, pred = pred, m =
+        100, printFlag = FALSE)
```

The object imp.2l.pan of class mids can now be used for further analysis in R (Sect. 5.7) or other software packages, for example, to fit the growth curve ZIP model from Sect. 5.2.2.[23]

Inclusion of Non-linear Time Trends

As our analysis model (the growth curve ZIP model from Sect. 5.2.2) contains both a linear and quadratic TIME slope, the imputation model should include a linear and quadratic TIME trend, as well. We now want to demonstrate, how to add a quadratic TIME term into the imputation model. The most straightforward way to do this is to create a new variable—the square of the original variable TIME, which we label TIME2, and to include this variable into the imputation model:

```
> dat.long$TIME2 <- dat.long$TIME^2
```

To define the newly created variable TIME2 both as a fixed and random effect, we set the predictorMatrix entry for this variable to 2:

```
> ini <- mice(dat.long, maxit = 0)
> method <- ini$method
> pred <- ini$pred
> method["DELINQ"] <- "2l.pan"
> pred["DELINQ", ] <- c(1, 1, 1, 2, 0, -2, 2)
> print(pred)
```

[23]In the supplementary material of the book, we provide R code to extract the imputed data sets from the mids object and to write the data to disk for further analysis in M*plus*.

```
        FEMALE RE GY TIME DELINQ ID TIME2
FEMALE       0  0  0    0      0  0     0
RE           0  0  0    0      0  0     0
GY           0  0  0    0      0  0     0
TIME         0  0  0    0      0  0     0
DELINQ       1  1  1    2      0 -2     2
ID           0  0  0    0      0  0     0
TIME2        0  0  0    0      0  0     0
```

Imputation then works analogous to the example above. Note that in this example the linear time trend was completely observed. How to properly impute non-linear associations and interaction terms, when the variables used to form these terms are only partially observed, is discussed in Spiess et al. (in press).

5.6.3.2 `pan`—Multiple Imputation Under the Multivariate Linear Mixed-Effects Model

Creating multiple imputations with the joint modeling package `pan` is not as straightforward as in `mice.impute.2l.pan()` from package `mice`. We provide two functions `test.pan()` and `mi.pan()`, which we adapted from `mice.impute.2l.pan()`, to facilitate the imputation process.

`test.pan()` cycles through a predefined number of iterations (argument `paniter`) and stores the iteration history for convergence diagnostics. If convergence can be assumed, m imputations can then be generated using function `mi.pan()`. The latter function reads out a list of m completed data sets.

Both functions take the following input: `y` is a matrix of incomplete response variables in long format. All variables that need to be imputed have to be included in `y`. `x` is a numeric matrix (also in long format) of complete predictors. Note that `pan` does not allow for missing data in the predictors. Furthermore, the function will not handle categorical variables with more than two levels in an appropriate way. So users are advised to manually create dummy variables of such factors beforehand. `xcol` and `zcol` refer to the columns in `x` and indicate fixed and random effects, respectively (see our example below and the R documentation of function `pan()` for details). `group` is the class variable. In our case, measurement time points (level 1) are clustered in persons (level 2). The person identifier (variable `ID`) is the class variable. `paniter` sets the number of iterations the algorithm cycles through before each set of imputations is drawn. `mi.pan()` runs separate chains from different starting points to create the m imputations (default is $m = 5$). Finally, the `intercept` argument tells the function, whether or not to include a random intercept into the model. If `intercept=TRUE` (default), the function will include a column of ones at the first position of matrix `x`.

To assess convergence of the MCMC algorithm, Schafer (1997) recommends to inspect time series plots and autocorrelation functions. As already outlined in Sect. 5.5, time series (Fig. 5.8) should show an unsystematic up and down zig-zag-pattern without any longer lasting trends and autocorrelations (Fig. 5.9) should die down rapidly.

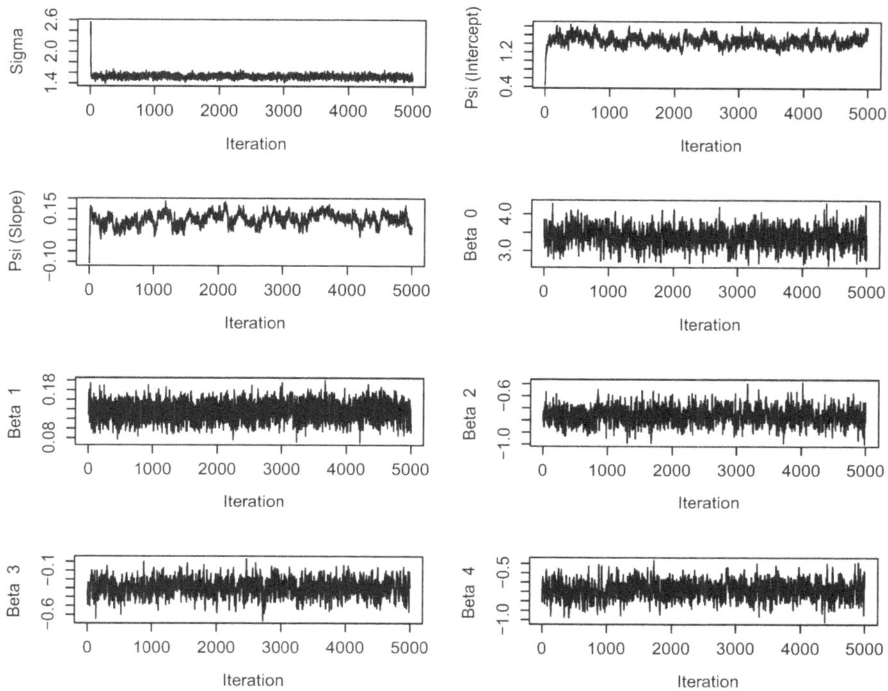

Fig. 5.8 Time series plots for the pan model parameters—'Sigma' refers to the individual level error term, 'Psi' to the random effects, and 'Beta' to the fixed effects: (Intercept), TIME, FEMALE, RE and GY

The following two code blocks produce Figs. 5.8 and 5.9:

```
> source("./functions/test.pan.R")
> set.seed(123456)
> pan.convergence <- test.pan(group = dat.long$ID, y =
+        matrix(dat.long$DELINQ, ncol = 1), x = dat.long[,
+        c("TIME", "FEMALE", "RE", "GY")], xcol = 1:5, zcol =
+        1:2, paniter = 5000)
```

In our example, we only have one dependent variable (the delinquency score in long format) to be imputed. So `y` is a numeric matrix with only one column. As predictors, we use the `TIME` variable, gender (`FEMALE`) and the two school type indicators (`RE` and `GY`): `x = dat.long[,c("TIME","FEMALE","RE","GY")]`. As `intercept = TRUE`, x has 5 columns, a column of ones for the intercept term, and variables `TIME`, `FEMALE`, `RE` and `GY`. We include all variables in the fixed part of the model, so `xcol = 1:5`. Furthermore, we set `zcol = 1:2` to have a random intercept and random `TIME` slope.

The `test.pan` function runs 5000 iterations and stores the results in object `pan.convergence`. The interesting output at this stage are objects `$sigma`,

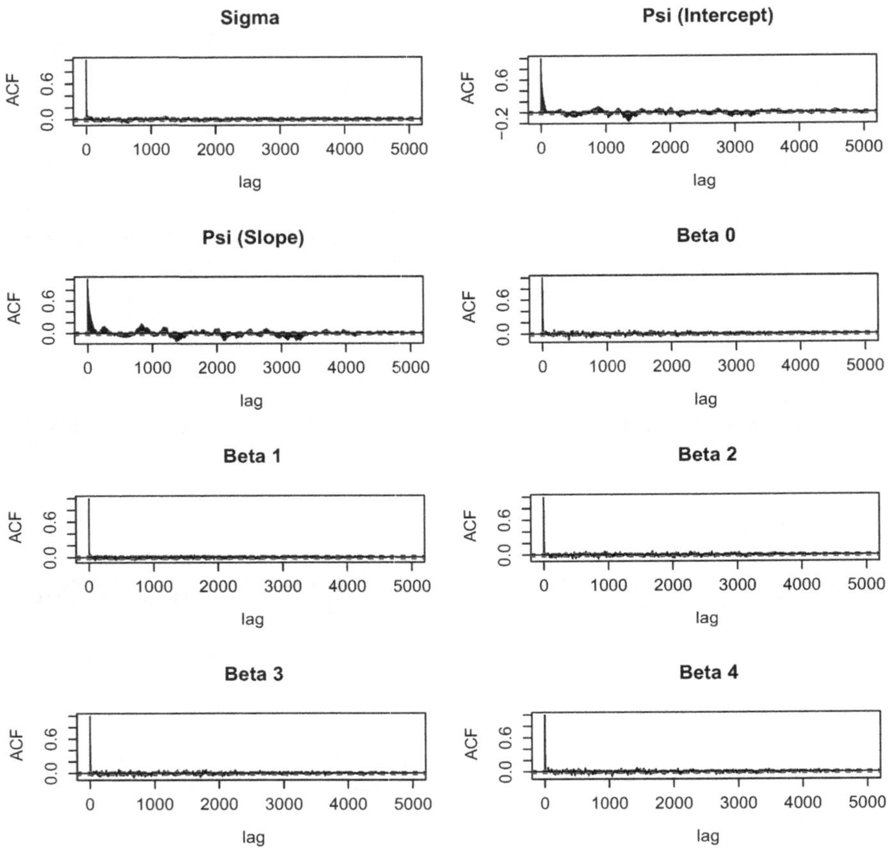

Fig. 5.9 Autocorrelation functions for the pan model parameters—'Sigma' refers to the individual level error term, 'Psi' to the random effects, and 'Beta' to the fixed effects: (Intercept), TIME, FEMALE, RE and GY

`$psi`, and `$beta`, which contain the simulated values of σ (the individual level errors), Ψ (random effects), and β (fixed effects) from all 5000 cycles. Using the generic `plot()` function and the `acf()` function, we create time series plots and ACF plots for these parameters:

```
> iter = 5000
> pdf(file = "./plots/panTS.pdf")
> par(mfrow = c(4, 2))
> plot(1:iter, pan.convergence$sigma[1, 1, ], type = "l", xlab =
+         "Iteration", ylab = "Sigma", main = "")
> plot(1:iter, pan.convergence$psi[1, 1, ], type = "l", xlab =
+         "Iteration", ylab = "Psi (Intercept)")
> plot(1:iter, pan.convergence$psi[2, 1, ], type = "l", xlab =
+         "Iteration", ylab = "Psi (Slope)")
```

```
> for (i in 1:5) {
+ plot(1:iter, pan.convergence$beta[i, 1, ], type = "l", xlab =
+         "Iteration", ylab = paste("Beta ", i - 1))
+ }
> dev.off()

> pdf(file = "./plots/panACF.pdf")
> par(mfrow = c(4, 2))
> acf(pan.convergence$sigma[1, 1, ], lag.max = iter, xlab =
+         "lag", main = "Sigma")
> acf(pan.convergence$psi[1, 1, ], lag.max = iter, xlab = "lag",
+         main = "Psi (Intercept)")
> acf(pan.convergence$psi[2, 1, ], lag.max = iter, xlab = "lag",
+         main = "Psi (Slope)")
> for (i in 1:5) {
+ acf(pan.convergence$beta[i, 1, ], lag.max = iter, xlab =
+         "lag", main = paste("Beta", i - 1))
+ }
> dev.off()
```

We observe no longer lasting trends in the time series, and the lag k autocorrelations also look sufficiently healthy. We therefore proceed with function `mi.pan()` to obtain the imputations.

```
> source("./functions/mi.pan.R")
> set.seed(123456)
> imp.pan <- mi.pan(group = dat.long$ID, y =
+         matrix(dat.long$DELINQ, ncol = 1), x = dat.long[,
+         c("TIME", "FEMALE", "RE", "GY")], xcol = 1:5, zcol =
+         1:2, m = 100, paniter = 5000)
```

Object `imp.pan` is a list of length m, containing the completed data sets. These can be used for further analysis either in R (Sect. 5.7) or other software packages like M*plus*, for example, (see the supplementary material for R and M*plus* code).

5.7 Repeated Data Analysis and Pooling of Results in R

In this section, we give various examples on repeated data analysis and pooling of results in R.

We show how to analyse and pool the data 'manually', and how to use the user friendly `with.mids()` function from package `mice` to automate this process.

For the examples in this section, we use object `imp.mice.mt` of class `mids`, which we have created in Sect. 5.4. Data are imputed by predictive mean matching using the donor selection variant `midastouch`. `imp.mice.mt` which is available from the supplementary material of the book and contains $m = 100$ imputations of the CrimoC data in wide format.

5.7.1 t-test

In our first example we are interested in a simple independent samples t-test. We want to test the hypothesis, that boys on average exhibit more versatile delinquent behaviours than girls at the first panel wave.

Recall, that MI is a three-step-process. In the first step, m completed data sets are created (which we have done in Sect. 5.4). Secondly, these data sets are analysed separately by any complete-data technique (like the t-test in this example). Thirdly, the m sets of model parameters and corresponding standard errors are integrated into an overall set of results.

Combining results from MI analyses can be done with function `miInference()` from package `norm2`. This function requires the M estimates based on the imputed data sets, and their standard errors. The standard errors are then squared to get the estimated variances which are needed for the combining rules proposed by Rubin (1987) (see Sect. 4.3.3). Note that using the standard errors of estimators instead of the estimated variance matrices implies that confidence intervals or test for linear combinations of single parameters cannot be conducted because the estimated covariances are ignored. To get an overall MI estimate, we need to run the t-test $m = 100$ times, store the set of 100 mean differences and corresponding standard error estimates, and combine these quantities using Rubin's (1987) formula (see Sect. 4.3.3).

However, as regular R users will know, the output of R's `t.test()` function (here for the first completed data set in `imp.mice.mt`) does not provide an estimate for the standard error:

```
> load("./Rworkspace/pmm_mt.Rdata")
> com <- complete(imp.mice.mt, 1)
> t.test(ACRIM ~ FEMALE, com)

        Welch Two Sample t-test

data:  ACRIM by FEMALE
t = 7.2876, df = 1877.2, p-value = 4.626e-13
alternative hypothesis: true difference in means is not equal to
0
95 percent confidence interval:
 0.3102192 0.5386714
sample estimates:
mean in group 0 mean in group 1
      0.8608445       0.4363992
```

The function reads out group means for boys (0.86) and girls (0.44), the t statistic, corresponding degrees of freedom, the p value and a 95% confidence interval for the mean difference, but no standard errors. We therefore need another solution to obtain the standard error for the mean difference.

Recall that a t-test is equivalent to fitting a linear model, in which the only predictor of a continuous dependent variable is a categorical variable with two levels. Unlike the `t.test()` function, `lm()` does read out standard errors:

```
> ttest <- lm(ACRIM ~ FEMALE, com)
> s <- summary(ttest)
> s$coefficients
              Estimate Std. Error   t value     Pr(>|t|)
(Intercept)  0.8608445 0.04111554 20.937206 2.049498e-88
FEMALE2     -0.4244453 0.05842993 -7.264176 5.296684e-13
```

In the output above, the (Intercept) estimate (0.86) is the group mean of the reference category (boys). The coefficient FEMALE (−0.42) gives the estimated mean difference between boys and girls. The sum of these two values gives the estimated average delinquency score for girls at wave one (an average of 0.44).

5.7.1.1 Repeated Data Analysis and Pooling of Results—Manual Approach

Now, to test the null hypothesis that the mean difference of delinquency between boys and girls is zero, we need to set up two empty list objects, one for the 100 mean differences, and one for the corresponding standard errors. We call these objects est and se:

```
> est <- se <- vector(length = imp.mice.mt$m, mode = "list")
```

The repeated data analysis can then be automated by a for loop. First, we extract the respective completed data set from the mids object. Secondly, we fit the linear model and store the estimate of the mean difference and its standard error in the respective slot of est and se. Finally, we use function miInference() from package norm2 for MI pooling:

```
> for (i in 1:imp.mice.mt$m) {
+ com <- complete(imp.mice.mt, i)
+ ttest <- lm(ACRIM ~ FEMALE, com)
+ s <- summary(ttest)
+ est[[i]] <- s$coefficients[2, 1]
+ se[[i]] <- s$coefficients[2, 2]
+ }
> library(norm2)
> miinf <- miInference(est, se)
> print(miinf)
          Est       SE Est/SE    df p Pct.mis
[1,] -0.44861 0.081134 -5.529 666.1 0    38.6
```

In our example, the combined MI estimate of the mean difference is −0.45. The null hypothesis that this parameter is zero can be rejected ($p < 0.001$). Pct.mis gives the estimated rate of missing information. This statistic ranges between 0 and 100% and indicates, how strongly the parameter estimate was affected by missing data. Large values mean that the quality of the estimate depends heavily upon a correct specification of the imputation model. If misspecifications have to be assumed, the estimate could be biased. Note again that MI is a method proposed to compensate for item nonresponse in situations with not more than 30–50% information lost due to missing values (Rubin 1987, 1996, see also Sect. 3.5.2).

Finally, a 95% confidence interval for the mean difference could be obtained by

```
> miinf$est + c(-1, 1) * qt(0.975, miinf$df) * miinf$std.err
[1] -0.6079149 -0.2892962
```

In our example, the lower and upper limits of the 95% confidence interval are −0.61 and −0.29.

5.7.1.2 Repeated Data Analysis and Pooling of Results Using Functions `with.mids()` and `pool()` from Package `mice`

In contrast to the manual approach, the `mice` package provides some convenient functions that facilitate repeated data analysis and pooling of results: `with.mids()` takes care of repeated data analysis and supports many of the commonly used statistical models like linear models, generalized linear models, analysis of variance. The `pool()` function then applies Rubin's formulae and the generic `summary()` function produces typical MI output.

```
> mira <- with(imp.mice.mt, lm(ACRIM ~ FEMALE))
> result <- summary(pool(mira))
> print(result[, 1:5])
                    est         se         t       df     Pr(>|t|)
(Intercept)  0.9027543 0.06217193 14.520287 304.7054 0.000000e+00
FEMALE2     -0.4486056 0.08113409 -5.529187 436.4569 5.548366e-08
> print(result[, 6:10])
                 lo 95      hi 95 nmis       fmi    lambda
(Intercept)  0.7804136  1.0250950   NA 0.4851961 0.4818282
FEMALE2     -0.6080677 -0.2891435   NA 0.3883069 0.3855103
```

Note that in the example above, the generic `with()` function automatically calls the appropriate function `with.mids()`. Again, we obtain an estimate for the mean difference of −0.45 ($p < 0.001$). Note, however, that while point estimate and combined standard error estimates are identical to the ones obtained by `miInference()`, degrees of freedom (`df`) and the resulting 95% confidence interval (`lo 95`, `hi 95`) are not. The two functions use different default settings: `miInference()` uses the normal approximation for large samples, described in Rubin (1987, Chap. 3), while `pool()` uses the correction for small samples proposed in Barnard and Rubin (1999).

Both approaches yield virtual identical results, when sample size is large. However, the latter one is more appropriate, when sample size is small (Sect. 4.3.5). In our example, results are highly similar (but not identical) due to the large sample of more than 2000 participants. Furthermore, in the output above, `fmi` refers to the fraction of missing information (ranging between 0 and 1). This corresponds to `Pct.mis`—the percentage of missing information in Schafer's `miInference` output. Finally, `lambda` is the proportion of the variation attributable to the missing data, defined as $(1+1/M)\hat{b}/\widehat{\text{var}}(\bar{\theta})$, where $\hat{b}$ and $\widehat{\text{var}}(\bar{\theta})$ are scalar versions of $\hat{\mathbf{B}}$ and $\widehat{\text{Var}}(\bar{\boldsymbol{\theta}})$ (for further details, see Sect. 4.3.5; note that the statistic was labeled γ_M in this section).

5.7.2 Linear Model

We have already used the `lm()` function to pool t-test results. In fact, a t-test is a very simple linear model with just one binary predictor variable. In this example, we want to extend the previous model and include further predictors.

Here, we want to predict delinquency at wave one by gender and school type. In addition to `FEMALE`, we now also include variables `RE` and `GY` into the analysis model. The steps to perform the repeated data analysis and to combine the results are analogous to the ones described in Sect. 5.7.1: (a) For the manual approach, we either set up empty list objects for estimates and standard errors and store the mth set of parameter estimates and standard errors in the mth slot of these list objects, or (b) we use the convenient functions from package `mice` to facilitate data analysis and pooling of outcomes.

Variant (a)—Manual Data Analysis

```
> est <- se <- vector(length = imp.mice.mt$m, mode = "list")
> for (i in 1:imp.mice.mt$m) {
+ com <- complete(imp.mice.mt, i)
+ model <- lm(ACRIM ~ FEMALE + RE + GY, com)
+ s <- summary(model)
+ est[[i]] <- s$coefficients[, 1]
+ se[[i]] <- s$coefficients[, 2]
+ }
> library(norm2)
> miinf <- miInference(est, se)
> print(miinf)
                  Est        SE Est/SE    df     p Pct.mis
(Intercept)  1.08090 0.095060 11.371 482.2 0.000    45.3
FEMALE2     -0.43670 0.080736 -5.409 669.7 0.000    38.4
RE2         -0.10744 0.110410 -0.973 588.3 0.331    41.0
GY2         -0.34564 0.099846 -3.462 777.4 0.001    35.7
```

Confidence intervals can be obtained by:

```
> lower <- miinf$est - 1 * qt(0.975, miinf$df) * miinf$std.err
> print(lower)
(Intercept)     FEMALE2          RE2          GY2
  0.8941223  -0.5952266  -0.3242914  -0.5416444
> upper <- miinf$est + 1 * qt(0.975, miinf$df) * miinf$std.err
> print(upper)
(Intercept)     FEMALE2          RE2          GY2
  1.2676880  -0.2781750   0.1094117  -0.1496448
```

Variant (b)—Repeated Data Analysis and Pooling of Results Using Functions from the `mice` Package

```
> mira <- with(imp.mice.mt, lm(ACRIM ~ FEMALE + RE + GY))
> result <- round(summary(pool(mira)), 3)
```

```
> print(result[, 1:5])
                  est    se       t      df Pr(>|t|)
(Intercept)  1.081 0.095 11.371 337.558    0.000
FEMALE2     -0.437 0.081 -5.409 438.104    0.000
RE2         -0.107 0.110 -0.973 396.250    0.331
GY2         -0.346 0.100 -3.462 489.762    0.001
> print(result[, 6:10])
              lo 95   hi 95 nmis   fmi lambda
(Intercept)  0.894  1.268   NA 0.456  0.453
FEMALE2     -0.595 -0.278   NA 0.387  0.384
RE2         -0.325  0.110   NA 0.413  0.410
GY2         -0.542 -0.149   NA 0.359  0.357
```

Note that repeated analysis and pooling of generalized linear models (GLM) works analogously. The `lm()` function simply has to be replaced by the `glm()` function or any other supported function.

5.7.3 Growth Model

In this section, we want to fit a model that is currently not supported by `mice`'s `with.mids()` function: a growth curve model defined by structural equations and fitted by R package `lavaan` (Rosseel, 2012).[24] Readers who are not familiar with growth curve models will find a very brief introduction in Sect. 5.2.2. Currently `lavaan` does not support any count data models, so we fit a 'normal' growth curve model to the CrimoC data.

In `lavaan`, latent variables are defined using the `=~` operator. Variances and covariances are specified using the `~~` operator. Fixing factor loadings, variances and covariances to certain values can be done by pre-multiplying the corresponding variable in the model formula by the desired numeric value. In the syntax code below, we define a latent intercept (labelled `i`, i.e., `ACRIM`–`DCRIM` are fixed to 1), a linear slope (`s`, with loadings being fixed to 0, 1, 2, and 3, respectively), and a quadratic slope `q` (here, loadings are fixed to 0, 1, 4, 9, respectively). The latent intercept gives the starting level (i.e., delinquency at time 1), the linear slope gives the linear change in delinquency over time. Furthermore the quadratic slope is needed to model the decline in delinquency rates later on (see Sect. 5.2.2).

By default, the `growth()` function from package `lavaan` estimates all variances and covariances of the growth factors. However, in our example, we set the variance of the quadratic term and its covariances to 0, otherwise the model is only weakly identified:

```
> library(lavaan)
> model <- '
+ i =~ 1*ACRIM + 1*BCRIM + 1*CCRIM + 1*DCRIM
```

[24]An introduction to the `lavaan` syntax may be found at Yves Rosseel's website http://lavaan.ugent.be/.

```
+ s =~ 0*ACRIM + 1*BCRIM + 2*CCRIM + 3*DCRIM
+ q =~ 0*ACRIM + 1*BCRIM + 4*CCRIM + 9*DCRIM
+ i ~~ 0*q
+ s ~~ 0*q
+ q ~~ 0*q
+ '
```

After specification of the `lavaan` model, the next steps are similar to those outlined in the previous sections: First, we set up empty list objects for the parameter estimates and the standard errors. Again, we make use of a `for` loop to automate the repeated data analysis. For the ith completed data set, $i \in \{1, \ldots, m\}$, we fit the `growth` model, store the ith set of coefficients and standard errors, and finally pool the results.[25]

There is only one difference in the code listed below compared to the examples from the previous sections: As multiple imputation is a simulation based approach, there is always—due to an unfortunate constellation of imputed data—a chance that some of the $m = 100$ growth curve models result in an error. We therefore set up an empty vector `fail` that lists, which of the m computations resulted in an error message. `fail` is `NULL`, when all computations ran through smoothly. `options(warn=2)` furthermore tells R not to abort, when an error occurs. Instead, R now treats an error as a warning and goes on with the next completed data set. If the number of failed computations is only minor, MI inference could be based on the available sets of results. Otherwise, the analysis model should be checked. A misspecification of the analysis model could result in error messages. In our example, all $m = 100$ models could be estimated:

```
> est <- se <- vector(length = 100, mode = "list")
> options(warn = 2)
> fail <- NULL
> for (m in 1:100) {
+ fit <- try(growth(model, data = complete(imp.mice.mt, m)))
+ if (any(class(fit) == "try-error")) {
+ fail <- c(fail, m)
+ next
+ }
+ s <- parameterEstimates(fit)
+ est[[m]] <- s$est
+ se[[m]] <- s$se
+ nam <- s[, 1:3]
+ }
> print(fail)
NULL
```

This means, we can proceed with the pooling of results

```
> miinf <- miInference(est, se)
```

[25] Another option would be to use functions from package `semTools`, which we introduce in Sect. 5.7.7.5.

Had some of the *m* data analyses failed, we could have excluded them by writing:

```
miinf <- miInference(est[-fail], se[-fail])
```

Instead of displaying the entire pooled `lavaan` output, we focus on those parts that are most essential to us: the estimates of the latent intercept, slope and quadratic slope, and the variances and covariances of the intercept and slope. These can be found in rows 27–29, and 20–22 of the output. Furthermore we round the numeric output to three decimal points:

```
> output <- data.frame(nam, Est = miinf$est, SE = miinf$std.err,
+ df = miinf$df, p = miinf$p, Pct.mis = miinf$mis.inf)
> output[, -3:-1] <- round(output[, -3:-1], 3)
> output[c(27:29, 20:22), ]
   lhs op rhs    Est    SE      df     p Pct.mis
27   i ~1      0.679 0.042 673.300 0.000   0.383
28   s ~1      0.643 0.053 742.907 0.000   0.365
29   q ~1     -0.166 0.017 683.656 0.000   0.381
20   i ~~   i  1.709 0.215 141.959 0.000   0.835
21   s ~~   s  0.306 0.044 146.736 0.000   0.821
22   i ~~   s -0.232 0.078 138.476 0.004   0.846
```

`lhs` is the 'left-hand side' of the `lavaan` model equation, `rhs` the 'right-hand side', and `op` is the operator (see http://lavaan.ugent.be/tutorial/index.html for details). `i~1` is the latent intercept, `s~1` is the linear and `q~1` is the quadratic slope, respectively. Variances and covariances are denoted by `~~`. `i~~i` is the variance of the intercept, `s~~s` is the variance of the linear slope and `i~~s` is the covariance between intercept and slope. The estimates reflect the typical age-crime curve: The average estimated delinquency score (across all school types and all participants) was 0.679 at Wave 1. Delinquency then increases by an average of 0.643 delinquent behaviours per panel wave. However, the negative quadratic slope indicates that delinquency flattens or decreases later on.

5.7.4 Generalized Linear Mixed-Effects Model

In this example, we use R package `glmmTMB`[26] to fit an unconditional generalized linear mixed-effects model, here a two-level Poisson model. Mixed-effects models estimate fixed effects and random effects standard deviations (or variances) and correlations (or covariances). In contrast to the previous examples, we now set up four empty list objects: (1) for the fixed effects coefficients, (2) for their corresponding standard errors, (3) for the random effects variances, and (4) for the random effects correlations. Typically, R functions do not generate standard errors for the random part of the model. MI estimates for the random part are thus obtained

[26]https://cran.r-project.org/package=glmmTMB.

by averaging the respective quantities (i.e., the MI estimate is the mean of the *m* sets of random effects variances and correlations respectively[27]).

We use a `for` loop to automate the repeated data analysis. For each of the *m* imputations, we extract the *m*th completed data set from the `mids` object and bring it to long format using R's `reshape()` function—which is the required input format for `glmmTMB()`.

Then we estimate the `glmmTMB` model. The `glmmTMB` model syntax follows the `lme4` style (cf. Gałecki & Burzykowski, 2013). In the code below, we predict delinquency (variable `DELINQ`, i.e., variables `ACRIM–DCRIM` in long format) by a linear and quadratic `TIME` factor `(TIME+I(TIME^2))`. Furthermore, we define both linear and quadratic terms as 'random' `(TIME+I(TIME^2)|ID)`. By default, the function treats the intercept both as a fixed and random factor. Finally, `family=poisson` tells the function to fit a linear mixed Poisson model that by default uses a log link.

We use the generic `summary` function to extract the model coefficients for the fixed part of the model. `glmmTMB` may also be used to fit zero-inflation models. The `$coefficients` slot of the model summary has two sub-slots: `$cond` for the conditional model, and a further slot for the zero-inflation part of the model. In this example, the latter one is empty, as we do not fit a zero-inflation model. Finally, random effects standard deviations and correlations can be extracted using function `VarCorr()`:

```
> est <- se <- rvar <- rcor <- vector(length = 100, mode =
+         "list")
> for (i in 1:100) {
+ cat(i, "\n")
+ com <- complete(imp.mice.mt, i)
+ com.l <- reshape(data = com, varying = list(c("ACRIM",
+         "BCRIM",  "CCRIM", "DCRIM")), direction = "long",
+         v.names = "DELINQ", times = 0:3, timevar = "TIME",
+         idvar = "ID")
+ com.l$ID <- as.factor(com.l$ID)
+ poissonmodel <- glmmTMB::glmmTMB(DELINQ ~ (TIME + I(TIME^2)) +
+         (TIME + I(TIME^2) | ID), data = com.l, family = poisson)
+ s <- summary(poissonmodel)
+ est[[i]] <- s$coefficients$cond[, 1]
+ se[[i]] <- s$coefficients$cond[, 2]
+ rvar[[i]] <-
+         attr(glmmTMB::VarCorr(poissonmodel)[[1]]$"ID","stddev")^2
+ rcor[[i]] <-
+         cor2fisher(attr(glmmTMB::VarCorr(poissonmodel)[[1]]$"ID",
+         "correlation"))
+ }
```

[27]More precisely, we average the Fisher-Z-transformed correlations and then, in a second step, bring the mean of these transformed correlations back to the original scale (see, for example, Schafer, 1997, for details on how to pool correlation coefficients). Functions `cor2fisher()` and `fisher2cor()`, which we use for the transformation and back-transformation are available from the supplementary material of the book.

Again, we use the `miInference()` function from package `norm2` to pool the fixed effects results.

```
> miInference(est, se)
                   Est       SE  Est/SE    df p Pct.mis
(Intercept) -1.57080 0.097067 -16.183 567.6 0    41.8
TIME         0.79664 0.110730   7.195 630.3 0    39.6
I(TIME^2)   -0.17426 0.032579  -5.349 577.6 0    41.4
```

The expected delinquency score for Wave 1 is $\exp(-1.57080) = 0.21$. Note that the time variable was coded 0, 1, 2, 3, so that the intercept reflects the starting level—the average delinquency score at Wave 1. Since the Poisson model uses a log link, we can obtain the expected value on the original scale by using the exponential function. An expected score of 0.21 is lower than the observed mean of variable `ACRIM` of 0.60: This implies that this unconditional model does not fit the empirical data well.

Again, the parameter estimates reflect the typical age-crime curve, although neglecting the zero-inflation in the empirical data resulted in a lack of fit. The log of the expected counts first increases over time (positive linear slope) and then decreases afterwards (negative quadratic slope).

In addition, we want to report the pooled random effects variances, which we combine using `apply()` in combination with the `abind()` function from package `abind`. The code below basically transforms the `list` of random effects variances `rvar` to a `matrix` with three rows (for the estimates of the `(Intercept)`, `TIME`, and `I(TIME^2)` coefficients) and 100 columns. The `apply()` function then applies the `mean()` function to the specified dimension of the `matrix` (here: 1 gives the row means):

```
> library(abind)
> apply(abind(rvar, along = 2), 1, mean)
(Intercept)        TIME   I(TIME^2)
 2.72093071  0.90054843  0.05848062
```

Analogously, we pool the random effects correlation matrix and round the output to three decimal places. `as.dist()` produces a nicer output of the correlation matrix, displaying only the lower triangle.[28]

```
> as.dist(round(fisher2cor(apply(abind(rcor, along = 3), c(1,
+         2), mean)), 3))
            (Intercept)   TIME
TIME             -0.285
I(TIME^2)         0.059 -0.923
```

The negative correlation between the random intercept and linear slope (`TIME`) indicates that students who show a more versatile delinquent behaviour at wave one tend to have a lower linear slope coefficient (i.e., they show less increase of delinquency over time) in comparison to students who reported less delinquent behaviour at wave one. Furthermore, the high negative correlation between the

[28] For further details, see the help files of functions `abind()` and `apply()`.

linear and quadratic slope (TIME^2) suggests that students who have a larger increase of delinquency over time, also show a larger decrease of delinquency later on.

5.7.5 *Two-Level Negative Binomial Hurdle Model*

In this example, we repeatedly fit and pool a negative binomial mixed-effects hurdle model for zero-inflated data using package glmmTMB. Hurdle models contain two model components: A zero model (e.g., a binomial generalized linear mixed-effects model), that determines if a case belongs to the zero or the count process, and a zero-truncated count model (e.g., a zero-truncated negative binomial mixed-effects model) that models the non-zero part of the dependent variable.

Here, we model delinquency (variable DELINQ in long format) over time using a linear and quadratic time factor. The intercept is allowed to vary across participants ('random effect'). Furthermore, we include FEMALE and GY as predictors in the conditional (count) part of the model. In the zero part of the model (argument zi), we estimate an intercept term and include TIME, FEMALE, and GY as predictors. The zero part in our example is a binomial model with a logit link (without any random effects). The count part is a zero-truncated negative binomial model with a log link (using the NB2 parametrization; for details see Hilbe, 2011). The glmmTMB model formula for this example is:

```
> glmmTMB(DELINQ ~ (TIME+I(TIME^2)+FEMALE+GY) + (1|ID), zi =
+         ~(TIME+FEMALE+GY), data = com.l, family = list(family =
+         "truncated_nbinom2", link = "log")
```

In the first step, we repeatedly fit the model (which will take some time) and save the model output for further use later on:

```
> dir.create("./Routput/mira/")
> library(glmmTMB)
> options(warn = 1)
> for (i in 1:100) {
+ cat(i, "\n")
+ com <- complete(imp.mice.mt, i)
+ com.l <- reshape(data = com, varying = list(c("ACRIM",
+         "BCRIM", "CCRIM", "DCRIM")), direction = "long",
+         v.names = "DELINQ", times = 0:3, timevar = "TIME",
+         idvar = "ID")
+ com.l$ID <- as.factor(com.l$ID)
+ twolevel.hnbmodel <- try(glmmTMB(DELINQ ~ (TIME + I(TIME^2) +
+         FEMALE + GY) + (1 | ID), zi = ~(TIME + FEMALE + GY),
+         data = com.l, family = list(family =
+         "truncated_nbinom2", link = "log")))
+ save(twolevel.hnbmodel, file =
+         paste0("./Routput/mira/twolevel.hnbmodel", i))
+ }
```

We set `options(warn=1)` so that warning messages will be printed to the console immediately when they occur and we can see straight away if one of the repeated data analyses runs into estimation problems.

However, in our example, the estimation ran smoothly and we received neither warning nor error messages. In case of warnings, `vignette('trouble shooting')` gives helpful information regarding (a) why these warnings occurred, and (b) gives some advice on what can be done to improve the model.

In the next step, we set up empty lists for estimates and standard errors for the zero and count parts of the model, respectively, and for the random effect standard deviations. We store the information of the repeated data analyses in the respective slots of these objects. `est.cond` and `se.cond` contain the parameter estimates and corresponding standard errors of the count part of the model, `est.zi` and `se.zi` contain the same estimates for the zero inflation part of the model. `theta` is the list of m overdispersion parameters. Finally, `rvar` is the list of random effects variances.

```
> est.cond <- est.zi <- se.cond <- se.zi <- theta <- rvar <-
+        vector(length = 100, mode = "list")
> for (i in 1:100) {
+ load(paste0("./Routput/mira/twolevel.hnbmodel", i))
+ s <- summary(twolevel.hnbmodel)
+ est.cond[[i]] <- s$coefficients$cond[, 1]
+ est.zi[[i]] <- s$coefficients$zi[, 1]
+ se.cond[[i]] <- s$coefficients$cond[, 2]
+ se.zi[[i]] <- s$coefficients$zi[, 2]
+ theta[[i]] <- s$sigma
+ rvar[[i]] <- attr(VarCorr(twolevel.hnbmodel)[[1]]$ID,
+        "stddev")^2
+ }
```

Note that in the parametrization used by the `nbinom2` family,[29] larger `theta` values correspond to a lower variance, which is $(\mu + \mu^2/\theta)$, where μ is the location parameter (i.e., the mean) of the negative binomial distribution (Hilbe, 2011). We use the `miInference` function from package `norm2` to pool the estimates of the conditional part of the model.

```
> miInference(est.cond, se.cond)
                 Est        SE Est/SE     df p Pct.mis
(Intercept)  0.37889 0.074329  5.097  651.4 0    39.0
TIME         0.50359 0.072491  6.947  594.0 0    40.8
I(TIME^2)   -0.14462 0.021236 -6.810  712.2 0    37.3
FEMALE1     -0.54118 0.068259 -7.928 2356.5 0    20.5
GY1         -0.40392 0.068947 -5.858 2538.7 0    19.7
```

The expected count for boys from Hauptschule or Realschule at time one is exp(.37889) = 1.46. Again the positive linear slope (`TIME`) and the negative quadratic slope (`TIME^2`) reflects the age-crime curve. Furthermore, girls on average are expected to have $\exp(-0.54118) = 0.58$ less delinquent behaviours

[29] https://github.com/glmmTMB/glmmTMB/blob/master/glmmTMB/R/family.R

in comparison to the reference group and students from Gymnasium on average are expected to show $\exp(-0.40392) = 0.67$ less delinquent behaviours than the reference group. Again we use the `miInference` function from package `norm2` to pool the estimates of the zero-inflation part of the model:

```
> miInference(est.zi, se.zi)
                  Est        SE  Est/SE    df     p Pct.mis
(Intercept)  0.15195 0.063454   2.395 540.0 0.017    42.8
TIME        -0.22476 0.027716  -8.109 515.6 0.000    43.8
FEMALE1      0.73715 0.059133  12.466 665.6 0.000    38.6
GY1          0.49950 0.057016   8.761 960.3 0.000    32.1
```

The estimated odds of not being delinquent decrease over time. Furthermore, estimated odds of not being delinquent at wave one are significantly higher for girls and for students attending Gymnasium in comparison to Realschule and Hauptschule. The pooled overdispersion parameter is:

```
> mean(unlist(theta))
[1] 6.517848
```

Finally, like in the previous example, package `abind` is used to calculate the pooled variance of the random intercept:

```
> library(abind)
> randomvar <- apply(abind(rvar, along = 2), 1, mean)
> randomvar
(Intercept)
  0.5916271
```

5.7.6 Correlation Coefficients

Normal theory multiple imputation inference of correlation coefficients is not straightforward, since these are not normally distributed. Applying Rubin's (1987) formulae to pool correlation coefficients requires some normalizing transformations before the pooling and back-transformation afterwards. The `miceadds` package[30] provides a convenient function to do this. Function `mi.combine.cor()` takes a `mids` object as input (i.e., a data set that has been imputed by the `mice` package) and reads out the combined correlations for the specified variables, Fisher Z transformed correlations, corresponding standard errors and typical MI output (i.e., a statistical test that the correlation is zero), the estimated fraction of missing information, and a 95% confidence interval for the Fisher-Z-transformed correlation. Argument `variables` specifies the variables (position in the data set), for which correlations shall be computed and combined. In our case, `ACRIM–`

[30]https://cran.r-project.org/package=miceadds.

DCRIM are the first four variables in the completed data sets, so we specify variables=1:4:

```
> library(miceadds)
> correlations <- micombine.cor(imp.mice.mt, variables = 1:4,
+          method = "pearson")
> print(correlations[, 1:6], digits = 3)
   variable1 variable2     r    rse fisher_r fisher_rse
1      ACRIM     BCRIM 0.529 0.0357    0.588     0.0495
2      ACRIM     CCRIM 0.409 0.0365    0.435     0.0439
3      ACRIM     DCRIM 0.329 0.0361    0.342     0.0405
4      BCRIM     CCRIM 0.634 0.0263    0.748     0.0440
5      BCRIM     DCRIM 0.494 0.0338    0.542     0.0448
6      CCRIM     DCRIM 0.624 0.0266    0.731     0.0436
7      BCRIM     ACRIM 0.529 0.0357    0.588     0.0495
8      CCRIM     ACRIM 0.409 0.0365    0.435     0.0439
9      DCRIM     ACRIM 0.329 0.0361    0.342     0.0405
10     CCRIM     BCRIM 0.634 0.0263    0.748     0.0440
11     DCRIM     BCRIM 0.494 0.0338    0.542     0.0448
12     DCRIM     CCRIM 0.624 0.0266    0.731     0.0436
> print(correlations[, c(1, 2, 7:11)], digits = 3)
   variable1 variable2   fmi     t        p lower95 upper95
1      ACRIM     BCRIM 0.805 11.88 1.59e-32   0.455   0.595
2      ACRIM     CCRIM 0.751  9.91 3.88e-23   0.335   0.478
3      ACRIM     DCRIM 0.707  8.45 3.03e-17   0.257   0.398
4      BCRIM     CCRIM 0.752 17.02 5.92e-65   0.580   0.683
5      BCRIM     DCRIM 0.761 12.10 1.11e-33   0.425   0.558
6      CCRIM     DCRIM 0.747 16.78 3.58e-63   0.569   0.673
7      BCRIM     ACRIM 0.805 11.88 1.59e-32   0.455   0.595
8      CCRIM     ACRIM 0.751  9.91 3.88e-23   0.335   0.478
9      DCRIM     ACRIM 0.707  8.45 3.03e-17   0.257   0.398
10     CCRIM     BCRIM 0.752 17.02 5.92e-65   0.580   0.683
11     DCRIM     BCRIM 0.761 12.10 1.11e-33   0.425   0.558
12     DCRIM     CCRIM 0.747 16.78 3.58e-63   0.569   0.673
```

A correlation matrix can be extracted using the attribute "r_matrix":

```
> print(attr(correlations, "r_matrix"), digits = 3)
      ACRIM BCRIM CCRIM DCRIM
ACRIM 1.000 0.529 0.409 0.329
BCRIM 0.529 1.000 0.634 0.494
CCRIM 0.409 0.634 1.000 0.624
DCRIM 0.329 0.494 0.624 1.000
```

5.7.7 *Further Useful Tools for Multiple Imputation Inference*

We want to draw attention to special MI inference tools from packages mice, miceadds, and semTools, which may be useful in practice (for an overview, see Table 5.9). These are: pooling of R^2-values, comparing nested models fitted to multiply imputed data sets, pooling F statistics and analysis of variance tables, and pooling χ^2-statistics.

Table 5.9 Special MI pooling

Statistic/procedure	Package	Function
Explained variance (R^2)	`mice`	`pool.r.squared`
Model comparison	`mice`	`pool.compare`
Analysis of variance	`miceadds`	`mi.anova`
F	`miceadds`	`micombine.F`
χ^2/SEM model fit	`semTools`	`runMI`

5.7.7.1 Pooling Explained Variance in a Linear Model

The `pool.r.squared()` function from package `mice` can be used to combine R^2 or adjusted R^2 statistics from (multiple) regression analysis (see also Harel, 2009). Input is an object of class `mira`, produced by `with.mids()` with `lm` as modeling function. The function first Fisher-Z-transforms the obtained R^2 values from the `lm` model output, performs MI pooling on the Fisher-Z-transformed values and then reads out the pooled results on the original scale.

In the example below, delinquency at wave one was predicted by gender and school type:

```
> pool.r.squared(with(imp.mice.mt, lm(ACRIM ~ FEMALE + RE +
+         GY)))[, "est"]
[1] 0.03414674
```

To get the adjusted R^2 value, argument `adjusted` has to be set to `TRUE`:

```
> pool.r.squared(with(imp.mice.mt, lm(ACRIM ~ FEMALE + RE +
+         GY)), adjusted = TRUE)[, "est"]
[1] 0.03273072
```

5.7.7.2 Comparison of Two Nested Models Fitted to Imputed Data

Function `pool.compare()` from package `mice` is extremely helpful during the early exploratory stages of the data analysis process: The procedure is based on Meng and Rubin (1992) and allows comparisons of nested linear models or generalized linear models using the `"Wald"` or `"likelihood"` methods described in Meng and Rubin (1992), respectively. It takes two objects of class `mira` (see Sect. 5.4), produced by `with.mids()` as input: `fit1` and `fit0`. `fit0` is a submodel of `fit1` (see `?pool.compare` for details). In the example below, at first delinquency (at Wave 1) is predicted by gender, and then by the two indicators of school type (`RE` and `GY`):

```
> fit1 <- with(imp.mice.mt, lm(ACRIM ~ FEMALE))
> fit2 <- with(imp.mice.mt, lm(ACRIM ~ FEMALE + RE))
> fit3 <- with(imp.mice.mt, lm(ACRIM ~ FEMALE + RE + GY))
> comp1 <- pool.compare(fit2, fit1, method = "Wald")
> print(comp1$pvalue, digits = 3)
```

```
        [,1]
[1,] 0.197
```

Comparison of models using the Wald method is appropriate for normal linear models. It tests the null hypothesis that all extra parameters of the larger model are zero: A comparison of the first two models yields a p-value of 0.197. The null hypothesis that the coefficient of RE is zero cannot be rejected at the $\alpha = 0.05$ level. On the other hand, when we compare models two and three, we get a p-value of < 0.001, which indicates that GY is a significant predictor for delinquency at wave one:

```
> comp2 <- pool.compare(fit3, fit2, method = "Wald")
> print(comp2$pvalue, digits = 2)
        [,1]
[1,] 0.00057
```

5.7.7.3 Combination of F-Values

We have demonstrated how to pool regression coefficients, how to compare nested linear models, and how to obtain a combined estimate for the variance explained by a linear model. In this and the following section, we want to focus on pooling analysis of variance (ANOVA) results (i.e., F-values). Formulae for pooling F-values are based on Enders (2010, Chap. 8).

In our first example, we pool the omnibus F-statistic for the linear model from the previous section. We predicted delinquency at wave one by gender and school type. The omnibus ANOVA tests the null hypothesis that the coefficients of all predictors in the model are zero.

To pool F-values, we use the micombine.F() function from package miceadds. The function takes a vector of length m of F-values and the degrees of freedom of the numerator (equal to the number of predictors in the model) as input. In our example, we have three predictors (FEMALE, RE, and GY) and thus three degrees of freedom. For the m F-values, we set up an empty vector of length 100 (labelled fvalues in the R code below). Then we use a for loop to fit the model to the 100 completed data sets. We extract the respective F-value from the model output and store it in the respective slot of vector fvalues:

```
> fvalues = vector(length = imp.mice.mt$m)
> for (i in 1:imp.mice.mt$m) {
+ com <- complete(imp.mice.mt, i)
+ model <- lm(ACRIM ~ FEMALE + RE + GY, com)
+ s <- summary(model)
+ fvalues[i] <- s$fstatistic["value"]
+ }
> micombine.F(fvalues, 3)
Combination of Chi Square Statistics for Multiply Imputed Data
Using 100 Imputed Data Sets
F(3, 913.06)=16.192     p=0
```

We obtain a combined F-statistic of 16.192, $p < .001$, which means that at least one of the predictors seems to be not zero ($\alpha = 0.05$).

5.7.7.4 Analysis of Variance

Basically, linear regression and analysis of variance (ANOVA) is the same model class: We can view an ANOVA model as a linear model, in which the factor is usually effect coded. Each group mean is compared to the grand mean or overall mean, while in most typical regression settings, dummy coding is used. Dummy coding means that we compare the fitted mean of a reference group against the means of the other groups.

We want to show two different ways of pooling ANOVA models in R: (1) using `micombine.F()` and (2) using `mi.anova()` from package `miceadds`.

The data file `crim4a.csv` is used for this example (available from the supplementary material of the book). `crim4a.csv` is identical to `crim4.dat`, which we have used so far—with one exception: School type is stored as a single categorical variable `SCHOOL` in `crim4a.csv`, while `crim4.dat` has separate dummy coded school type indicators. First, we load `crim4a.csv` using R's `read.csv2()` function, which reads csv files, in which a ',' is the decimal character and ';' is the field separator. We then impute missing data by `mice`'s default method predictive mean matching (although an imputation method for count data, which we will introduce in Chap. 6, might be the better choice).

```
> crim4a <- read.csv2("./data/crim4a.csv", row.names = 1)
> set.seed(123456)
> imp.mice.pmm.crim4a <- mice(crim4a, m = 100, maxit = 20,
+         printFlag = FALSE)
> save(imp.mice.pmm.crim4a, file =
+         "./imputations/pmm/imp.mice.pmm.crim4a.Rdata")
```

Next, we repeatedly fit an analysis of variance model to the data, in which we predict delinquency at wave one by school type, gender and the interaction between school type and gender. The `mi.anova` function takes a `mids` object and a model formula, which is supplied as a string vector, as input.

```
> result <- mi.anova(imp.mice.pmm.crim4a, "ACRIM~FEMALE*SCHOOL")
> round(result$r.squared, 3)
[1] 0.039
> colnames(result$anova.table)[7] <- "p.eta2"
> round(result$anova.table, 3)
                   SSQ df1     df2 F value Pr(>F)  eta2 p.eta2
FEMALE         119.993   1 709.878  34.353  0.000 0.026  0.026
SCHOOL          53.964   2 705.791   7.449  0.001 0.012  0.012
FEMALE:SCHOOL    5.826   2 885.707   0.559  0.572 0.001  0.001
Residual      4454.138  NA      NA      NA     NA    NA     NA
```

The `mi.anova` function reads out a pooled R^2 statistic, pooled F-values, as well as η^2 (`eta2`) and partial η^2-values (`p.eta2`), which are typical measures of effect size used in ANOVA type analyses. We see significant differences in delinquency between boys and girls in wave one ($F = 34.353$, $p < 0.001$), and also between the three different school types ($F = 7.449$, $p = 0.001$). Furthermore, the interaction between gender and school type ($F = 0.559$, $p = 0.572$) is not significant.

In addition to the `mi.anova()` function, we also could have used the `micombine.F()` function from the previous section to combine the F-values of the respective terms: First, we set up an empty object in which we store the sets of F-values. Then we repeatedly fit the models and extract the F-values from the model output. Finally, we use `micombine.F()` with the corresponding degrees of freedom of the numerator to pool the results.

```
> fvalues <- vector(length = imp.mice.pmm.crim4a$m, mode =
+         "list")
> for (i in 1:imp.mice.pmm.crim4a$m) {
+ com <- complete(imp.mice.pmm.crim4a, i)
+ model <- lm(ACRIM ~ FEMALE * SCHOOL, com)
+ a <- anova(model)
+ fvalues[[i]] <- a$'F value'
+ }
> library(abind)
> fvalues <- abind(fvalues, along = 2)
> micombine.F(fvalues[1, ], 1)
Combination of Chi Square Statistics for Multiply Imputed Data
Using 100 Imputed Data Sets
F(1, 709.88)=34.353      p=0
> micombine.F(fvalues[2, ], 2)
Combination of Chi Square Statistics for Multiply Imputed Data
Using 100 Imputed Data Sets
F(2, 705.79)=7.449      p=0.00063
> micombine.F(fvalues[3, ], 2)
Combination of Chi Square Statistics for Multiply Imputed Data
Using 100 Imputed Data Sets
F(2, 885.71)=0.559      p=0.5722
```

Combined F-statistics for factors `FEMALE`, `SCHOOL` and their interaction are identical to the output obtained by `mi.anova()`.

5.7.7.5 Combination of χ^2-Values and Other Model Fit Statistics

We have previously used M*plus* to fit the growth curve ZIP model from Sect. 5.2.2 to the various sets of imputed data for two reasons: First of all, ZIP models are currently not supported by R package `lavaan` for structural equation modelling. Secondly, M*plus* also automatically combines important statistics for model evaluation like the χ^2 statistic. In R, the `lavaan` package currently does not support automated analysis of multiply imputed data sets. However, the `semTools` package does and can produce results that are usually very close, or even identical to the ones obtained by M*plus*.[31]

To illustrate this, we re-analyse the example from Sect. 5.7.3. Now, however, we use function `growth.mi()` from package `semTools` to facilitate repeated data analysis and pooling of results.

`growth.mi()` takes the following main arguments as input: `model`, a `lavaan` model formula, and `data`, a list of imputed data sets. For further options, see `?growth.mi`. The generic `summary()` function then displays the model results. Argument `fit.measures = TRUE` lists pooled fit measures (including the pooled χ^2 statistic). Argument `fmi = TRUE` displays estimates for the fraction of missing information for the model parameters. `ci = TRUE` gives 95% confidence intervals for the model parameters. `asymptotic = TRUE` tells the function to use Rubin's (1987) combining rules for large samples, i.e., the degrees of freedom are assumed to be sufficiently large for the t statistic to follow a normal distribution. We used this option to get inferences that are identical to the ones reported in Sect. 5.7.3.

R code as well as the parts of the model output regarding the pooled χ^2-statistic and other model fit indices are listed below:

```
> implist <- vector(length = 100, mode = "list")
> for (i in 1:100) {
+ implist[[i]] <- complete(imp.mice.mt, i)
+ }
> growth.res <- growth.mi(model, implist)
> summary(growth.res, fit.measures = TRUE, fmi = TRUE, ci = TRUE,
+ asymptotic = TRUE)

Convergence information:
The model converged on 100 imputed data sets

Model Test User Model:

  Test statistic                                    81.042
  Degrees of freedom                                     4
  P-value                                            0.000

Model Test Baseline Model:

  Test statistic                                   538.821
  Degrees of freedom                                     6
  P-value                                            0.000

User Model versus Baseline Model:

  Comparative Fit Index (CFI)                        0.855
  Tucker-Lewis Index (TLI)                           0.783
```

[31]For further information, see option `mimic="Mplus"` in `lavaan` (https://cran.r-project.org/web/packages/lavaan/lavaan.pdf).

```
Root Mean Square Error of Approximation:

  RMSEA                                          0.097
  90 Percent confidence interval - lower         0.079
  90 Percent confidence interval - upper         0.115
  P-value RMSEA <= 0.05                          0.000

Standardized Root Mean Square Residual:

  SRMR                                           0.091
```

The combined χ^2-statistic is 81.042, $p < 0.001$, which indicates a bad model fit. Also the other fit statistics indicate that the 'normal' growth model does not fit the data well. According to Hu and Bentler (1999), CFI and TLI should be larger than 0.95, and RMSEA, as well as SRMR should be below 0.05 and 0.08, respectively.

Fitting the same model in M*plus* gives identical estimates of the model fit statistics, except for SRMR. Here, `lavaan` and M*plus* use different formulae by default. An SRMR estimate that is identical to the one given by M*plus* could be obtained by using the `fitmeasures()` function, and setting argument `fit.measures="srmr_mplus"` (see the supplementary material for details):

```
Chi-Square Test of Model Fit

          Value                               81.042
          Degrees of Freedom                       4
          P-Value                             0.0000

RMSEA (Root Mean Square Error Of Approximation)

          Estimate                             0.097
          90 Percent C.I.                      0.079  0.115
          Probability RMSEA <= .05             0.000

CFI/TLI

          CFI                                  0.855
          TLI                                  0.783

Chi-Square Test of Model Fit for the Baseline Model

          Value                              538.821
          Degrees of Freedom                       6
          P-Value                             0.0000

SRMR (Standardized Root Mean Square Residual)

          Value                                0.081
```

Combined parameter estimates, standard errors, as well as estimated fractions of missing information obtained by function `growth.mi` (not shown here) are furthermore identical to the ones reported in Sect. 5.7.3. `semTools` is thus a very useful package to facilitate repeated data analysis and pooling of results of `lavaan` models.

5.7.7.6 `datlist2mids`

In the previous sections, we have shown, how functions from packages `mice` and `miceadds` can be used to facilitate repeated data analysis and pooling of results. Typically, however, these functions require an object of class `mids` as input. In cases where data have been imputed by other packages (e.g., `norm2` or `Amelia`), the `datalist2mids()` function from package `miceadds` can be used to convert a `list` of imputed data sets to `mids` format. The code below illustrates this conversion. In the supplementary material of the book, readers will find a set of 100 data files (`imp1.dat`—`imp100.dat`), which are imputed by `norm2` and were written to disk in ASCII format.

In the first step, we create an empty `list` of length 100 and store these 100 completed data sets in the respective slot of this `list`. We then use the `datlist2mids()` function to convert the `list` to an object of class `mids`:

```
> implist <- vector(length = 100, mode = "list")
> for (i in 1:100) {
+ implist[[i]] <-
+        read.table(paste0("./imputations/other/norm2/imp", i,
+        ".dat"), col.names = c("id", "FEMALE", "RE", "GY",
+        "ACRIM", "BCRIM", "CCRIM", "DCRIM"))
+ }
> implist.mids <- miceadds::datlist2mids(implist)
```

Now, the resulting `mids` object can be used for repeated data analysis and pooling of results in R (here a Poisson model):

```
> mira <- with(implist.mids, glm(ACRIM ~ FEMALE + RE + GY,
+        family = poisson))
> result <- summary(pool(mira))
> round(result[, 1:5], 3)
               est    se      t      df Pr(>|t|)
(Intercept)  0.183 0.076  2.418 217.162    0.016
FEMALE      -0.619 0.077 -8.041 298.497    0.000
RE          -0.197 0.102 -1.933 201.791    0.055
GY          -0.530 0.095 -5.581 252.806    0.000
> round(result[, 6:10], 3)
             lo 95  hi 95 nmis   fmi lambda
(Intercept)  0.034  0.333   NA 0.587  0.583
FEMALE      -0.771 -0.468    0 0.491  0.488
RE          -0.397  0.004    0 0.611  0.607
GY          -0.717 -0.343    0 0.540  0.536
```

We want to draw attention to the relatively large fractions of missing information in this example, which suggests that results should be interpreted with caution. FMI is estimated from the completed data and therefore also depends on the chosen imputation model. Large FMI values could stem from a large number of missing values, but could also be an indicator that the imputation model was not adequate.

5.8 Diagnostic Tools

Model checking is an important step in the multiple imputation process that should not be neglected. A recent overview on different tools for MI model checking has been given by Nguyen, Carlin, and Lee (2017). Here, we focus on simple (descriptive and graphical) tools that can easily be applied in R.

In a first step we can inspect the imputed values either by means of histograms or boxplots, or by looking at descriptive summary statistics (cf. Sect. 2.6). This gives an idea of the plausibility of the imputations and also helps to identify extreme values. Nguyen et al. (2017) argue that 'judgements about the plausibility of the imputed data should be made with respect to subject matter knowledge' (p. 4). This means: Do the obtained imputations make sense from a theoretical point of view?

Furthermore, it is usually not problematic, if some of the imputed values are outside the range of the observed ones. However, extreme values which lie far outside the observed range can be a result of non-convergence of the imputation algorithm or a result of a misspecified imputation model.

5.8.1 Inspection of Imputed Values Using the `boxplot()` Function

To illustrate the process of MI model checking, we create a set of imputations using function `mice.impute.norm()`—i.e., Bayesian linear regression. The function assumes normally distributed error terms like any normal linear regression model. In our application, where the dependent variable was a zero-inflated count variable, this assumption is clearly violated. We use the data set `dat3` from Sect. 5.5.1, where we have split `ACRIM`–`DCRIM` into two separate variables: binary zero versus non-zero indicators, and zero-truncated count variables, respectively. Thus, the multivariate distribution of the integer-valued variables should be closer to a normal distribution. `acrim.c` is the zero-truncated count variable derived from variable `ACRIM`.

```
> load("./data/dat3.Rdata")
> ini <- mice(dat3, maxit = 0)
> method <- ini$method
> method[1:8] <- "norm"
> set.seed(123456)
> imp.mice.norm = mice(dat3, method = method, m = 100, maxit =
+         20, printFlag = FALSE)
> save(imp.mice.norm, file =
+         "./imputations/other/micenorm/imp.mice.norm.Rdata")
```

The resulting R object `imp.mice.norm` is of class `mids`. The imputations are stored in slot `$imp` of the `mids` object.

Now, we want to get an overview of the resulting imputations. We extract the set of imputations of variable `acrim.c` and store them in a `data.frame` object. This object has 1679 rows and 100 columns, which are labelled `X1–X100`:

```
> imp.acrim.c <- data.frame(imp.mice.norm$imp$acrim.c)
> head(imp.acrim.c[, 1:5])
          X1        X2         X3         X4        X5
3 -0.1445456 -1.964864  2.5769738  1.6483557 3.0036571
4  3.5863059  4.550958  2.4053458  3.9716251 1.0772613
5  3.3826765  6.064686  0.4019897 -2.3923536 0.5345809
6  1.5444311  1.499977  3.9302237  3.5210123 1.6605954
7  1.8778471  4.448703  0.4870001  2.2394383 3.0187463
9  1.7594917  2.227205 -1.7148685  0.4660177 2.1895376
```

We bring these data into long format and produce boxplots for the first 20 imputations:

```
> imp.acrim.c.long <- reshape(imp.acrim.c, varying =
+        list(c(paste0("X", 1:100))), direction = "long",
+        v.names = "acrim.c", times = 1:100, timevar = "IMP",
+        idvar = "ID")
> sub <- subset(imp.acrim.c.long, imp.acrim.c.long$IMP <= 20)
> pdf("./plots/plausibility1.pdf")
> boxplot(acrim.c ~ IMP, sub, xlab = "Imputation number", ylab =
+        "acrim.c", pch = 20, col = "gray80")
> dev.off()
```

`acrim.c` is the name of the variable in long format, `IMP` gives the imputation number. The `boxplot()` function is used to produce the boxplots. Formula `acrim.c~ IMP` produces separate boxplots of variable `acrim.c` for a `subset` (`sub`) of the $m = 100$ imputations. Figure 5.10 displays the resulting boxplots for the first 20 imputations of variable `acrim.c` based on the Bayesian normal linear regression model. As can be seen, imputations have a range between approximately -5 and 10 with a median around 1 and 2. The distributions appear to be symmetric. The figure indicates that the distribution of the imputed values does not fit the distribution of the original empirical data, because values below zero are not observed and negative counts of delinquent behaviours do not make any sense from an applied point of view.

To fit a Poisson model to the data, imputations would have to be rounded to non-negative integer values before the analysis, which could introduce bias (Horton et al., 2003), although according to Horton et al. (2003) the expected bias may be small because consequences of rounding seem to be strongest if the categorical discrete variable is binary or has only a few different possible values, and may be small in the case of discrete variables with a large number of possible realizations.

In the next section, we show how to use histograms for a direct comparison of the distributions of observed and imputed values.

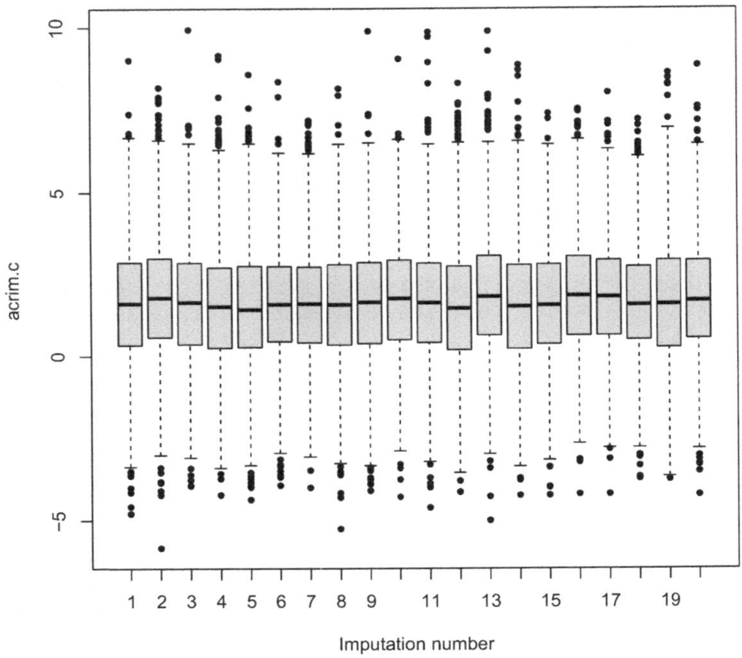

Fig. 5.10 Boxplots of the first 20 imputations of variable `acrim.c` obtained by `mice.impute.norm()`

5.8.2 *Comparison of the Distributions of Observed and Imputed Values Using the* `hist()` *Function*

To explore the similarity of the distribution of imputed values to the distribution of the observed part of the data, we can overlay histograms for the observed and imputed part of the data. In this example we use `mids` object `mice.impute.mt` from Sect. 5.4.

As already outlined, the different sets of imputations are stored in slot `$imp` of the `mids` object. We extract the different sets of imputations of variable `ACRIM` and store them in a data frame:

```
> imp.acrim <- data.frame(imp.mice.mt$imp$ACRIM)
> head(imp.acrim[, 1:15])
    X1 X2 X3 X4 X5 X6 X7 X8 X9 X10 X11 X12 X13 X14 X15
259  0  0  0  0  0  0  0  0  0   0   0   1   1   0   0
270  0  0  0  0  0  0  0  1  0   2   0   0   0   0   0
271  0  0  0  0  1  4  0  0  1   1   0   2   2   0   0
282  1  2  8  7  0  3  5  0  2   1   3   1   2   1   2
284  1  0  0  1  2  0  1  1  0   0   0   0   0   1   0
285  0  1  0  4  0  0  1  0  0   5   0   0   0   0   3
```

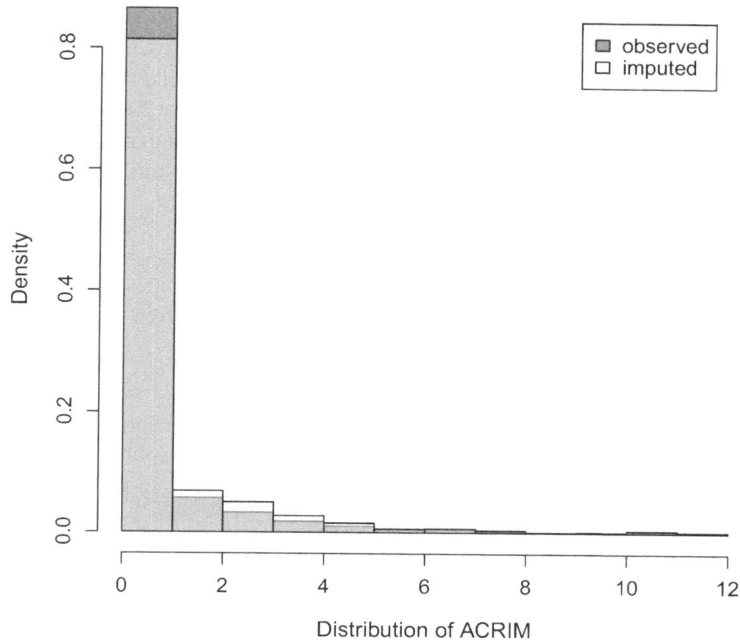

Fig. 5.11 Histograms of observed and imputed values of variable `ACRIM` obtained by `mice.impute.midastouch()`

`imp.acrim` has 689 rows (`ACRIM` had 689 missing values) and 100 columns (we created $m = 100$ imputations).

Analogous to the previous section, we bring this `data.frame` into long format. We extract the subsets of cases with observed and missing delinquency scores at wave one and use the `hist()` function to overlay the histograms of observed and imputed `ACRIM` scores. Argument `add=TRUE` tells R to plot the second histogram over the first one. We define light gray and dark gray colour (with transparency `alpha`) to distinguish between imputed and observed data, respectively (see Fig. 5.11).

```
> imp.acrim.long <- reshape(imp.acrim, varying =
+         list(c(paste0("X", 1:100))), direction = "long",
+         v.names = "ACRIM", times = 1:100, timevar = "IMP",
+         idvar = "ID")
> sub.com = subset(dat, !is.na(dat$ACRIM))
> pdf("./plots/plausibility2.pdf")
> hist(sub.com$ACRIM, col = gray(0.1, alpha = 0.5), freq =
+         FALSE, xlab = "Distribution of ACRIM", main = "")
> hist(imp.acrim.long$ACRIM, col = gray(0.8, alpha = 0.5), freq
+         = FALSE, add = TRUE, breaks = 0:12)
> legend("topright", legend = c("observed", "imputed"), fill =
+         c(gray(0.1, alpha = 0.5), gray(0.8, alpha = 0.5)))
> dev.off()
```

As can be seen, less zeros are imputed in comparison to the observed data. From a theoretical point of view, imputations are not implausible. We have explored that male students and students from Hauptschule are more likely to have missing delinquency scores (Sections 5.2.1, 5.3.2, Reinecke & Weins, 2013). Furthermore, both gender and school type predict delinquency, so we might expect less zeros and more non-zero imputations among the subgroup of participants with unobserved delinquency at wave one.

5.8.3 *Comparison of Observed and Imputed Values Using the `stripplot()` Function*

Another method to compare the distributions of observed and imputed data is the `stripplot()` function from package `mice` (van Buuren & Groothuis-Oudshoorn, 2011)—see Fig. 5.12. While histograms give a more global picture,

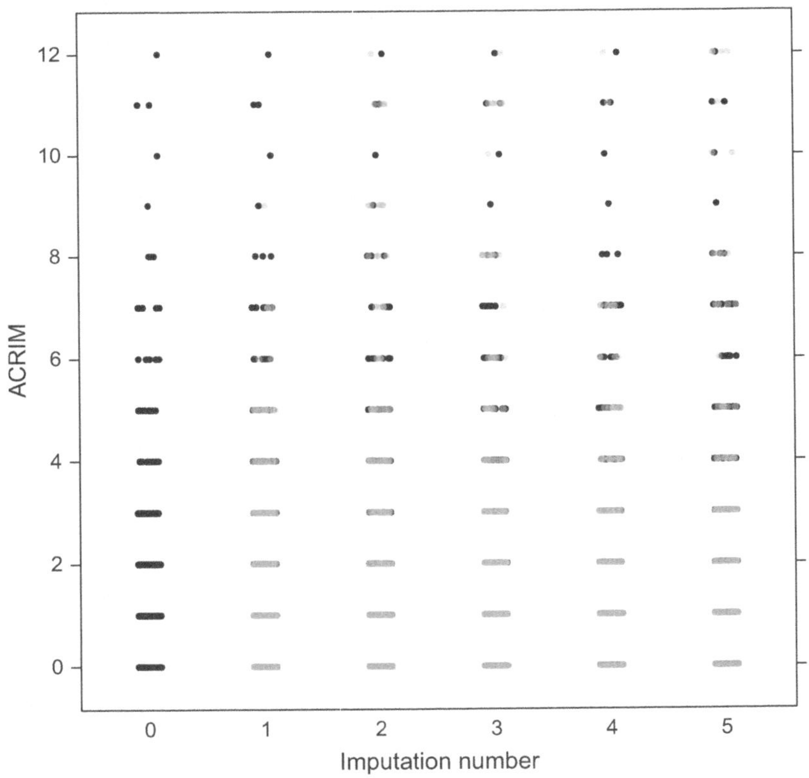

Fig. 5.12 Stripplot of observed (black) and imputed (gray) values for the first 5 imputations of variable `ACRIM` obtained by `mice.impute.midastouch()`

stripplots are extremely helpful to obtain more detailed information. With stripplots we can inspect if imputations can be found across the whole range of the distribution of the observed cases, or if imputations are clustered in certain regions, or may not be found at all in certain regions. If the latter cases are true, applied researchers are advised to reflect, if absence or clustering of imputations in certain regions makes sense from a theoretical perspective, if a selective missing data mechanism is plausible, or if the result may reflect a shortcoming of the applied imputation method.

In our example, we again use `mids` object `imp.mice.mt` from Sect. 5.4. However, we do not want to create a plot for the entire set of $m = 100$ imputations—the plot would be too dense and we would not be able to see any systematic pattern in the plot. Instead we inspect only the first five imputations of variable `ACRIM`. The easiest way to achieve this is to make a copy of `imp.mice.mt` and overwrite the `$m` slot. Next, we load the required `lattice` package and produce the stripplot:

```
> imp.mice.mt.copy <- imp.mice.mt
> imp.mice.mt.copy$m <- 5
> library(lattice)
> pdf("./plots/plausibility3.pdf")
> stripplot(imp.mice.mt.copy, data = ACRIM ~ .imp, col =
+         c("black", gray(0.6, alpha = 0.5)), pch = 20)
> dev.off()
```

We overwrite the default colour settings and use black and gray colour for observed and imputed data, respectively. The first strip in Fig. 5.12 shows the slightly jittered observed data points of variable `ACRIM`, the other strips show observed *and* imputed values. We used slightly transparent gray colour to be better able to distinguish the distributions. We see gray data points across the whole range of delinquency scores from 0 to 12. Furthermore there are many more data points in the lower regions than in the upper regions of the distribution, reflecting the fact that the majority of participants reported no or very few offences in the previous year.

In the next paragraph, we discuss descriptive statistics that help to get an even more detailed picture about the distributions of observed and imputed data.

5.8.4 Comparison of Observed and Imputed Values Using `compare.percent.count()`

The `compare.percent.count()` function, which is available from the supplementary material of the book, reads in three arguments: `orig`, `imp`, and `counts`. `imp` is an object of class `mids`, a multiply imputed data set created by the `mice` package.[32] Furthermore, argument `orig` is a `data.frame` containing the original

[32]The transformation of imputed data lists that were created by other packages to an object of class `mids` is described in Sect. 5.7.

incomplete data. Finally, counts is a string vector giving the names of the count variables in the data set.

The function compares percentages of observed and imputed counts for the variables specified in counts. In the example below, we compare observed and imputed percentages of counts for variables ACRIM and BCRIM. Imputations were created by mice.impute.midastouch(), as outlined in Sect. 5.4.

```
> source("./functions/compare.percent.count.R")
> result <- compare.percent.count(orig = dat, imp = imp.mice.mt,
+ counts = c("ACRIM", "BCRIM"))
> result$ACRIM[, 1:11]
             0     1    2    3    4    5    6    7    8    9   10
imputed  64.96 16.48 6.86 5.03 2.74 1.55 0.57 0.66 0.36 0.09 0.14
observed 72.00 14.62 5.67 3.27 1.82 1.02 0.51 0.51 0.22 0.07 0.07
> result$BCRIM[, 1:11]
             0     1    2    3    4    5    6    7   8    9   10
imputed  51.88 19.64 7.72 6.57 4.47 3.68 1.71 1.41 0.8 0.48 0.44
observed 60.65 17.28 7.32 4.68 3.36 2.58 1.26 0.96 0.6 0.36 0.24
```

As argued before, two explanations for discrepancies between the observed and imputed counts are possible: Firstly, differences between observed and imputed counts can stem from the underlying MAR mechanism. For example, we have argued before that boys as well as students from Hauptschule have higher missingness probabilities. Furthermore, as gender and school type is related to delinquency, it makes sense from a theoretical point of view, that the observed part of the data set contains more zeros than the imputed part.

Secondly, differences could also indicate a misspecified imputation model. In our case, the function output does not suggest any severe model misspecifications. However, using PMM in this case might not be unproblematic (due to the underlying normal linear regression model), as we have argued before. For a general discussion of predictive mean matching, see Sect. 4.5.7.

5.8.5 Comparison of Observed and Imputed Values Using compare.obs.imp()

The compare.obs.imp() function, which is available from the supplementary material of the book reads in the original incomplete data (argument orig) and a mids object created by mice (argument imp). It reads out summary statistics (obtained by the summary() function) for the observed and imputed parts of the data. In the example below, we use mids object imp.mice.mt, which we have created in Sect. 5.4:

```
> source("./functions/compare.obs.imp.R")
> result <- compare.obs.imp(dat, imp.mice.mt)
> print(result, digits = 3)
$ACRIM
```

```
         Min. 1st Qu. Median  Mean 3rd Qu. Max.
imputed     0       0      0 0.834       1   12
observed    0       0      0 0.604       1   12

$BCRIM
         Min. 1st Qu. Median Mean 3rd Qu. Max.
imputed     0       0      0 1.41       2   15
observed    0       0      0 1.06       1   15

$CCRIM
         Min. 1st Qu. Median Mean 3rd Qu. Max.
imputed     0       0      1 1.53       2   16
observed    0       0      0 1.29       2   16

$DCRIM
         Min. 1st Qu. Median Mean 3rd Qu. Max.
imputed     0       0      1 1.39       2   16
observed    0       0      0 1.00       1   16
```

From the output above, we can see that the range of imputations created by `mice.impute.midastouch()` matches the range of the original data. When looking at the quantiles and the means, we see that the distributions differ quite a bit. The medians of variables `CCRIM` and `DCRIM` are larger for the imputed part in comparison to the observed part. Additionally, third quartiles of variables `BCRIM` and `DCRIM` are larger for the imputed part. Finally, all means are larger for the imputed in comparison to the observed part. As already discussed in the previous section, these differences both make sense from a theoretical perspective.

5.8.6 Assessing the Suitability of the Imputation Method by Means of Monte Carlo Simulation

We have discussed multiple imputation theory and the criteria regarding properness of imputation methods in Chaps. 3 and 4. Recall that if the imputation method is proper, inferences tend to be valid.

Many imputation methods require parametric assumptions such as (multivariate) normality to be met. In practice, however, these parametric assumptions are seldomly (entirely) met. Furthermore, systematic Monte Carlo simulations are often scarce regarding the robustness of a given imputation method towards violated assumptions in a particular scenario.

To get at least a rough idea, if an imputation method is suitable for the empirical data at hand in a certain scenario, we can run simulations based on the complete cases. The general idea is

1. to create a set of complete Bootstrap samples from the completely observed cases,
2. estimate a statistical model of interest using these Bootstrap samples,
3. delete values from the complete-data sets,

4. impute the data and re-estimate the models and
5. compare complete-data estimates with estimates based on the imputed data sets.

Note that the true distribution of the observed and unobserved part of the data, the true missing data mechanism and the true parameters are unknown. With the simulation method we cannot assess, how well the imputation method can estimate these unknown parameters. We can, however, get an idea about whether the chosen imputation method can reproduce the estimates based on the simulated complete data under the assumed missing data process. An imputation method may be regarded as suitable for the problem at hand, if model estimates based on MI are close to the complete-data estimates.

Let us illustrate this with an example: We sample with replacement $N = 2064$ cases (the original sample size) from the completely observed cases (which we label `cc`) and replicate this process 1000 times.

```
> cc <- dat[complete.cases(dat), -1]
> cdata <- vector(length = 1000, mode = "list")
> set.seed(123456)
> for (i in 1:1000) {
+ s <- sample(1:nrow(cc), nrow(dat), replace = TRUE)
+ cdata[[i]] <- cc[s, ]
+ }
```

The 1000 (complete) bootstrap samples are stored in object `cdata`. Recall that variable `ACRIM` had around 33% missing data. In the next step, we want to impose a simple MCAR mechanism and create 33% missing data in `ACRIM`. Note that even under MCAR, MI can produce biased results, if the imputation model is misspecified.[33] The resulting 1000 incomplete data sets are stored in `list` object `mdata`:

```
> set.seed(123456)
> mdata <- cdata
> for (i in 1:1000) {
+ s <- sample(1:nrow(dat), round(0.33 * nrow(dat)), replace =
+         FALSE)
+ mdata[[i]][s, "ACRIM"] <- NA
+ }
```

Now we have to perform the analyses on the complete data 1000 times. The overall set of estimates is then obtained by averaging the respective estimates across the 1000 replications.

In this example, we want to fit the growth model from Sect. 5.7, using package `lavaan`:

```
> library(lavaan)
> model <- '
```

[33]Instead of a simple MCAR mechanism, applied researchers could also simulate more complex and more realistic MAR or MNAR mechanisms that are believed to be present in the empirical data.

```
+ i =~ 1*ACRIM + 1*BCRIM + 1*CCRIM + 1*DCRIM
+ s =~ 0*ACRIM + 1*BCRIM + 2*CCRIM + 3*DCRIM
+ q =~ 0*ACRIM + 1*BCRIM + 4*CCRIM + 9*DCRIM
+ i ~~ 0*q
+ s ~~ 0*q
+ q ~~ 0*q
+ '
```

The set of 1000 estimates are stored in `list` object `cd.est`:

```
> cd.est <- vector(length = 1000, mode = "list")
> for (i in 1:1000) {
+ fit <- growth(model, data = cdata[[i]])
+ s <- parameterEstimates(fit)
+ cd.est[[i]] <- s$est
+ }
```

Next, we extract the coefficients that interest us the most from the model output: the latent intercept factor (`I`), linear and quadratic slope (`S` and `Q`), intercept variance (`Ivar`), slope variance (`Svar`), and the covariance between intercept and slope (`IS`). `Q` is the `vector` of complete-data estimates, the average of the respective quantities across the 1000 replications:

```
> library(abind)
> cd.est.matrix <- abind(cd.est, along = 2)
> cd.est.matrix <- cd.est.matrix[c(20, 21, 22, 27, 28, 29), ]
> Q = apply(cd.est.matrix, 1, mean)
> names(Q) = c("Ivar", "Svar", "IS", "I", "S", "Q")
```

We intend to compare the complete-data estimates with estimates obtained by multiple imputation. So, we set up an empty list object `imp` for the 1000 sets of imputations. Then we impute the data (here: using PMM in `mice`):

```
> imp <- vector(length = 1000, mode = "list")
> library(mice)
> set.seed(123456)
> for (i in 1:1000) {
+ imp[[i]] <- mice(mdata[[i]], printFlag = FALSE)
+ }
```

Repeatedly fitting the `lavaan` models works analogous to the steps described above. The only difference is that we now have two `for` loops: the outer loop for the 1000 replications and the inner loop for the m imputed data sets within each of the 1000 replications. To pool the m results, respectively, we use function `miInference` from package `norm2`. Point estimates are stored in `list` `mi.est`, lower and upper bounds of a normal theory confidence interval are stored in `list` objects `lo` and `hi`:

```
> library(norm2)
> mi.est <- lo <- hi vector(length = 1000, mode = "list")
> for (i in 1:1000) {
+ est <- se <- vector(length = imp[[i]]$m, mode = "list")
+ for (m in 1:imp[[i]]$m) {
+ fit <- growth(model, data = complete(imp[[i]], m))
```

```
+ s <- parameterEstimates(fit)
+ est[[m]] <- s$est
+ se[[m]] <- s$se
+ }
+ miinf <- (miInference(est, se))
+ mi.est[[i]] <- miinf$est
+ lo[[i]] <- miinf$est -1 * qt(.975,miinf$df) * miinf$std.err
+ hi[[i]] <- miinf$est +1 * qt(.975,miinf$df) * miinf$std.err
+ }
```

The next steps are analogous to the complete-data steps described above. We extract the model parameters of interest and average the MI parameter estimates across the replications:

```
> mi.est.matrix <- abind(mi.est, along = 2)
> mi.est.matrix <- mi.est.matrix[c(20, 21, 22, 27, 28, 29), ]
> Qhat <- apply(mi.est.matrix, 1, mean)
> names(Qhat) <- c("Ivar", "Svar", "IS", "I", "S", "Q")
```

We define bias as the difference between the average complete-data estimate and the average estimate based on imputation.

```
> Bias <- Q - Qhat
> round(Bias, 3)
  Ivar   Svar     IS      I      S      Q
 0.020 -0.004  0.000 -0.007  0.008 -0.002
> PBias = abs(((Q - Qhat)/Q) * 100)
> round(PBias, 3)
 Ivar  Svar    IS     I     S     Q
2.178 2.433 0.498 1.639 2.572 2.947
```

Bias can also be expressed in relative terms (bias relative to the complete-data estimates). Regarding this particular analysis, all relative biases are below 3% and can be deemed sufficiently small. In this scenario, predictive mean matching performed well (with regards to MI point estimates).

Additionally, one could look at further evaluation criteria such as coverage rates of the 95% confidence intervals. Note again that this illustration was based on the complete cases of the CrimoC data and on missing values being MCAR. The true distribution of observed and missing data, as well as the true missing data mechanism is unknown. This simulation can thus only be taken as a rough approximation of the true missing data problem, but it can help identify possible problems of the selected imputation method.

References

Allison, P. D. (2001). *Missing data*. Thousand Oaks, CA: Sage.

Andridge, R. R. (2011). Quantifying the impact of fixed effects modeling of clusters in multiple imputation for cluster randomized trials. *Biometrical Journal, 53*(1), 57–74.

Barnard, J., & Rubin, D. B. (1999). Small-sample degrees of freedom with multiple imputation. *Biometrika, 86*(4), 948–955.

Bodner, T. E. (2008). What improves with increased missing data imputations? *Structural Equation Modeling, 15*(4), 651–675.

Boers, K., Reinecke, J., Seddig, D., & Mariotti, L. (2010). Explaining the development of adolescent violent delinquency. *European Journal of Criminology, 7*(6), 499–520.

Bollen, K. A., & Curran, P. J. (2006). *Latent curve models: A structural equation perspective*. New York, NY: Wiley.

Bryk, A. S., & Raudenbush, S. W. (1992). *Hierarchical linear models*. Newbury Park, CA: Sage.

Carpenter, J. R., Goldstein, H., & Kenward, M. G. (2011). REALCOM-IMPUTE software for multilevel multiple imputation with mixed response types. *Journal of Statistical Software, 45*(5), 1–14.

Collins, L. M., Schafer, J. L., & Kam, C. M. (2001). A comparison of inclusive and restrictive strategies in modern missing data procedures. *Psychological Methods, 6*(4), 330–351.

Dahl, F. A. (2007). Convergence of random k-nearest-neighbour imputation. *Computational Statistics & Data Analysis, 51*(12), 5913–5917.

de Jong, R., van Buuren, S., & Spiess, M. (2016). Multiple imputation of predictor variables using generalized additive models. *Communications in Statistics – Simulation and Computation, 45*(3), 968–985.

Drechsler, J. (2015). Multiple imputation of multilevel missing data—Rigor versus simplicity. *Journal of Educational and Behavioral Statistics, 40*(1), 69–95.

Enders, C. K. (2010). *Applied missing data analysis*. New York, NY: Guilford.

Enders, C. K., Mistler, S. A., & Keller, B. T. (2016). Multilevel multiple imputation: A review and evaluation of joint modeling and chained equations imputation. *Psychological Methods, 21*(2), 222–240.

Gaffert, P., Meinfelder, F., & Bosch, V. (2016). *Towards an MI-proper predictive mean matching* (Discussion Paper). https://www.uni-bamberg.de/fileadmin/uni/fakultaeten/sowi_lehrstuehle/statistik/Personen/Dateien_Florian/properPMM.pdf.

Gałecki, A., & Burzykowski, T. (2013). *Linear mixed-effects models using R: A step-by-step approach*. Heidelberg/New York, NY: Springer.

Graham, J. W. (2009). Missing data analysis: Making it work in the real world. *Annual Review of Psychology, 60*, 549–576.

Graham, J. W., Olchowski, A. E., & Gilreath, T. D. (2007). How many imputations are really needed? Some practical clarifications of multiple imputation theory. *Prevention Science, 8*(3), 206–213.

Grund, S., Lüdtke, O., & Robitzsch, A. (2016). Multiple imputation of missing covariate values in multilevel models with random slopes: A cautionary note. *Behavior Research Methods, 48*(2), 640–649.

Harel, O. (2009). The estimation of r^2 and adjusted r^2 in incomplete data sets using multiple imputation. *Journal of Applied Statistics, 36*(10), 1109–1118.

He, Y., & Raghunathan, T. E. (2009). On the performance of sequential regression multiple imputation methods with non normal error distributions. *Communications in Statistics – Simulation and Computation, 38*(4), 856–883.

Hilbe, J. M. (2011). *Negative binomial regression* (2nd ed.). Cambridge, UK: Cambridge University Press.

Hill, M. (1997). *SPSS missing value analysis 7.5*. Chicago, IL: SPSS.

Horton, N. J., Lipsitz, S. R., & Parzen, M. (2003). A potential for bias when rounding in multiple imputation. *The American Statistician, 57*(4), 229–232.

Hox, J. J. (2010). *Multilevel analysis: Techniques and applications* (2nd ed.). New York, NY: Routledge.

Hu, L.-t., & Bentler, P. M. (1999). Cutoff criteria for fit indexes in covariance structure analysis: Conventional criteria versus new alternatives. *Structural Equation Modeling: A Multidisciplinary Journal, 6*(1), 1–55.

Kleinke, K. (2017). Multiple imputation under violated distributional assumptions—a systematic evaluation of the assumed robustness of predictive mean matching. *Journal of Educational and Behavioral Statistics, 42*(4), 371–404.

Kleinke, K. (2018). Multiple imputation by predictive mean matching when sample size is small. *Methodology, 14*(1), 3–15.
Kleinke, K., Stemmler, M., Reinecke, J., & Lösel, F. (2011). Efficient ways to impute incomplete panel data. *Advances in Statistical Analysis, 95*(4), 351–373.
Lally, J. R., Mangione, P. L., & Honig, A. S. (1988). The Syracuse University Family Development Research Program: Long-range impact of an early intervention with low-income children and their families. In D. R. Powell (Ed.), *Parent education as early childhood intervention: Emerging directions in theory, research and practice* (pp. 79–104). Norwood, NJ: Ablex.
Lambert, D. (1992). Zero-inflated Poisson regression, with an application to defects in manufacturing. *Technometrics, 34*(1), 1–14.
Lüdtke, O., Robitzsch, A., & Grund, S. (2017). Multiple imputation of missing data in multilevel designs: A comparison of different strategies. *Psychological Methods, 22*(1), 141–165.
Mariotti, L., & Reinecke, J. (2010). *Wachstums- und Mischverteilungsmodelle unter Berücksichtigung unbeobachteter Heterogenität: Empirische Analysen zum delinquenten Verhalten Jugendlicher in Duisburg* [Growth models, mixture models, and unobserved heterogeneity: Empirical analyses of juvenile delinquent behaviors in Duisburg.] Münster, Germany: Institut für sozialwissenschaftliche Forschung e.V.
McCord, J. (1978). A thirty-year follow-up of treatment effects. *American Psychologist, 33*(3), 284–289.
Meng, X.-L. (1994). Multiple-imputation inferences with uncongenial sources of input. *Statistical Science, 9*(4), 538–558.
Meng, X.-L. & Rubin, D. B. (1992). Performing likelihood ratio tests with multiply-imputed data sets. *Biometrika, 79*(1), 103–111.
Moffitt, T. E. (1993). Adolescence-limited and life-course-persistent antisocial behavior: A developmental taxonomy. *Psychological Review, 100*(4), 674–701.
Morris, T. P., White, I. R., & Royston, P. (2014). Tuning multiple imputation by predictive mean matching and local residual draws. *BMC Medical Research Methodology, 14*(1), 75–87.
Muthén, L. K. & Muthén, B. O. (2017). *Mplus user's guide* (8th ed.). Los Angeles, CA: Muthén & Muthén.
Nguyen, C. D., Carlin, J. B., & Lee, K. J. (2017). Model checking in multiple imputation: An overview and case study. *Emerging Themes in Epidemiology, 14*(8), 1–12.
Pöge, A. (2005). Persönliche Codes bei Längsschnittstudien. Ein Erfahrungsbericht. *ZA-Nachrichten, 56*, 50–69.
Pöge, A. (2008). Persönliche Codes 'reloaded'. *Methoden—Daten—Analysen, 2*(1), 59–70.
Reinecke, J., & Seddig, D. (2011). Growth mixture models in longitudinal research. *AStA Advances in Statistical Analysis, 95*(4), 415–434.
Reinecke, J., & Weins, C. (2013). The development of delinquency during adolescence: A comparison of missing data techniques. *Quality & Quantity, 47*(6), 3319–3334.
Rosseel, Y. (2012). `lavaan`: An R Package for structural equation modeling. *Journal of Statistical Software, 48*(2), 1–36.
Rubin, D. B. (1987). *Multiple imputation for nonresponse in surveys*. New York, NY: Wiley.
Rubin, D. B. (1996). Multiple imputation after 18+ years. *Journal of the American Statistical Association, 91*(434), 473–489.
Schafer, J. L. (1997). *Analysis of incomplete multivariate data*. London, UK: Chapman & Hall.
Schafer, J. L. (1999b). NORM users guide (version 2) [Computer software manual]. University Park, PA: The Methodology Center, The Pennsylvania State University. https://www.methodology.psu.edu/training/missing-data/.
Schafer, J. L. (2016). `norm2`: Analysis of incomplete multivariate data under a normal model [Computer software manual]. https://CRAN.R-project.org/package=norm2 (R Package Version 2.0.1).
Schafer, J. L. & Graham, J. W. (2002). Missing data: Our view of the state of the art. *Psychological Methods, 7*(2), 147–177.
Schafer, J. L., & Olsen, M. K. (1998). Multiple imputation for missing-data problems: A data analyst's perspective. *Multivariate Behavioral Research, 33*(4), 545–571.

Schafer, J. L., & Olsen, M. K. (1999). *Modeling and imputation of semicontinuous survey variables*. https://citeseerx.ist.psu.edu/viewdoc/summary?doi=10.1.1.159.7891

Schafer, J. L., & Yucel, R. M. (2002). Computational strategies for multivariate linear mixed-effects models with missing values. *Journal of Computational and Graphical Statistics, 11*(2), 437–457.

Schenker, N., & Taylor, J. M. G. (1996). Partially parametric techniques for multiple imputation. *Computational Statistics & Data Analysis, 22*(4), 425–446.

Siddique, J., & Belin, T. R. (2008). Multiple imputation using an iterative hot-deck with distance-based donor selection. *Statistics in Medicine, 27*(1), 83–102.

Speidel, M., Drechsler, J., & Sakshaug, J. W. (2018). Biases in multilevel analyses caused by cluster-specific fixed-effects imputation. *Behavior Research Methods, 50*(5), 1824–1840.

Spiess, M., Kleinke, K., & Reinecke, J. (in press). Proper multiple imputation of clustered or panel data. In P. Lynn (Ed.), *Advances in longitudinal survey methodology*. New York, NY: Wiley. https://www.wiley.com/en-us/Advances+in+Longitudinal+Survey+Methodology-p-9781119376934

Su, Y.-S., Gelman, A., Hill, J., & Yajima, M. (2011). Multiple imputation with diagnostics (mi) in R: Opening windows into the black box. *Journal of Statistical Software, 45*(2), 1–31.

van Buuren, S. (2011). Multiple imputation of multilevel data. In J. J. Hox & J. K. Roberts (Eds.), *Handbook of advanced multilevel analysis* (pp. 173–196). New York, NY: Taylor & Francis.

van Buuren, S. (2012). *Flexible imputation of missing data*. Boca Raton, FL: Chapmann & Hall/CRC.

van Buuren, S. (2013). *Multiple imputation of multilevel data*. Paper presented at the Conference on Recent Advances in Multiple Imputation, with Emphasis on Dealing with Deviations from MAR or Exchangeability, Utrecht, the Netherlands.

van Buuren, S., & Groothuis-Oudshoorn, K. (2011). `mice`: Multivariate imputation by chained equations in R. *Journal of Statistical Software, 45*(3), 1–67.

Venables, W. N., & Ripley, B. D. (2002). *Modern applied statistics with* `S` (4th ed.). New York, NY: Springer.

Vink, G., Lazendic, G., & van Buuren, S. (2015). Partitioned predictive mean matching as a large data multilevel imputation technique. *Psychological Test and Assessment Modeling, 57*(4), 577–594.

Weins, C., & Reinecke, J. (2007). Delinquenzverläufe im Jugendalter: Eine methodologische Analyse zur Auswirkung von fehlenden Werten im Längsschnitt [Development of Juvenile Delinquency: An analysis of the effects of missing data]. *Monatsschrift für Kriminologie und Strafrechtsreform, 90*(5), 418–437.

Yu, L. M., Burton, A., & Rivero-Arias, O. (2007). Evaluation of software for multiple imputation of semi-continuous data. *Statistical Methods in Medical Research, 16*(3), 243–258.

Chapter 6
Multiple Imputation: New Developments

6.1 Overview

In this chapter, we discuss new developments in the field of multiple imputation. Our focus will be on non-standard missing data problems, i.e., we focus on situations, where distributional assumptions of standard MI approaches (for example, multivariate normality or homoscedasticity) are violated, and outline solutions to these problems.

When incomplete data are counts, which are typically skewed, the `countimp` package has solutions to create imputations based on the Poisson or the negative binomial model, but also based on zero-inflation models, hurdle models, and two-level generalized linear mixed-effects count models (Sect. 6.2). In addition to parametric models that do not rely on normality, we also discuss semi- and nonparametric imputation procedures like the R-package `ImputeRobust` (Sect. 6.3), which creates imputations based on generalized additive models for location, scale and shape. R-package `Qtools` (Sect. 6.4) furthermore has functions to create imputations based on nonparametric quantile regression. At the moment, functions from packages `Qtools` and `ImputeRobust` do not yet support multilevel imputation models. Robust methods for multilevel data are still scarce. One approach that might be useful in this context is an extension of semi-parametric predictive mean matching to two-level data (Sect. 6.5). Although systematic evaluations are to our best knowledge not yet available, two-level predictive mean matching should be more robust against violations of distributional assumptions than the fully parametric multilevel multiple imputation functions from Chap. 5. Finally, in Sect. 6.6, we apply these methods to the longitudinal CrimoC data and discuss, to what extent the respective imputation method influences results of the growth curve ZIP model from Sect. 5.2.2.

Note that all of these methods build upon (and extend) the multiple imputation by chained equations framework and work hand in hand with R-package `mice` (see

K. Kleinke et al., *Applied Multiple Imputation*,
Statistics for Social and Behavioral Sciences,
https://doi.org/10.1007/978-3-030-38164-6_6

Chap. 5). Empirical researchers, who are already familiar with `mice`, will find it quite easy to apply these methods.

6.2 Parametric Multiple Imputation of Incomplete Count Data

Count data are non-negative integer values and give the frequency of occurrences of an event or a certain behaviour, often within a given timespan, e.g., the number of delinquent behaviours within one year or the number of days a patient spends in hospital. Count data distributions are skewed in many applications and should therefore not be analysed by standard data analysis techniques that rely on the normal model like standard ordinary least squares (OLS) regression (Erdman, Jackson, & Sinko, 2008). The same is true for multiple imputation models. If it has to be assumed that the conditional distribution of the count variable to be imputed conditional on predictors is skewed, then the variable should not be imputed by methods that are based on the normal model (Kleinke, 2017; Yu et al., 2007).

Hence, in case of incompletely observed count variables and under the assumption that this variable conditional on the relevant predictors follows a distribution for count variables, a corresponding imputation model should be chosen. Unfortunately, most standard multiple imputation packages either do not provide count data imputation models or they support only very basic count models: `IVEware`[1], for example, currently supports an ordinary Poisson model. R-package `mi` (Sect. 5.5) allows to create multiple imputations based on a quasi-Poisson imputation model (see Sect. 6.2.1 for an overview on count models). `ice` for Stata supports imputation based on a Poisson or negative binomial model. Typically, zero-inflation models or multilevel count models are not supported by any of the standard MI packages.

This is problematic, because as discussed in Chap. 4, a misspecified imputation method may imply an improper imputation method and invalid inferences. For example, regarding misspecified count imputation models, see Kleinke and Reinecke (2013b) or de Jong et al. (2016). Kleinke and Reinecke (2013a) have provided additional `mice` imputation functions based on the most commonly used count data models: Package `countimp` supports multivariate (wide format) imputation of incomplete count data under the classical Poisson model, the quasi-Poisson model, the negative Binomial model, the zero-inflated Poisson or negative binomial model, or the Poisson or negative binomial hurdle model. Additionally, long format two-level count data can be imputed by a generalized linear mixed-effects Poisson or negative Binomial model. Zero-inflation in multilevel data is also supported. For a very comprehensive introduction to count data models, see Hilbe (2011). A brief introduction is given in the following section.

[1] https://www.src.isr.umich.edu/software/.

6.2.1 Count Data Modeling in a Nutshell

The most basic count model is the Poisson generalized linear model (GLM). Here, the probability of observing a certain count y_i for unit i given covariates $\mathbf{x}_i$ is

$$P(y_i \mid \mathbf{x}_i) = \frac{e^{-\lambda_i}\lambda_i^{y_i}}{y_i!}, \quad y_i = 0, 1, 2, \ldots , \tag{6.1}$$

where $E(y_i \mid \mathbf{x}_i) = \lambda_i = \exp(\mathbf{x}_i^T \boldsymbol{\beta})$, $\text{var}(y_i \mid \mathbf{x}_i) = \lambda_i$ and the skewness is given by $1/\sqrt{\lambda_i}$. Skewness increases with decreasing λ. Thus, with decreasing λ, the normal model becomes less appropriate for these data (cf. Kleinke, 2017).

Note furthermore that the Poisson model assumes equidispersion, which means that the variance of the count variable has to be equal to its mean. This assumption is often violated in empirical data because very often the variance is larger than the mean, i.e., the data are *overdispersed*. Using a standard Poisson model for the analysis of overdispersed data can lead to underestimated standard errors and therefore to too liberal test statistics, i.e., hypothesis tests are rejected too often and confidence intervals are too short (cf. Zeileis, Kleiber, & Jackman, 2008).

Both the quasi-Poisson model and the negative binomial model (NB) estimate an extra parameter that represents the amount of overdispersion in the data. The quasi-Poisson model estimates Pearson dispersion δ

$$\hat{\delta} = \frac{\sum_{i=1}^{n} R_{pi}^2}{\text{df}_{\text{resid}}} , \tag{6.2}$$

with $R_{pi} = (y_i - \hat{\lambda}_i)/\hat{\lambda}_i^{1/2}$ being the Pearson residuals. $\hat{\lambda}_i$ is the estimated mean of y_i conditional on $\mathbf{x}_i$ and df_{resid} are the residual degrees of freedom. $\hat{\delta}$ is then used to correct the standard error (se) from the Poisson regression model (Hilbe, 2011):

$$\text{se}_{\text{corrected}} = \text{se}\sqrt{\hat{\delta}} . \tag{6.3}$$

The NB model estimates a dispersion parameter $\alpha > 0$, which represents the random variation in y_i that is not fully accounted for by $\mathbf{x}_i$. For different parametrizations of the model, see Hilbe (2011). Conditionally on $\mathbf{x}_i$, y_i is distributed as

$$P(y_i \mid \mathbf{x}_i) = \frac{\theta^\theta \mu_i^{y_i} \Gamma(\theta + y_i)}{\Gamma(y_i + 1)\Gamma(\theta)(\mu_i + \theta)^{\theta + y_i}}, \tag{6.4}$$

with conditional mean $\mu_i = E(y_i \mid \mathbf{x}_i) = \exp(\mathbf{x}_i^T \boldsymbol{\beta})$ and variance $\text{var}(y_i \mid \mathbf{x}_i) = \mu_i(1 + \alpha\mu_i)$, where $\alpha = \theta^{-1} > 0$. Note that the mean of $y_i \mid \mathbf{x}_i$ is the same as in the Poisson model but the variance is larger. Further, the NB distribution converges to a Poisson distribution, when $\alpha \to 0$.

Sometimes, empirical count data are *zero-inflated*, which means that the empirical data contain more zero counts than one would expect under both the standard Poisson or the negative binomial model. In our juvenile delinquency example from Chap. 5, most participants did not report to have committed any punishable offence in the previous year. Models that address an excess number of zero counts are so-called zero-inflation models (Lambert, 1992) and hurdle models (Mullahy, 1986). Both model classes are mixture models and assume that the outcome is a mixture of two data-generating processes: the zero-process and the count process. The zero model (e.g., a binomial GLM) determines if an observation belongs to the zero-inflation process or to the count process. The count model typically is a Poisson or negative binomial model. The difference between zero-inflation and hurdle models is that the former allow two possible sources of zeros, while the latter assume only one source of zeros. Hurdle models use a zero-truncated Poisson or negative binomial model for the count part, i.e., models for variables with positive integer values only, while zero-inflation models use an ordinary Poisson or negative binomial model for the count part. In the latter case, zeros could stem both from the zero-inflation or from the count process. Whether zero-inflation models or hurdle models are more appropriate depends on theoretical considerations, namely if it makes sense from a theoretical perspective that there could be two possible sources of zeros: In our delinquency example, we might assume a subgroup of participants who *could* have shown some delinquent behaviours in the previous year, but nevertheless reported zero delinquent behaviours, for example, because they are closely monitored by their parents after the first offence the year before. In this case a zero-inflation model would be appropriate. On the other hand, with the assumption that offenders and non-offenders are very distinct groups without any overlaps, a hurdle model would have been the better choice.

Finally, these models could also be fitted as generalized linear mixed-effects versions (see Sect. 5.6.1 for a brief introduction to GLMM).

6.2.2 The `countimp` Package

`countimp` is an extension to the `mice` package and provides `mice` imputation functions based on various count data models. The general approach realized in `mice` was described in Sects. 4.4.2, 4.4.3, 4.4.4, and 4.4.6. Example 4.3 in Sect. 4.4.2 describes the imputation of continuous and binary variables. An overview of imputation functions that are currently available in `countimp` is given in Table 6.1. The most recent version of `countimp` can be installed from GitHub using `install_git()` from package `devtools`:

```
> devtools::install_git(url =
+         "https://github.com/kkleinke/countimp", branch =
+         "master")
```

Table 6.1 `countimp`—overview of count data imputation functions and models

Imputation function	Model
`mice.impute.poisson`	Poisson
`mice.impute.quasipoisson`	Quasi-Poisson
`mice.impute.nb`	Negative binomial
`mice.impute.zip`	Zero-inflated Poisson
`mice.impute.zinb`	Zero-inflated negative binomial
`mice.impute.hp`	Hurdle Poisson
`mice.impute.hnb`	Hurdle negative binomial
`mice.impute.2l.poisson`[a]	Two-level Poisson
`mice.impute.2l.nb`[a]	Two-level negative binomial
`mice.impute.2l.hp`[a]	Two-level hurdle Poisson
`mice.impute.2l.hnb`[a]	Two-level hurdle negative binomial
`mice.impute.2l.zip`[a]	Two-level zero-inflated Poisson
`mice.impute.2l.zinb`[a]	Two-level zero-inflated negative binomial

[a]Note that all two-level imputation functions require the data to be in long format

In the following subsections, we give a brief introduction to these imputation methods, outline in which scenarios they can be applied, and give practical examples and advice regarding how to use these functions.

Most functions listed in Table 6.1 are available as *Bayesian regression* (Rubin, 1987, p. 169) and *bootstrap regression MI* variants. For the bootstrap version, prior distributions for parameters $\boldsymbol{\theta}_l$, $l = 1, \ldots, q$ (see Sect. 4.4.2) need not to be specified and the random draws of the parameters from their posterior distributions are replaced by selecting bootstrap samples from the corresponding subsamples and by obtaining model estimates from these bootstrap samples. Algorithms 6.1 and 6.2 summarize the steps involved in creating the imputations following the two approaches: Let $\mathbf{U}$ be an $n \times p$ matrix with n independent observations of p variables. $\mathbf{u}_j$ is an incomplete count variable in data set $\mathbf{U}$. Vectors $\mathbf{u}_{j,(1)}$ and $\mathbf{u}_{j,(0)}$ refer to the observed and missing observations in $\mathbf{u}_j$, respectively, and $\mathbf{U}_s$ is a completely observed or already imputed subset of the data set that includes a selection of variables (except from $\mathbf{u}_j$) that is used to predict missing information in $\mathbf{u}_j$. Parameter vectors $\boldsymbol{\theta}_l$, $l = 1, \ldots, q$, include regression parameters $\boldsymbol{\beta}$ and, if necessary, additional scale parameters. For the Bayesian approach flat priors are chosen.

6.2.2.1 Imputation of Incomplete Poisson Distributed Variables

Function `mice.impute.poisson()` imputes univariate missing data based on a Bayesian Poisson GLM (cf. Kleinke et al., 2011). Appending `.boot` to the

Algorithm 6.1 Bayesian regression

1. fit a regression model to $(\mathbf{u}_{j,(1)} \mid \mathbf{U}_{s,(1)})$,
2. find $\hat{\boldsymbol{\beta}}$, the posterior mean, and $\hat{\mathbf{V}}$, the posterior variance of model parameters $\boldsymbol{\beta}$,
3. simulate parameter values $\tilde{\boldsymbol{\beta}}$ from $N(\hat{\boldsymbol{\beta}}, \tilde{\mathbf{V}})$ if $\hat{\mathbf{V}}$ depends on additional scale parameters in $\boldsymbol{\theta}$, where $\tilde{\mathbf{V}}$ is a function of the scale parameters selected from their posterior distribution, and from $N(\hat{\boldsymbol{\beta}}, \hat{\mathbf{V}})$ otherwise (see Example 4.3),
4. generate the imputations based on the model from step 1 and new parameter values $\tilde{\boldsymbol{\theta}}$,
5. perform steps (1)–(4) M times to obtain the M imputations.

Algorithm 6.2 Bootstrap regression

1. draw a bootstrap sample B from $(\mathbf{u}_{j,(1)}\ \mathbf{U}_{s,(1)})$,
2. fit a regression model to this bootstrap sample B and obtain bootstrap estimates $\tilde{\boldsymbol{\beta}}$ for model parameters $\boldsymbol{\beta}$, and if necessary additional scale or dispersion parameter estimates,
3. generate the imputations based on these bootstrap estimates,
4. perform steps (1)–(3) M times to obtain the M imputations.

function name calls the bootstrap regression variant. For details, see

```
> library(countimp)
> help("mice.impute.poisson")
```

As research by Kleinke et al. (2011), Kleinke and Reinecke (2013b) and Kleinke (2017) suggests, the method yields valid statistical inferences, when the distribution of the empirical count variable conditional on the predictors is approximately Poisson. Biased estimators are to be expected, when the Poisson model is not appropriate (e.g. when empirical data are overdispersed or zero-inflated). Bias—inter alia—can be expected to increase with increasing departures from the Poisson model and with increasing missing data percentages even in large samples.

6.2.2.2 Application

Creating multiple imputations with package `countimp` works analogous to the steps outlined in Sect. 5.4. `countimp` automatically loads the `mice` package and the imputations are created by the `mice()` function. However, applied researchers should use the wrapper function `countimp()` instead of `mice()` to create the imputations. `countimp()` basically has the same arguments as `mice()`, but ensures that the respective arguments are handled correctly, since some of our functions depart a little bit from the standard `mice` architecture.

For the examples in this chapter, we use the same data as in Chap. 5. The CrimoC data (see Sect. 5.2) are included in package `countimp` and can be loaded using the `data()` command:

```
> data(crim4w)
> data(crim4l)
```

Letters `w` and `l` indicate the format of the data set: wide format and long format, respectively. Analogous to Sect. 5.4, `mice()` can be used to set up `method` and `predictorMatrix`:

```
> ini <- mice(crim4w, maxit=0)
> meth <- ini$method
> pred <- ini$predictorMatrix
```

In this example, we want to impute variables `ACRIM–DCRIM`, the repeatedly measured delinquency scores, by a Bayesian Poisson regression model:

```
> meth[6:9] <- "poisson"
```

Furthermore, to avoid multicollinearity problems, we use only one other panel wave (either an earlier or later panel wave) to predict missing values in the respective delinquency score:

```
> pred["ACRIM",c("CCRIM","DCRIM")] <-0
> pred["BCRIM",c("ACRIM","DCRIM")] <-0
> pred["CCRIM",c("BCRIM","DCRIM")] <-0
> pred["DCRIM",c("BCRIM","CCRIM")] <-0
```

Additionally, we exclude the participant identifier and dummy variable `HA` from the imputation models, since *Hauptschule* is the reference category in our models:

```
> pred[,"id"] <- 0
> pred[,c("HA")] <- 0
```

Imputations are finally generated by the `countimp()` function:

```
> set.seed(123456)
> imp.poisson <- countimp(data = crim4w, method = meth, m = 100,
+         predictorMatrix = pred, maxit = 20, print = FALSE)
```

The resulting object is of class `mids`—a multiply imputed data set. Useful `mice` functions, for example, `plot.mids()`, `with.mids()`, or `complete()` can be applied to this object, as outlined in Sect. 5.4.

6.2.2.3 Imputation of Overdispersed Count Data

`countimp` has two methods to impute overdispersed count data in wide format:

1. imputation based on a quasi-Poisson model, and
2. imputation based on a negative binomial model.

Both methods can be used when the equidispersion assumption of the standard Poisson model is violated, i.e., when the variance of the count variable is larger in comparison to its mean. Method `"quasipoisson"` (Kleinke et al., 2011) imputes univariate missing data based on a Bayesian quasi-Poisson GLM using the standard R function `glm.fit` with `family = quasipoisson(link = log)`. Method `"nb"` fits a negative binomial model using function `glm.nb` from package `MASS`. Again, appending `.boot` to the function name calls the bootstrap variants. Both methods draw the imputations from a negative binomial distribution to ensure an adequate amount of overdispersion in the imputed data. In our experience, both methods lead to virtually identical results. However, estimation of the `quasipoisson` GLM appears to be more efficient and stable in comparison to the NB model.

6.2.2.4 Application

We assume that readers have run the example from Sect. 6.2.2.2 and that objects `meth` and `pred` are still in the R workspace. To impute missing data in variables `ACRIM–DCRIM` by the Bayesian quasi-Poisson method, one simply has to change the corresponding slots in `method`:

```
> set.seed(123456)
> meth[6:9] <- "quasipoisson"
> imp.quasipoisson <- countimp(data = crim4w, method = meth, m =
+         100, predictorMatrix = pred, maxit = 20, print = FALSE)
```

Using the bootstrap variant works analogously:

```
> set.seed(123456)
> meth[6:9] <- "quasipoisson.boot"
> imp.qp.boot <- countimp(data = crim4w, method = meth, m = 100,
+         predictorMatrix = pred, maxit = 20, print = FALSE)
```

The resulting `mids` objects can then be used for further data analysis as outlined in Chap. 5.

6.2.2.5 Imputation of Count Data with an Excess Number of Zero Counts

Methods `"zip"` and `"zinb"` impute missing data based on a zero-inflated Poisson or NB model, respectively, (for details, see Kleinke & Reinecke, 2013b). Methods `"hp"` and `"hnb"` use a hurdle Poisson or NB model. In practice, the zero-process and the count process are often determined by quite different sets of predictors. To be able to specify both model components separately via `mice`'s `predictorMatrix` argument, we use entries apart from zero and one[2]: Analogous to other `mice` imputation functions, a '0' still means that the variable is not included in either imputation model. A '1' specifies variables that will be included in both the zero and the count model. '2' furthermore identifies a count model predictor and a '3' a zero model predictor.

---

[2]See Chap. 5 for details on how to specify imputation models in `mice`.

6.2.2.6 Application

Again we assume that readers have run the example from Sect. 6.2.2.2 and that objects `meth` and `pred` are still available in the R workspace. We now want to impute variables `ACRIM`–`DCRIM` by a negative binomial hurdle model. Such a model would be appropriate if we assumed offenders and non-offenders to be highly distinct groups with quite different sets of predictors. We set the respective slots of `method` to `"hnb"`. In our first example, we want to include all predictors in both the zero and the count part of the model. In this case we do not need to make any adjustments to the `predictorMatrix`. We can simply run `countimp()` to obtain the imputations:

```
> set.seed(123456)
> meth[6:9] <- "hnb"
> imp.hnb <- countimp(data = crim4w, method = meth, m = 100,
+          predictorMatrix = pred, maxit = 20, print = FALSE)
```

To use certain predictors only for the count part of the model, we need to set the corresponding entry in the `predictorMatrix` to '2'. In the following example, we use `FEMALE`, `RE` and `GY` only as count model predictors:

```
> pred[c("ACRIM", "BCRIM", "CCRIM", "DCRIM"), c("FEMALE", "RE",
+          "GY")] <- 2
> set.seed(123456)
> imp.hnb2 <- countimp(data = crim4w, method = meth, m = 100,
+          predictorMatrix = pred, maxit = 20, print = FALSE)
```

In the last example, we want to define `FEMALE`, `RE` and `GY` only as zero model predictors:

```
> pred[c("ACRIM", "BCRIM", "CCRIM", "DCRIM"), c("FEMALE", "RE",
+          "GY")] <- 3
> set.seed(123456)
> imp.hnb3 <- countimp(data = crim4w, method = meth, m = 100,
+          predictorMatrix = pred, maxit = 20, print = FALSE)
```

The resulting objects of class `mids` can then be analysed as outlined in Chap. 5.

6.2.2.7 Imputation of Two-Level Poisson Distributed Data

`mice.impute.2l.poisson()` imputes missing information based on a generalized linear mixed effects Poisson model. As the function name suggests, currently only a two-level model can be fitted. The function is described in detail in Kleinke and Reinecke (2015a). The estimation technique is penalized quasilikelihood (PQL), which in comparison to other methods is quite fast. For a discussion of different GLMM estimation methods, see Bolker et al. (2009). To specify the imputation model, we use the same coding scheme as other two-level imputation functions in `mice` (see Chap. 5). Allowed entries in the `predictorMatrix` are: '0', the variable is not included in the imputation model; '1', the variable is included as a fixed effect; '2', the variable is included as a fixed *and* random effect. Finally, '−2' defines the class variable. Note that the intercept is always treated as a fixed and random factor. If this is not desired, the `.noint` variant of the function could be used, which treats the intercept only as a fixed, but not as a random effect. Furthermore, the `.boot` variants of the function use bootstrap regression rather than Bayesian regression. Here, we resample clusters rather than individual cases. For details about the variants of the function, see `help("mice.impute.2l.poisson")`.

6.2.2.8 Application

Recall from Chap. 5 that multilevel multiple imputation functions in `mice` require the data to be in long format. We have included a long format version of our example data set from Chap. 5 in package `countimp`. The data file is called `crim4l`. To set up `method` and `predictorMatrix`, we start with an initial run of `mice()`. In `crim4l`, the repeatedly measured delinquency scores are stored in one single variable `DELINQ`. We set the imputation method for variable `DELINQ` to `"2l.poisson"`. Furthermore, we define variables `FEMALE`, `RE` and `GY` as fixed effects, `TIME` as a fixed and random factor and its quadratic term `TIME2` as a fixed factor (see Sect. 5.6.3.1). Finally, we define `ID` as class variable:

```
> data(crim4l)
> crim4l$TIME2 <- crim4l$TIME^2
> ini <- mice(crim4l, maxit = 0)
> meth <- ini$method
> pred <- ini$predictorMatrix
> meth["DELINQ"] <- "2l.poisson"
> pred["DELINQ", ] <- c(1, 1, 1, 2, 0, -2, 1)
> options(warn = 1)
```

Imputations are finally generated using the wrapper function `countimp()`:

```
> set.seed(123456)
> imp.2l.poisson <- countimp(data = crim4l, m = 100, method =
+         meth, predictorMatrix = pred, maxit = 20)
```

The resulting object `imp.2l.poisson` is of class `mids` and can be analysed as outlined in Chap. 5.

6.2.2.9 Imputation of Overdispersed Two-Level Count Data

When two-level data are overdispersed, using method `"2l.nb"` is preferable over `"2l.poisson"` (for details, see Kleinke & Reinecke, 2015b). Again, appending `.boot` to the function name calls the bootstrap regression version of the function. Here, we resample clusters rather than individual cases. Also, we provide `.noint` versions of the functions, which define the intercept as a fixed effect and exclude the intercept from the random part of the model. For details, see `help("mice.impute.2l.nb")`.

6.2.2.10 Application

We assume that readers have run the example from Sect. 6.2.2.8 and that objects `meth` and `pred` are still in the R workspace.

To select the two-level NB imputation method, we need to change the corresponding entry in `meth` to `"2l.nb"` and run `countimp()`. Specification of the imputation model works analogous to other two-level imputation functions in `mice` (e.g. `mice.impute.2l.poisson()`, see Sect. 6.2.2.8). Like in the previous example, we want to include `FEMALE`, `RE` and `GY` as fixed effects, `TIME` as a fixed and random factor and `TIME2` as a fixed factor. `ID` again is the class variable. Therefore, we do not need to make any adjustments to `pred`.

```
> meth["DELINQ"] <- "2l.nb"
> set.seed(123456)
> imp.2l.nb <- countimp(data = crim4l, method = meth, m = 100,
+         predictorMatrix = pred, maxit = 20)
```

Repeated data analysis and pooling of results can be done as outlined in Chap. 5.

6.2.2.11 Imputation of Zero-Inflated Two-Level Count Data

Methods `"2l.hp"` and `"2l.hnb"` impute zero-inflated two-level count data based on a two-level hurdle model, either using the Bayesian regression or the bootstrap regression approach (appendix: `.boot`). Analogously, methods `"2l.zip"` and `"2l.zinb"` create imputations based on a two-level ZIP or ZINB model, respectively. The `.noint` variants of the functions treat the intercept only as a fixed, but not as a random effect. It may be specified, if the intercept is excluded from the random part of the zero model (`.noint.zero`), the random part of the count model (`.noint.count`) or from the random part of both models (`.noint.both`). For details, see `help("mice.impute.2l.hnb")`.

Since applied researchers might want to specify different sets of predictors for the zero and count parts of the model, we use entries in the `predictorMatrix` apart from 0, 1, 2, −2. Allowed entries are:

−2	Class variable
0	Not included
1	Fixed effect (zero and count model)
2	Fixed and random effect (zero and count model)
3	Fixed effect (count model only)
4	Fixed and random effect (count model only)
5	Fixed effect (zero model only)
6	Fixed and random effect (zero model only)

6.2.2.12 Application

We assume that readers have run the example from Sect. 6.2.2.8. Again, we use objects `meth` and `pred` from that example. To select the hurdle NB model to impute missing values in variable `DELINQ`, we set the corresponding slot in `meth` to `"2l.hnb"`. In case we do not make any changes to `pred` (see the example in Sect. 6.2.2.8), information about gender (`FEMALE`) and school type (`RE` and `GY`) will be treated-as-fixed effects and `TIME` as fixed and random effect in both model components. Finally, the quadratic time trend will be modeled only as a fixed effect.

```
> meth["DELINQ"] <- "2l.hnb"
> set.seed(123456)
> imp.2l.hnb <- countimp(data = crim4l, method = meth, m = 100,
+         predictorMatrix = pred, maxit = 20)
```

6.2.3 Discussion

In this section, we have demonstrated the application of multiple imputation procedures for count data with R-package `countimp`. This package supports imputation of ordinary, overdispersed, zero-inflated and multilevel count data.

We want to emphasize that thorough data exploration and statistical modeling is essential to be able to select imputation methods that are adequate for the problem at hand. As with parametric imputation models in general, if the chosen imputation model is not appropriate for the situation at hand, like choosing a Poisson imputation model—although, for example, a zero-inflation negative binomial model would be more appropriate, then imputations will not be proper and inferences might be invalid. Thus the imputation model should be chosen carefully. This is particularly important if the variable to be imputed enters the model of applied-scientific interest as a predictor variable. In this case, one must have in mind that the unconditional distribution of the incompletely observed variable to be imputed and the conditional distribution that has to be modeled for the imputation task, are different in general (see, for example, de Jong, 2012; de Jong et al., 2016, and the discussions in Sects. 3.3.2 and 4.4.6).

6.3 `ImputeRobust`—Imputation Based on Generalized Additive Models for Location, Scale and Shape

Standard regression based MI procedures like the ones from package `countimp` generate imputations by modeling the conditional distribution of the incomplete variable given certain complete (or previously completed) predictors. Validity of statistical inferences—inter alia—depends on to what extent model assumptions

Table 6.2 GAMLSS imputation models that are currently supported by ImputeRobust

Imputation function	Model distribution
mice.impute.gamlss	Normal
mice.impute.gamlssBI	Binomial
mice.impute.gamlssGA	Gamma
mice.impute.gamlssJSU	Johnson's SU
mice.impute.gamlssPO	Poisson
mice.impute.gamlssTF	Student's t
mice.impute.gamlssZIBI	Zero-inflated binomial
mice.impute.gamlssZIP	Zero-inflated Poisson

like normality of errors or homoscedasticity are met. If model assumptions of the adopted imputation models are violated, it is advisable to use robust semi-parametric or nonparametric imputation procedures.

De Jong (2012) and de Jong et al. (2016) propose a robust MI procedure based on a class of semi-parametric generalized additive models for location, scale and shape (i.e., GAMLSS, Rigby & Stasinopoulos, 2005; Stasinopoulos & Rigby, 2007; Stasinopoulos, Rigby, Heller, Voudouris, & De Bastiani, 2017), which allows flexible modeling not only of the location (e.g. the mean) of the distribution of the incomplete dependent variable, but also of the scale (e.g. variance), and the shape (e.g., skewness and kurtosis) of the distribution. Salfrán and Spiess (2017) implemented these ideas in R-package ImputeRobust. ImputeRobust extends the functionality of the mice package (see Chap. 5). Imputation methods and models can be specified in mice and the imputations are then created by mice. For an overview of models that are currently available, see Table 6.2. Section 6.3.1 gives a brief introduction to the theoretical underpinnings of the imputation method. Section 6.3.2 demonstrates the application in R. In Sect. 6.3.3, we discuss advantages and disadvantages of the GAMLSS imputation approach and give practical advice in which situations functions from package ImputeRobust could or should be used.

6.3.1 ImputeRobust in a Nutshell

Package ImputeRobust can be installed from CRAN (the comprehensive R archive network) using the install.packages() command, or from GitHub:

```
> devtools::install_git(url =
+         "https://github.com/dsalfran/ImputeRobust", branch =
+         "master")
```

A detailed description of the imputation method and its theoretical underpinnings may be found in Salfrán and Spiess (2018) and Salfrán (2018). Further information about GAMLSS is given in Rigby and Stasinopoulos (2005), Stasinopoulos and Rigby (2007) and Stasinopoulos et al. (2017).

GAMLSS assume that given predictor variables $\mathbf{x}$ the response variable y follows a parametric distribution $y \sim D(\mu, \sigma, \nu, \tau)$, where μ and σ are the location and scale parameters, and ν and τ are the shape parameters—depending on the type of distribution $D(\cdot)$ specified by the user. An overview of model distributions supported by `ImputeRobust` is given in Table 6.2.

To highlight that in the missing data context variables may have to be imputed that enter the model of applied-scientific interest as predictor variables, we will use $\mathbf{u}_j = (u_{1,j}\ u_{2,j} \cdots u_{n,j})^T$ to denote the variable to be imputed, with indices j for the jth variable and $i = 1, \ldots, n$ for the units. All remaining variables are collected in the $(n \times p)$-matrix $\mathbf{U}_{-j}$. For each $u_{i,j}$ we assume that $u_{i,j} \sim D(\theta_{i,j}^{(1)}, \theta_{i,j}^{(2)}, \theta_{i,j}^{(3)}, \theta_{i,j}^{(4)})$, where $\theta_{i,j}^{(1)} = \mu_{i,j}$, $\theta_{i,j}^{(2)} = \sigma_{i,j}$, $\theta_{i,j}^{(3)} = \nu_{i,j}$ and $\theta_{i,j}^{(4)} = \tau_{i,j}$. If we collect all the individual specific parameters in $\boldsymbol{\theta}_j^{(k)} = (\theta_{1,j}^{(k)} \cdots \theta_{n,j}^{(k)})^T$, the model for the jth variable to be imputed can be written as

$$g_k(\boldsymbol{\theta}_j^{(k)}) = \mathbf{U}_k \boldsymbol{\beta}_k + \sum_{l=1}^{L_k} h_{k,l}(\mathbf{u}_{k,l}) \,, \tag{6.5}$$

where $g_k(\cdot)$ is the link function relating the vector of individual parameters of the corresponding location, scale or shape parameter to predictor variables in $\mathbf{U}$. $\mathbf{U}_k$ is a design matrix that does not include $\mathbf{u}_j$ but whose effects are assumed to be linear additive, $\boldsymbol{\beta}_k$ is the vector of these unknown effects and $h_{k,l}(\mathbf{u}_{k,l})$ are unknown smoothing functions of the explanatory variables $\mathbf{u}_{lk} = (u_{1,k,l} \cdots u_{n,k,l})^T$ which are from $\mathbf{U}_{-j}$ but are not necessarily elements from $\mathbf{U}_k$. Actually, $\mathbf{U}_k$ and $\mathbf{u}_{k,l}$ may have no elements in common. Functions h implemented in package `gamlss` include cubic smoothing splines, penalized splines and local regression. `ImputeRobust` uses penalized B-splines with 20 knots, a third-degree piecewise polynomial, a second order penalty and automatic selection of the smoothing parameter using the local maximum likelihood criterion (for a discussion, see Eilers & Marx, 1996).

Sometimes, the automatic smoothing selection of parameters can fail—for example, if sample size is too small in relation to the number of model parameters to be estimated. In those cases, the imputation method automatically reduces the order of the piecewise polynomial or the penalty, and in the most extreme case, falls back to a normal linear model.

Furthermore, users can restrict the number of parameters to be modeled by specifying the `n.ind.par` argument of the respective imputation function. The argument is to be included in the `mice` call and will be automatically passed down by `mice` to the `ImputeRobust` imputation sub-function. Setting `n.ind.par` can be useful in some scenarios, for example, to improve the stability of the imputation process (see the example below for details on how to use this argument). Imputations are then created as outlined in Algorithm 6.3.

As before, let $\mathbf{u}_j$ be the incompletely observed variable to be imputed, let $\mathbf{u}_{j,(1)}$ and $\mathbf{u}_{j,(0)}$ refer to the observed and missing part in $\mathbf{u}_j$, respectively, and let $\mathbf{u}_s$ be a subset of $\mathbf{U}_{-j}$ that includes a selection of variables (except from $\mathbf{u}_j$)

Algorithm 6.3 `ImputeRobust`

1. Fit the GAMLSS imputation model based on the observed part of the data $(\mathbf{u}_{j,(1)}, \mathbf{u}_{s,(1)})$ by (penalized) maximum likelihood estimation.
2. Replace the observed values of the variable to be imputed by predictions from the fitted model from step one (which we label $\mathbf{u}_{j*,(1)}$) and create a parametric bootstrap sample $B = (\mathbf{u}^T_{j*,(1)}\ \mathbf{u}^T_{s,(1)})$ to approximate draws of parameters from their posterior distribution.
3. Refit the model based on this bootstrap sample B and estimate the model parameters.
4. Draw imputations for $\mathbf{u}_{j*,(0)}$ from the assumed distribution using the predicted parameters from step 3.
5. Perform steps 2–4 m times to generate m imputations for each missing value.

used to predict missing information in $\mathbf{u}_j$. In addition, let $\mathbf{u}_{s,(1)}$ be that part of $\mathbf{u}_s$, observed or already imputed, corresponding to those units for which u_j is observed and, correspondingly $\mathbf{u}_{s,(0)}$ be that part of $\mathbf{u}_s$, observed or already imputed, corresponding to those units for which u_j is missing. Since `gamlss` does not support Bayesian inference, draws from the posterior predictive distribution are approximated by the bootstrap predictive distribution (Harris, 1989),

$$f^*(\mathbf{u}_{j,(0)} \mid \mathbf{u}_{j,(1)}, \mathbf{u}_s) = \int f(\mathbf{u}_{j,(0)} \mid \tilde{\eta}, \mathbf{u}_{s,(0)}) f(\tilde{\eta} \mid \hat{\eta}(\mathbf{u}_{j,(1)} \mid \mathbf{u}_{s,(1)}))\, d\tilde{\eta}, \tag{6.6}$$

where $\tilde{\eta}$ denotes the possible values of the imputation model parameters, $\hat{\eta}(\mathbf{u}_{j,(1)} \mid \mathbf{u}_{s,(1)})$ is an estimator of such parameters and $f(\tilde{\eta} \mid \hat{\eta}(\mathbf{u}_{j,(1)} \mid \mathbf{u}_{s,(1)}))$ is the sampling distribution of the imputation parameters evaluated at the estimated values. The sampling distribution is simulated with a parametric bootstrap acting as a replacement for the posterior distribution of the imputation parameters.

It should be noted that the GAMLSS framework proposed by Rigby and Stasinopoulos (2005) is much more general: The conditional distributions of the dependent variable can be chosen from a large class of distributions (for an overview, see https://www.gamlss.com). `ImputeRobust` currently supports only a small portion of the functionality offered by `gamlss`, but will be extended in future versions.

6.3.2 Application

Like in the previous examples, we want to demonstrate the application of package `ImputeRobust` using the data from Sect. 5.2. The data file for this example is available from package `countimp` and can be loaded using the `data()` command. We impute the longitudinal CrimoC data in wide format because in the current version of `ImputeRobust` the multilevel structure of the panel data cannot be explicitly modeled. We use methods `gamlss` (two-parameter normal imputation model), `gamlssPO` (Poisson model) and `gamlssZIP` (zero-inflated Poisson model). Analogous to Sect. 5.4, `mice()` can be used to set up `method` and `predictorMatrix`:

```
> ini <- mice(crim4w, maxit=0)
> meth <- ini$method
> pred <- ini$predictorMatrix
```

At first, we want to impute the repeatedly measured delinquency scores, (variables `ACRIM–DCRIM`) by the default method `"gamlss"`, which denotes the two-parameter normal model with location and scale parameter:

```
> meth[6:9] <- "gamlss"
```

Similar to Sect. 6.2.2.2 we use only one other panel wave to predict missing values in the respective delinquency score to avoid problems due to multicollinearity. Again, this can be an earlier or later panel wave:

```
> pred["ACRIM",c("CCRIM","DCRIM")] <-0
> pred["BCRIM",c("ACRIM","DCRIM")] <-0
> pred["CCRIM",c("BCRIM","DCRIM")] <-0
> pred["DCRIM",c("BCRIM","CCRIM")] <-0
```

Additionally, we exclude the participant identifier and dummy variable `HA` from the imputation models, since *Hauptschule* is the reference category in our models:

```
> pred[,"id"] <- 0
> pred[,c("HA")] <- 0
```

Finally imputations are generated by the `mice()` function:

```
> set.seed(123456)
> library(ImputeRobust)
> imp.gamlss <- mice(data = crim4w, method = meth, m = 100,
+         predictorMatrix = pred, maxit = 20, print = FALSE)
```

In case of estimation problems, imputation models can be simplified by restricting the number of parameters to be estimated. By setting `n.ind.par = 1`, only the individual means will be modeled, while the scale parameters are restricted to be the same for all units, meaning the scale parameter is modeled as a constant value.

```
> imp.gamlss.1par <- mice( data = crim4w, method = meth, m =
+         100, predictorMatrix = pred, maxit = 20, n.ind.par = 1,
+         print = FALSE)
```

Using methods `"gamlssPO"` and `"gamlssZIP"` works analogously:

```
> meth[6:9] <- "gamlssPO"
> imp.gamlssPO <- mice( data = crim4w, method = meth, m = 100,
+         predictorMatrix = pred, maxit = 20, print = FALSE)

> meth[6:9] <- "gamlssZIP"
> imp.gamlssZIP <- mice( data = crim4w, method = meth, m = 100,
+         predictorMatrix = pred, maxit = 20, print = FALSE)
```

The resulting objects `imp.gamlss`, `imp.gamlssPO`, `imp.gamlssZIP` and `imp.gamlss.1par` are of class `mids` and can be analysed as outlined in Chap. 5.

6.3.3 Discussion

Rigby, Stasinopoulos, and Voudouris (2013) argue that 'for data with more than say 1000 observations, regression models beyond the mean should be the norm, not the exception' (p. 335). When sample size is sufficiently large, GAMLSS models allow far greater modeling flexibility than standard approaches. Using functions from package `ImputeRobust` is especially worthwhile in situations in which assumptions of standard fully parametric models are violated. For example, standard parametric imputation techniques can produce invalid inferences when there are outliers in the data, or in the case of skewed, heavy-tailed or multi-modal distributions (e.g., He & Raghunathan, 2012; Yu et al., 2007). The `gamlss.dist` package provides more than 80 distributions for continuous, discrete or mixed response variables. Any distribution can be truncated to the left, to the right or both. Furthermore, data can be censored (Rigby, et al., 2013). `ImputeRobust` can be extended to support these distributions. However, great modeling flexibility also comes with a price, namely the choices empirical researchers have to make from an abundance of options and settings: e.g., regarding the GAMLSS family that (supposedly) has the best fit to the empirical data, regarding the link functions, and the number of parameters. This is not trivial but does not really differ from current practice: By choosing any parametric imputation model, a certain model including the distribution family, e.g., the normal, a link function, e.g., the identity link, and the number of predictors included into the model defines the richness of the model. The difference lies mainly in the fact that more options are available and the applied researcher has to make a decision which is only seemingly not necessary if one of the standard imputation methods is chosen. However, empirical researchers are required to have a good understanding of GAMLSS and the respective models and are required to spend sufficient time on statistical modeling, model comparison and model checking. For a more comprehensive discussion of advantages and disadvantages of the GAMLSS approach, see, for example, Rigby, et al. (2013), Stasinopoulos et al. (2017) or Salfrán (2018). Also, `ImputeRobust` at the moment does not support multilevel imputation models. This will be an interesting avenue for future software development.

6.4 Quantile Regression Based Multiple Imputation

Standard regression based MI approaches create imputations by estimating the conditional mean of the response variable given certain predictors. GAMLSS models (Sect. 6.3) are more flexible and estimate the conditional mean, and—depending on the selected distribution—additional scale and shape parameters given certain predictors. GAMLSS models, however, still assume that the dependent variable has some kind of parametric distribution. Quantile regression (QR), on the other hand, has no parametric requirements except that the dependent variable has to be continuous. QR estimates either the conditional *median* or any other quantile p of the response variable given certain predictor variables (see, for example, Koenker, 2005; Koenker & Hallock, 2001). Recent simulations have shown that quantile-based imputations can have some appreciable benefits when the sample size is sufficiently large (Geraci & McLain, 2018).

Similar to OLS regression, the p-quantile regression model assumes a linear (additive) predictor for the p-quantiles of a variable y_i conditional on predictor variables $\mathbf{x}_i$. The pth conditional quantile function depending on p-specific regression parameter $\boldsymbol{\beta}_p$ is modeled as

$$Q_{y_i|\mathbf{x}_i}(p) = \mathbf{x}_i^T \boldsymbol{\beta}_p \ .$$

Parameter estimates of this model, $\hat{\boldsymbol{\beta}}_p$, are obtained by minimizing the mean of functions of $(y_i - \mathbf{x}_i^T \boldsymbol{\beta}_p)$ and p over $i = 1, \ldots, n$ with respect to $\boldsymbol{\beta}_p$ (for details see Koenker, 2005). This is done for all p-quantiles of interest. The assumed data generating process for all i underlying this model is

$$y_i = \mathbf{x}_i^T \boldsymbol{\beta}_p + \epsilon_{p,i} \ , \quad \epsilon_{p,i} \sim F_{p,i} \quad \text{and} \quad F_{p,i}^{-1}(p) = 0 \ ,$$

where $F_{p,i}$ is some distribution function and $F_{p,i}^{-1}$ is its inverse, so that if q is a quantile such that $p = F_{p,i}(q)$, we have $q = F_{p,i}^{-1}(p)$. The weak assumptions about the distribution of the errors and the fact that quantiles of the conditional distribution of y_i's are modeled implies that this method has its advantages over restrictive parametric methods if strong distributional assumptions cannot be justified, and in the presence of valid outliers. In addition, it allows to account explicitly for heteroscedasticity (see Koenker, 2005). On the other hand, because for each quantile all parameters are estimated, this method may not be identified or may only be weakly identified, when sample size is too small.

Geraci (2016b) implemented quantile regression based MI in R-package `Qtools` (see also Bottai & Zhen, 2013; Geraci, 2016a). Like the functions from packages `countimp` or `ImputeRobust`, Geraci's functions work as an add-on to the multiple imputation package `mice` (see Chap. 5). The imputation function is called `mice.impute.rq()` and works as follows. Let $\mathbf{u}$ denote an incompletely observed vector of independent variables where the values of the first $i = 1, \ldots, n_{(1)}$ units are observed and the remaining $i = n_{(1)} + 1, \ldots, n$ are not observed. Let $\mathbf{u}_{(1)}$ denote the observed and $\mathbf{u}_{(0)}$ be the missing part of $\mathbf{u}$. Individual elements are $u_{i,(1)}$ and $u_{i,(0)}$, respectively. For each i, let furthermore $\mathbf{v}_{i,(1)}$ be a vector of observed or already imputed covariates corresponding to unit i with observed u_i and, correspondingly, $\mathbf{v}_{i,(0)}$ for unit i with u_i not observed.

In a first step a bootstrap sample from the completely observed or completed sample, $(u_{i,(1)} \ \mathbf{v}_{i(1)}^T)$, $i = 1, \ldots, n_{(1)}$, of size $n_{(1)}$ is selected with replacement. In the second step, $n_{(0)}$ pseudo-random values $p_1, \ldots, p_{n_{(0)}}$ are generated from a uniform distribution on [0, 1]. Based on these p-values and the bootstrap sample from the first step the parameters of the corresponding quantile regressions are estimated. Thus, $n_{(0)}$ parameter estimates $\tilde{\boldsymbol{\beta}}_p$ are calculated. For each missing value $u_{i,(0)}$ an imputation is generated by plugging in the corresponding observed predictor variable $\mathbf{v}_{i,(0)}$ and the estimated parameter $\tilde{\boldsymbol{\beta}}_{p_i}$ into the conditional quantile function. This method is generalized in Geraci and McLain (2018) to generate multiple imputations for bounded variables.

6.4.1 Application

Again, we want to demonstrate the application of QR-based imputation using the CrimoC data set from Sect. 5.2. We assume that readers have run the examples from Sect. 6.2.2.8 and that the data set `crim4l`, as well as objects `ini`, `meth` and `pred` are still available in the R workspace. The imputation function that we are going to use is `mice.impute.rq()`, which can be called like any other `mice` imputation function by setting the respective slot in `meth` to `rq`. In contrast to the `countimp`-functions, quantile regression imputation is not (yet) able to explicitly model the multilevel structure of the panel data. Users need to bear this in mind when using our example with long format data. Some bias especially in the random part of the model is to be expected.

In addition, we demonstrate the use of `mice`'s post-processing functionality. If we want to fit the growth curve ZIP model from Sect. 5.2.2, the imputed values have to be non-negative integers. The `round()` function rounds the imputations to integer values. If theoretical arguments or strong empirical results imply a certain possible range of the data, one may restrict imputations to this admissible interval by the `squeeze()` function. It replaces values outside the admissible range by the specified bounds. Because the delinquency scores in our example data set can range between 0 (no delinquency) and 16 (largest variety of delinquency), the imputed values are squeezed into this range. The function `squeeze()` replaces imputed values below zero by 0, and values above 16 by 16. From the discussion in Sect. 4.5.1 it should be clear that both ad-hoc techniques should be applied very cautiously and if no theoretically better justified technique is available. In our application imputing integer values with `Qtools` is not possible, but we need integer values as the dependent variables in the growth curve ZIP model of applied-scientific interest. Otherwise, if these variables would enter the model of interest as covariates, inferences could be expected to be valid even if imputations are generated from a continuous distribution (e.g., de Jong et al., 2016). Restricting possible values to the range from 0 to 16 allows generating imputations from an imperfect model given the known admissible range of the variable.

The `post` argument in `mice` is a vector of strings telling `mice` what to do during the post processing. In our example, we post-process imputations of variable `DELINQ` using functions `round()` and `squeeze()`. The expression `imp[[j]][,i]` in the definition of `post["DELINQ"]` denotes the vector that is used internally by mice to store the imputations (cf. van Buuren & Groothuis-Oudshoorn, 2011).

```
> library(Qtools)
> meth["DELINQ"] <- "rq"
> post=ini$post
> post["DELINQ"] <- "imp[[j]][, i] <- round(squeeze(imp[[j]][,
+         i], c(0, 16)))"
> imp.rq <- mice( data = crim4l, method = meth,  m = 100,
+         predictorMatrix = pred, maxit = 20, post = post, print
+         = FALSE)
```

imp.rq is of class mids and can be analysed as outlined in Chap. 5.

6.4.2 *Discussion*

In this application, we have used method "rq" to impute the CrimoC data in long format. Note that this imputation method fits an ordinary quantile regression model, which ignores the clustered structure of the data. This has some disadvantages, as outlined in Chap. 5. Although there are extensions of the quantile regression framework to longitudinal data sets (see, for example, Geraci, 2014; Koenker, 2004), imputation procedures based on these methods are currently not yet available. We deem this an interesting (and necessary) avenue for future research and software development. Note furthermore that systematic simulation studies comparing quantile regression imputation with other available imputation methods are still scarce not only with respect to robustness against misspecifications of the imputation model and the missing data mechanism, but also with respect to the relative efficiency of estimators and test statistics of applied-scientific interest. In addition, quantile regression based MI will produce imputations that are continuous, and also negative values might occur. If the model of applied-scientific interest is a count model, the values of the dependent variable must be non-negative integers. As argued before, generating continuous imputations which are then rounded and trimmed may lead to invalid inferences. On the other hand, since rounding can be expected to cause much less bias if applied to a discrete variable with many levels (see the discussion in Horton et al., 2003) it would be interesting to adopt the quantile-based imputation procedure for bounded variables proposed by Geraci and McLain (2018), round the imputed values to integers and compare this method with other imputation methods in various situations for count variables. Although there is a lack of such evaluations at the time being, quantile regression based MI may be an alternative to standard linear imputation models, for situations where assumptions of a normal linear regression based imputation model are grossly violated and sample size is sufficiently large.

6.5 Two-Level Predictive Mean Matching

6.5.1 The General Idea

We have discussed flat-file or wide-format predictive mean matching approaches in Sect. 5.4. PMM is the default method in `mice` for continuous data. Van Buuren (2013) lists wide-format PMM as an alternative to multilevel multiple imputation procedures, since many of the currently available parametric procedures appear to be quite sensitive towards violations of their model assumptions. In 2013, multilevel PMM approaches were not yet available. Since then, several solutions to extend the classical PMM idea to multilevel models have emerged (for an overview, see Table 6.3).

The procedure by Kleinke (2016) fits a two-level linear mixed-effects model, which is specified via `mice`'s `predictorMatrix` argument analogous to other two-level imputation functions in `mice` (see Chap. 5). The estimation is done by package `nlme` (whereas method `"2l.pmm"` from `miceadds` uses `lme4`). The method then follows the classical Bayesian regression steps (see Chap. 4). Matching is finally done by function `.pmm.match()` from package `mice`. Donors are selected from the whole sample and are not restricted to the cluster where the respective incomplete case stems from. The size of the donor pool can be adjusted by the `donors` argument.

Function `mice.impute.2l.2stage.pmm()` from package `micemd` creates imputations based on a two-level heteroscedastic model. The method was designed to be used for situations where both single observations and whole clusters are unobserved. Estimation methods (argument `method_est`) include restricted maximum likelihood (`"reml"`) and the method of moments (`"mm"`, cf. Resche-Rigon & White, 2016). Their two-stage approach is described in Audigier et al. (2017): At stage one, a linear regression model is fitted to each observed cluster. Then, estimates obtained from each cluster are combined according to a linear random effects model. Unlike the other approaches, method `"2l.2stage.pmm"` supports two donor selection strategies: Argument `incluster` defines if the donor is chosen from the cluster of the case that is to be imputed or from all clusters. Argument `k` defines the size of the donor pool.

Table 6.3 Two-level predictive mean matching approaches

Method	Package	Model	Reference
`2l.pmm`	`countimp`	Gaussian homoscedastic	Kleinke (2016)
`2l.pmm`	`miceadds`	Gaussian homoscedastic	Robitzsch, Grund, and Henke (2017)
`2l.2stage.pmm`	`micemd`	Gaussian heteroscedastic	Audigier and Resche-Rigon (2018)

6.5.2 Application

We would like to demonstrate the application of method "2l.pmm" from package miceadds. Note that when package countimp is already loaded, calling miceadds produces the following warning:

```
> library(miceadds)

* miceadds 2.8-24 (2017-11-20 19:47:38)
Attaching package: miceadds
The following object is masked from
package:countimp:mice.impute.2l.pmm
```

This warning appears because both packages have a function called mice.impute.2l.pmm(). The question now is: How can we make sure that the right one is called? When we look at R's search path, we see the order R is using to find functions:

```
> search()

[1] ".GlobalEnv" "package:miceadds" "package:MplusAutomation"
[4] "package:micemd" "package:xtable" "package:countimp"
```

Since we have loaded miceadds after countimp, it appears earlier in the search path, so the two-level PMM function from package miceadds will be used. Apart from that, the imputation process works analogous to other two-level imputation functions in mice (see, for example, Sect. 6.2.2.7):

```
> data(crim4l)
> crim4l$TIME2 <- crim4l$TIME^2
> ini <- mice(crim4l, maxit=0)
> meth <- ini$method
> meth["DELINQ"] <- "2l.pmm"
> pred <- ini$predictorMatrix
> pred["DELINQ",] <- c(1,1,1,2,0,-2,1)
> imp.2l.pmm <- mice( data = crim4l, method = meth, m = 100,
+          predictorMatrix = pred, maxit = 20, print = FALSE)
```

Object imp.2l.pmm is of class mids and can be analysed as outlined in Chap. 5.

6.5.3 Discussion

Two-level predictive mean matching might be a fruitful addition to the methodological toolbox, especially in situations where assumptions of fully parametric imputation models are violated. The major theoretical problem is to adapt standard k-NN techniques like PMM to the special structure of multilevel data in such a way that the final inferences can be assumed to allow (approximately) valid inferences. In particular, two-level PMM approaches need to successfully address the bias/variance trade-off problems discussed in the literature (see Sect. 4.5.7).

Note that little is yet known about the properties of existing two-level predictive mean matching approaches, and sound recommendations cannot yet be made in which scenarios the method may safely be applied. Systematic Monte Carlo Simulations and comparisons to existing procedures are very scarce. Kleinke (2016), for example, has demonstrated that two-level PMM may produce unbiased valid inferences and seems to work as well as standard two-level approaches in situations, where all model assumptions of the multilevel models are met. Kleinke (2016), however, only examined situations with a minimum of 50 clusters of size 30 or more. In situations, where both the number of clusters and the sample size per cluster are sufficiently large, the method appears to allow valid inferences. However, in panel data sets cluster sizes are typically small (e.g., 5 panel waves). It is plausible that two-level PMM might produce biased estimates of cluster effects, when sample size per cluster is small.

Generally, bias can be expected to depend on the availability of suitable donor cases (Dahl, 2007; Schenker & Taylor, 1996). The smaller the sample, the less likely it becomes that suitable donor cases can be selected. Consequently, with small level-1 and level-2 sample sizes, other methods might be a better option. At the moment, practical guidelines are not yet available regarding whether to adopt PMM at all for multilevel data, and which donor selection strategy to choose in which scenario. All methods listed in Table 6.3 only support classical PMM matching based on a donor pool of constant size k. Future research should explore, if and how more flexible solutions like the strategy of Siddique and Belin (2008) adopted in `midastouch` can fruitfully be adapted to generate imputations for clustered data (see also Sect. 4.5.7 and Chap. 5).

Finally, one disadvantage of PMM is that for very large data sets, the method can become quite slow (as classical PMM involves comparisons of the predicted means of each donee to the predicted means of all potential donor cases) in each iteration for each of the m sets of imputations. Vink et al. (2015) have proposed some ideas to increase the efficiency of PMM algorithms, when data sets are very large. These ideas can be easily implemented in the functions listed in Table 6.3.

6.6 The Growth Curve ZIP Model Revisited

Throughout the book, we have used the CrimoC data to illustrate the application of various MI methods. Like in Chap. 5, we want to fit the growth curve ZIP model from Reinecke and Weins (2013) to the imputed data sets to demonstrate, to what extent statistical inferences can be affected by the respective imputation method. We have discussed several imputation procedures in Chaps. 5 and 6, which seem to be more or less appropriate for the empirical problem at hand (here: a growth curve model with a zero-inflated dependent count variable). In this section, we want to compare results obtained by more recently proposed MI approaches.

Table 6.4 Comparison of the distributions of the observed and imputed parts of variable DELINQ

	Min.	1st Qu.	Median	Mean	3rd Qu.	Max.	0%	1%	2%	3%	4%	5%
Observed	0.00	0.00	0.00	1.01	1.00	16.00	60.71	17.43	8.07	5.04	3.12	1.97
2l.poisson	0.00	0.00	0.00	0.77	1.00	16.00	56.85	23.19	10.43	5.79	3.41	0.13
2l.nb	0.00	0.00	0.00	0.77	1.00	16.00	56.86	23.32	10.47	5.66	3.36	0.14
2l.zip	0.00	0.00	0.00	0.91	2.00	15.00	63.17	10.28	10.51	7.99	5.02	2.89
2l.zinb	0.00	0.00	0.00	0.91	2.00	15.00	63.15	10.37	10.62	7.88	5.05	2.79
2l.hnb	0.00	0.00	0.00	0.79	1.00	16.00	58.50	18.84	12.14	6.63	3.56	0.18
2l.pmm	0.00	0.00	0.00	1.03	1.00	16.00	60.32	17.54	8.09	5.04	3.22	1.99

Note. The table displays the minimum, quartiles, maximum, as well as the percentages of counts from 0 to 5 for the observed and imputed parts of variable DELINQ

Table 6.4 contrasts descriptive statistics of variable DELINQ in long format based on observed information alone with the distributions of the imputed values created by functions from packages countimp and miceadds. Note that the hierarchical structure of the panel data can at the moment not explicitly be modeled with robust imputation methods from packages Quantreg and ImputeRobust. Therefore these techniques are not considered in the following comparisons. Also note that the CrimoC data are empirical panel data obtained from survey questionnaires and, if the missing values are not MCAR or the imputation model is misspecified, the distribution of the imputed values can be expected to differ from the distribution of the observed part of the data set. If there are striking differences in the distributions, when the imputed values are heavily clustered in extreme areas or if they exhibit exaggerated variation, then the adopted imputation model should receive more attention. If imputations are generated using more flexible imputation models and the descriptive results and inferences from analyses of applied-scientific interest remain roughly unchanged, then one might argue that the imputation method based on more restrictive models seems not to be misspecified with respect to the specific analyses, at least given the class of imputation models adopted and thus given the underlying assumptions. Finally, if the assumption is warranted that the majority of missing values may not be MNAR, the amount of missing information due to missing values being possibly MNAR is low and there is no evidence of grossly misspecified imputation models, then cautious interpretation of the results are justified.

As can be seen in Table 6.4, distributions differ to some extent. The majority of the observed part of the sample (about 96%) has delinquency scores between 0 and 5. That means, only around 4% of all scores range between 6 and 16 (the latter being the maximum of the scale).

We first look at the main part of the distribution (i.e., delinquency between 0 and 5). The procedure that overall generated imputations with a distribution closest to the distribution of the observed delinquency scores is two-level predictive mean matching. Although the imputation model of method "2l.pmm" assumes a two-level model with continuous normal distributions (for matching the potential donor cases to the donees), imputations seem to preserve the distribution of the (observed) empirical data. Note that predictive mean matching always imputes an actual observed value. This result, however, does *not* imply that inferences are valid: If the missing data mechanism is ignorable but missing values are not MCAR, then it may well happen that missing values are not a subset of the observed values or may be outside the range of the observed part of the data set. Predictive mean matching approaches cannot make any extrapolations beyond the set of observed values (see also van Buuren, 2012). Assuming that the range of the complete cases—for example—is between 0 and 10, it would not have been possible to obtain any imputations above 10. Furthermore, PMM approaches also tend to fail, when model assumptions are severely violated or when the number of possible donors to choose from is inappropriate (Dahl 2007; de Jong et al. 2016; Kleinke 2017, Schenker & Taylor 1996).

Methods `"2l.poisson"` and `"2l.nb"` imputed less zeros in comparison to the complete part of the data. These functions create counts based on a Poisson or negative binomial model, respectively. As these models do not assume zero-inflation in the data, the number of imputed zeros can be expected to be less in comparison to both the distribution of the empirical variable and in comparison to results obtained by dedicated zero-inflation imputation models (e.g. `"2l.zip"`, `"2l.zinb"` or `"2l.hnb"`, see also simulation results by Kleinke & Reinecke, 2013b).

Now, let us explore the more extreme cases of juvenile delinquency (scores between 6 and 16, not shown in Table 6.4). An observed delinquency score of 16 indicates the highest possible versatility in criminal activity. Note again that the majority of the sample reported either no punishable offence or only very few offences. Only less than one percent (0.91%) of the observed part of the sample has a delinquency score larger than 9. However, the extreme observations (which in this case are very much of interest to applied researchers focusing on juvenile delinquency) can affect model results quite noticeably and we need to establish, how the respective imputation methods fare to create a sufficient number of values in this part of the distribution.

In fact, using the default settings, methods `"2l.poisson"`, `"2l.nb"`, `"2l.zip"`, `"2l.zinb"` and `"2l.hnb"` produce only very few extreme imputations above a score of 9 with a maximum of only 0.04%. Note that by default functions from package `countimp` try to avoid extreme imputations.[3] We encourage applied researchers to think about how to properly handle outliers in their data for the respective analysis at hand.

Table 6.5 shows the model fit statistics of the growth curve ZIP model based on the different imputed data sets. Models are estimated in M*plus* using R's

[3]Usually imputations of extreme values are not desired and can bias parameter estimates and statistical inferences. Users can turn this feature off by setting argument `EV` (i.e., extreme values) to `FALSE`. For details, see, for example, `help("mice.impute.2l.poisson")`.

Table 6.5 Results of the growth curve ZIP model under different robust imputation procedures (fit statistics)

	LL_Mean	LL_SD	AIC_Mean	AIC_SD	BIC_Mean	BIC_SD	aBIC_Mean	aBIC_SD
2l.poisson	−11069.92	39.74	22187.84	79.48	22323.02	79.48	22246.77	79.48
2l.nb	−11070.97	42.07	22189.95	84.13	22325.12	84.13	22248.88	84.13
2l.zip	−10992.82	61.52	22033.65	123.03	22168.83	123.03	22092.58	123.03
2l.zinb	−10991.77	61.73	22031.54	123.45	22166.72	123.45	22090.47	123.45
2l.hnb	−11012.74	44.40	22073.48	88.81	22208.66	88.81	22132.41	88.81
2l.pmm	−11570.28	85.984	23188.56	171.96	23323.74	171.96	23247.49	171.96

Note. Abbreviations are explained in the text

`MplusAutomation` package.[4] R code to reproduce the results may be found in the supplementary material of the book. For each imputation technique and for each of the $m = 100$ imputed data sets, log-likelihood (LL) as well as several information criteria (Akaike Information Criteria (AIC); Bayesian Information Criteria (BIC); adjusted BIC (aBIC)) are calculated (see further explanations in Appendix A.3.3).

The mean and standard deviations of the respective fit statistics across the $m = 100$ sets of imputations are displayed in Table 6.5 and are labelled $*$_Mean and $*$_SD, respectively, where $*$ represents LL or one of the information criteria. Generally, the lower the values of the information criteria, the better the model fit. Imputations with `"2l.zinb"`, `"2l.zip"` and `"2l.hnb"` lead to the lowest mean values of AIC, BIC and aBIC. All three methods consider the excess number of zeros in the data. Here, model assumptions of both the imputation and the subsequent analysis model are more in agreement in comparison to the other techniques.

Two-level predictive mean matching lead to the worst model fits. The procedure is based on a two-level model assuming a continuous normal distributed variable. Previous research has shown that using normal model predictive mean matching for highly skewed data could yield biased inferences (e.g. Kleinke, 2017; Yu et al., 2007).

To what extent the different imputation methods lead to differences in parameter estimates and their standard errors is summarized in Table 6.6. The table displays the pooled results. For details about the model, see Sect. 5.2.2, for details about MI inference, see Chap. 4.

The upper part of Table 6.6 lists estimated growth curve parameters of the count part (I, S, Q) and the zero-inflation part (II, SI, QI) of the model, respectively. The lower part of Table 6.6 displays the estimated regression coefficients. Here, growth factors are regressed on dichotomous variables gender (`FEMALE`) and school type (`RE` and `GY`).[5] Recall that for identification purposes the intercept of the zero part (II) is always fixed to zero (Reinecke & Weins, 2013). We compare results obtained by the various MI methods against FIML estimates from Reinecke and Weins (2013), which we use as a benchmark. Since in this particular application missing data are only present in the dependent variable, we can expect FIML results to be valid given that our assumption holds that the missing data are MAR, that missingness in fact only depends on the predictors included in the model, and given that the growth curve ZIP model by Reinecke and Weins (2013) is not misspecified.

Intercept estimates (I) in Table 6.6 give the mean value of delinquency at the beginning of the panel study (on the log scale). The values range between 0.72 (`"2l.poisson"`, `"2l.nb"`) and 0.94 (`"2l.pmm"`). The FIML estimate by

---

[4] `MplusAutomation` is an R package that facilitates the creation, management, execution and interpretation of latent variable analyses using M*plus*; see https://CRAN.R-project.org/package=MplusAutomation. For more information see Hallquist and Wiley (2019).

[5] In Reinecke and Weins (2013) the respective school types are labelled 'Medium' (`RE`) and 'High' (`GY`). The school type 'Low' (`HA`) was the reference category, see Sect. 5.2.

Table 6.6 Results of the growth curve ZIP model under different two-level imputation procedures (parameter estimates)

	2l.poisson		2l.nb		2l.zip		2l.zinb		2l.hnb		2l.pmm	
	Est.	S.E.	Est.	S.E.	Est.	S.E.	Est.	S.E.	Est.	S.E.	Est.	S.E.
Growth factors												
I	0.72	0.07	0.72	0.07	0.92	0.06	0.91	0.07	0.78	0.07	0.94	0.08
S	0.60	0.10	0.60	0.10	0.42	0.09	0.43	0.09	0.58	0.09	0.41	0.11
Q	−0.18	0.03	−0.18	0.03	−0.13	0.03	−0.13	0.03	−0.17	0.03	−0.12	0.03
II	0.00	0.00	0.00	0.00	0.00	0.00	0.00	0.00	0.00	0.00	0.00	0.00
SI	−0.70	0.21	−0.70	0.22	−0.88	0.20	−0.89	0.20	−0.72	0.22	−0.73	0.21
QI	0.16	0.07	0.16	0.07	0.21	0.06	0.21	0.06	0.16	0.07	0.20	0.07
Regressions												
I ON FEMALE	−0.37	0.09	−0.38	0.09	−0.38	0.09	−0.38	0.09	−0.37	0.09	−0.29	0.10
I ON RE	−0.24	0.10	−0.25	0.10	−0.22	0.09	−0.22	0.09	−0.25	0.10	−0.20	0.11
I ON GY	−0.25	0.10	−0.25	0.10	−0.32	0.09	−0.31	0.09	−0.29	0.10	−0.29	0.10
S ON FEMALE	−0.18	0.12	−0.18	0.12	−0.15	0.12	−0.15	0.12	−0.18	0.12	−0.23	0.13
S ON RE	0.08	0.13	0.10	0.13	0.09	0.12	0.09	0.12	0.10	0.12	0.05	0.14
S ON GY	−0.06	0.13	−0.06	0.13	0.04	0.12	0.02	0.13	−0.03	0.13	−0.01	0.14
Q ON FEMALE	0.07	0.04	0.06	0.04	0.06	0.03	0.06	0.04	0.06	0.04	0.08	0.04
Q ON RE	−0.01	0.04	−0.02	0.04	−0.02	0.04	−0.02	0.04	−0.02	0.04	−0.01	0.04
Q ON GY	−0.01	0.04	−0.01	0.04	−0.03	0.04	−0.03	0.04	−0.02	0.04	−0.02	0.04
II ON FEMALE	0.47	0.14	0.47	0.15	0.53	0.14	0.53	0.13	0.50	0.14	0.37	0.14
II ON RE	−0.04	0.18	−0.06	0.18	0.03	0.16	0.00	0.17	−0.03	0.18	0.07	0.18
II ON GY	0.42	0.17	0.41	0.17	0.33	0.15	0.33	0.16	0.35	0.17	0.38	0.16
SI ON FEMALE	0.05	0.21	0.06	0.21	0.05	0.20	0.04	0.20	0.04	0.21	0.15	0.20
SI ON RE	0.36	0.27	0.39	0.27	0.30	0.24	0.33	0.25	0.35	0.26	0.30	0.26
SI ON GY	0.39	0.25	0.39	0.25	0.46	0.23	0.46	0.24	0.43	0.25	0.39	0.24
QI ON FEMALE	0.02	0.06	0.01	0.07	0.01	0.06	0.01	0.06	0.01	0.07	−0.03	0.06
QI ON RE	−0.12	0.08	−0.13	0.08	−0.11	0.08	−0.12	0.08	−0.12	0.08	−0.12	0.08
QI ON GY	−0.16	0.08	−0.16	0.08	−0.17	0.08	−0.17	0.08	−0.17	0.08	−0.16	0.08

Note. I is the intercept, S and Q the linear and quadratic slopes in the count part of the model. II, SI and QI are the respective counterparts in the zero-inflation part of the model. The growth factors of both parts are regressed on FEMALE (the gender indicator), RE and GY (the school type indicators)

Reinecke and Weins (2013) is 0.96. Two-level predictive mean matching as well as the two-level zero-inflation imputation techniques from package `countimp` produced estimates that are close to the FIML estimate.

Linear slope estimates (S) show the mean value of the linear development of delinquency throughout the period of the study. Positive estimated values reflect an average increase of delinquency. Estimates range between 0.41 (`"2l.pmm"`) and 0.60 (`"2l.poisson"`, `"2l.nb"`). The FIML estimate is 0.42. Again, the two-level zero-inflation models from package `countimp` as well as two-level PMM produced close estimates.

The quadratic slope (Q) gives the estimated mean value of the quadratic development of delinquency throughout the period of the study. Negative values reflect a weakening or even inversion of the positive time trend in reported delinquency. The estimates range between −0.12 (`"2l.pmm"`) and −0.18 (`"2l.poisson"`, `"2l.nb"`). The FIML estimate is −0.12. Again, the zero-inflation methods `"2l.zip"` and `"2l.zinb"` as well as two-level PMM yielded close estimates.

Note that because we considered only data from four panel waves, the estimates of Q are considerably smaller than the values of the linear slope S. The four panel waves do not show the complete trend of the curvilinear development of delinquency in adolescence. Nevertheless, parameter estimates of I, S and Q reflect the curvilinear development which is described as the *age-crime curve* in criminological research (e.g. Seddig & Reinecke, 2017).

Coefficients of the linear slope of the inflation part of the model (SI) vary between −0.70 (`"2l.poisson"`, `"2l.nb"`) and −0.89 (`"2l.zinb"`). Quadratic slopes (QI) range between 0.16 (`"2l.poisson"`, `"2l.nb"`, `"2l.hnb"`) and 0.21 (`"2l.zip"`, `"2l.zinb"`). The FIML estimates by Reinecke and Weins (2013) are −0.89 (SI) and 0.22 (QI), respectively. Again, the zero-inflation imputation models, as well as two-level PMM yielded the closest estimates to the FIML results.

Standard errors of all growth curve parameters are very similar across the imputation techniques.

Regression estimates regarding the intercept (`I ON FEMALE`, `RE` and `GY`) are all negative. The values range between −0.20 (`"2l.pmm"`) and −0.38 (`"2l.nb"`, `"2l.zip"` and `"2l.zinb"`). The FIML estimates by Reinecke and Weins (2013) are −0.42 (for `FEMALE`), −0.31 (`RE`) and −0.36 (`GY`). Substantially, the negative values reflect that female students and students attending either the intermediate or top-level branch of the German educational system have a lower estimated average starting level of delinquency.

Regression estimates regarding the slope (`I ON FEMALE`, `RE` and `GY`) are negative for gender. Values range between −0.15 (`"2l.zip"`, `"2l.zinb"`) and −0.23 (`"2l.pmm"`), whereas absolute estimated coefficients for school type are not larger than 0.10. The FIML estimate is −0.17 for `FEMALE`, 0.19 for `RE` and −0.09 for `GY`. Noticeable differences between FIML estimates and the ones obtained here are only the regression coefficients of the slope on `RE`. Substantially the negative values of the regression coefficients of gender imply that male students—on average—exhibit a higher estimated increase in delinquency over time. Furthermore, the estimated increase in delinquency seems to be only partly affected by school type.

Absolute values of the regression estimates regarding the quadratic slope (`Q ON FEMALE`, `RE` and `GY`) are always lower in comparison to the values obtained for the linear slope. In addition, all estimates have values close to zero, and the variation between the imputation procedures is small. All in all, the decrease of delinquency appears to depend neither on gender nor on school type.

Regression coefficients regarding the intercept of the inflation part of the model (II) vary between 0.37 (`"2l.pmm"`) and 0.53 (`"2l.zip"`, `"2l.zinb"`) for gender. Regarding the intermediate school branch (`RE`), coefficients are close to zero. Furthermore, coefficients range between 0.33 (`"2l.zip"`, `"2l.zinb"`) and 0.42 (`"2l.poisson"`) for the top-level branch (`GY`). In comparison, the FIML estimate for `FEMALE` is 0.40, for `RE` 0.06 and for `GY` 0.37. Substantially, the positive values of the regression coefficients of gender imply that female students on average seem to have a higher probability of reporting zero delinquent behaviours at the first panel wave. Furthermore, students attending the top-level branch (`GY`) also on average have a higher estimated percentage of zeros at the first panel wave.

Regression estimates regarding the linear slope of the inflation part of the model (SI) vary between 0.04 (`"2l.zinb"`, `"2l.hnb"`) and 0.15 (`"2l.pmm"`) for gender. For school type, they range between 0.30 (`"2l.pmm"`) and 0.39 (`"2l.nb"`) for the intermediate branch (`RE`), and between 0.39 (`"2l.pmm"`, `"2l.nb"`, `"2l.pmm"`) and 0.46 (`"2l.zip"`, `"2l.zinb"`) for the top-level branch (`GY`). The FIML estimate for `FEMALE` is 0.15, for `RE` 0.39 and for `GY` 0.54. Substantially, the positive values of the regression coefficients regarding the linear slope reflect that the estimated probability of reporting zero delinquent behaviours decreases less over time for female students in comparison to male students, and for students from Realschule and Gymnasium in comparison to Hauptschule. These subgroups on average have a higher estimated amount of zeros across the whole period of the study. Interpretations in this regard have to be made with caution because of the relatively large standard errors (between 0.2 and 0.3). Note, however, that also the corresponding FIML estimates have large standard errors of between 0.20 and 0.25 (see Table 7 in Reinecke & Weins, 2013).

Like in the count part of the model, estimated regression coefficients regarding the quadratic slope of the inflation part (`QI ON FEMALE`, `RE` and `GY`) are also lower compared to the values obtained for the linear slope. They are close to zero for gender. For the intermediate school branch (`RE`) estimated values lie between −0.11 (`"2l.zip"`) and −0.13 (`"2l.nb"`). For the top-level branch (`GY`), values range between −0.16 and −0.17. The FIML estimate for `FEMALE` is −0.02, for `RE` −0.15 and for `GY` −0.21. Substantially, the estimated negative values of the regression coefficients regarding the quadratic slope reflect a turning point and decrease in delinquency later on in adolescence. The estimated probability of reporting zero delinquent behaviours increases again later on, and more so for female students in comparison to male students, and more so for students from Realschule and Gymnasium in comparison to Hauptschule.

To sum up the comparisons of the parameter estimates of the growth curve ZIP model, we see some variation in model results depending on the selected missing data method. Overall, zero-inflation procedures and also two-level predictive mean matching imputation methods yielded estimates that are close to the FIML estimates by Reinecke and Weins (2013). Imputation models, which did not consider the zero-inflation in the data yielded model results that differed to a larger degree from the results based on FIML.

Finally, we want to revisit substantive model results from Chap. 5 and compare them with results obtained from imputation procedures applied in Chap. 6. Comparisons of model fit statistics regarding the growth curve ZIP model introduced in Chap. 5 (Sect. 5.2.2) are displayed in Table 6.7.

In terms of both AIC, BIC and aBIC, imputation methods considering level information (`"2l.zinb"`, `"2l.zip"` and `"2l.pmm"`) yield better model fit statistics in comparison to wide format techniques (`"norm2"`, `"midastouch"`, `"pmm"`). Two-level PMM in comparison to ordinary PMM explicitly considered time and the negative quadratic time trend in the imputation model, whereas wide format PMM only implicitly considers information from other panel waves. However, both PMM variants are based on the normal model. Also `"norm2"` used the implausible multivariate normal model as imputation model. The procedure we have adopted in Chap. 5 (to split of the zero-inflated variables into zero vs. non-zero indicators and zero-truncated count variables)—however—was (at least partially) able to buffer bias introduced by implausible model assumptions. All in all, considering level information and count data distributional assumptions resulted in better model fit statistics of the growth curve ZIP model. Note that this comparison of model results is descriptive in nature, does not allow an evaluation of the imputation method and cannot be generalized beyond the specific data set. The claim of every method to compensate for missing values is to allow valid statistical inferences about population statistics or, as in our example, about model parameters. Based on one empirical data set (with unknown distribution), it is *not* possible to verify whether an adopted imputation method is proper or not. This is similar to statistical model-based analyses using completely observed data sets, where it is usually not possible to decide whether all assumptions are met and the chosen model is correct. In the presence of missing values, it is therefore worthwhile to carefully choose and design the imputation steps based on theoretical considerations and available empirical results. Once the imputations are generated it is always advisable to apply diagnostic instruments like summary statistics and plots of imputed and observed variables, not with the claim to find out whether the assumptions underlying the imputation strategy are correct, but trying to rule out that given the assumed missing data mechanism, imputation models are grossly misspecified. The importance of this strategy increases with the amount of missing information. In addition, if several imputation models can be justified and are available, and if the effort is reasonable, it is advantageous to generate imputations under these different imputation strategies. The analyst may then conduct a sensitivity analysis: Estimate the model of applied-scientific interest using the different sets of imputations and compare the results, i.e., estimates, standard errors, confidence intervals or results

Table 6.7 Results of the growth curve ZIP model—a comparison of wide and long format imputation methods with fitting and inappropriate distributional assumptions (fit statistics)

	LL_Mean	LL_SD	AIC_Mean	AIC_SD	BIC_Mean	BIC_SD	aBIC_Mean	aBIC_SD
2l.zip	−10992.82	61.52	22033.65	123.03	22168.83	123.03	22092.58	123.03
2l.pmm	−11570.28	85.98	23188.56	171.96	23323.74	171.96	23247.49	171.96
norm2	−11618.10	54.15	23284.20	108.30	23419.38	108.30	23343.13	108.30
midastouch	−11724.22	92.88	23496.45	185.76	23631.62	185.76	23555.37	185.76
pmm	−11811.05	79.22	23670.09	158.43	23805.27	158.43	23729.02	158.43

Note. Results are ordered by AIC_Mean. Abbreviations are explained in the text

from hypotheses tests. If the inferences do not lead to different inferences regarding the applied-scientific questions then, obviously, these results are robust with respect to the different imputation techniques given the assumed missing data mechanism, and the model of applied-scientific interest. Otherwise, the analyst should rethink the design and models to generate the imputations. If no justifiable reason to prefer one of the imputation techniques is available, then all the results should be reported and differing inferences should be discussed.

6.7 Future Research—Multiple Imputation After More Than Three Decades

We have seen that relatively simple workaround solutions like the one used in Reinecke and Weins (2013), i.e., multiple imputation of skewed count data based on the multivariate normal model in combination with data transformations and rounding may produce results that are not obviously implausible (but since we did not run systematic Monte Carlo simulations, it cannot be decided, if inferences are valid in this particular situation). Also, if we are interested in the fixed part of regression models alone, wide format techniques like predictive mean matching (especially the distance-aided donor selection approach `midastouch`) may produce valid results, as long as assumptions of the underlying model are not severely violated, although the theoretically most sound method would have been to use imputation models that are congenial to the model of applied-scientific interest—in our application a growth curve ZIP model.

Typically, in applied statistics, there is often not the one single method that fits best to all problems at hand, and for some problems suitable solutions do not yet exist. Even after more than three decades of multiple imputation research, there is still work to do. With faster computers, more flexible but also more complex statistical models can be estimated with more time-consuming estimation procedures. We can thus further explore the worlds beyond simple models that are based on the often implausible assumption of normality. With packages like `ImputeRobust` or `Qtools`, we will be able to specially tailor our MI models to the distribution of the empirical data at hand, and we can model not only the conditional mean or median of the incomplete variable given certain covariates, but also other conditional moments or quantiles, hopefully moving our imputation methods closer to being proper in the sense of Rubin (1987, 1996).

Secondly, in addition to using models with appropriate distributional assumptions, multiple imputation theory states that the imputation model should be compatible to the substantial model of applied-scientific interest (e.g. Rubin, 1996). This means, for example, that non-linear terms like interactions or higher-order polynomials have to be adequately included in the imputation model, as well. The often applied quick solutions like *passive imputation* or including these terms as *just another variable* into the imputation model either do not work at all or work only

Table 6.8 Overview of additional multiple imputation software/packages

Package/macro	Software	Framework
Blimp	standalone	FCS
mdmb	R	FCS
mitml	R	tools for multilevel MI with `pan` and `jomo`

Note. FCS fully conditional specification

in very special situations. Therefore, these quick solutions cannot be recommended (see Sect. 4.5.2). One focus of MI research at the moment is on what has come to be known as *substantive model compatible MI (smcmi)*—i.e., MI methods and models that explicitly support complex imputation models containing non-linear terms (e.g. Bartlett et al., 2015; Goldstein, Carpenter, & Browne, 2014).

Thirdly, with faster processors, we can expand MI research regarding complex survey data, which often have a clustered or multilevel structure. Currently most software packages support only two-level models. For example, M*plus*—the leading software for structural equation modeling—now allows three-level models as well (e.g. repeated measurements clustered in persons clustered in schools). In case the imputer has knowledge about the substantive model to be analysed, standard imputation models should allow for more hierarchical levels.

Another important point is that missing values may occur not only in the dependent variable but also in variables included as predictors into a model of applied scientific interest. Although imputing these variables is not structurally different from imputing variables that enter the model of interest as dependent variable, again, other imputation models are necessary, as the reverse regression from an independent variable on a dependent variable (the imputation model) is usually not the same as the regression from a dependent variable on the independent variable (the model of applied-scientific interest; cf. Sect. 4.4.1).

Along with theoretical developments in the field of MI, also software developments happen quite rapidly, and it is unclear, which of the newer packages will prevail and which methods will be absorbed into the more established packages. It is beyond the scope of this book to cover all MI packages that may be of interest. Our focus was on free and open source tools that work platform-independent on Mac, Linux and Windows systems, and that are available to a wide audience. Additional (free/open source) MI packages and tools that may be worth looking at are listed in Table 6.8.

Blimp[6] is a standalone package available for Mac, Windows and Linux operating systems. It is based on the conditional modeling MI framework and can do both single-level and multilevel imputation with mixtures of continuous, ordinal and nominal variables. Like `mdmb`, substantive model compatible MI is supported. The current version 1.1 also supports three-level models.

[6]http://www.appliedmissingdata.com/multilevel-imputation.html.

R-package `mdmb`[7]—i.e., model-based treatment of missing data supports substantive model compatible multilevel MI models with missing values in both the dependent variable and the covariates. Models can contain non-linear terms like interaction effects, quadratic terms or B-spline functions.

Finally, package `mitml` provides useful tools to facilitate fitting multilevel MI models with packages `pan` and `jomo`. The latter one also supports substantive model compatible MI based on the joint modeling framework.

There are several emerging fields where MI as a method to compensate for missing values would be a valuable tool, but only a few sound suggestions for MI methods exist. One area is big data analysis where large data sets have to be imputed, probably with (hundreds of) millions of units and hundreds or thousands of variables. Another characteristic of these data sets is that they may be very dynamic, changing (usually growing) within short time intervals, probably not rectangular and that the information about the same construct is gathered on various variable levels or scales, e.g., on an ordered categorical level with 3 and 5 point scales as well as on a nominal level. One very basic but nonetheless and often not explicitly addressed question in this context is whether statistical inference is of interest at all, or if statistical models and techniques are adopted to simply reduce dimension of and condense information. If MI is applied to the latter situation the concept of a proper multiple imputation method is not defined anymore, leading to the acceptance of criteria like the hit-rate criterion to evaluate (multiple) imputation methods. If, however, these data sets are used to answer questions based on statistical estimators, confidence intervals or test statistics, then the properties of these functions are of interest, and proper imputation methods are required. The first challenge is to develop flexible methods which are proper in many situations, but at the same time are fast and use memory efficiently.

Another field is network analysis (for an introduction to network analysis, see, for example, Epskamp, Borsboom, & Fried, 2018). In this case each unit is connected with a varying number of other units and these connections are varying in strength. A challenge in this context is, if statistical inference is of interest, to adapt or develop imputation methods which are able to deal with the complex relationships. Actually, there are some first ideas to use MI in network analysis (Huisman, 2009; Krause, Huisman, & Snijders, 2018), but results about the conditions under which these methods are proper are not yet available.

Finally, as a consequence of these different branches of MI, research focusing on different MI models and techniques, we now have a relatively great abundance of available MI software, not all of them realizing proper imputation methods, however. There is neither the one single MI package that gives practitioners all they will ever need nor do the available methods and techniques necessarily allow valid inferences. Thus the analyst needs to carefully choose the imputation method for his or her problem at hand and should be able to justify his or her choice. And the set

---

[7] https://CRAN.R-project.org/package=mdmb.

of available models and techniques is not exhaustive, i.e., it can be expected that an increasing number thereof will be available within the next years.

In this book, we have focused mainly on R-package `mice`, which currently seems to be one of the most open and flexible solutions and which has the great advantage compared to other software solutions that it is very easy for MI researchers to implement additional imputation functions as add-ons. However, this freedom comes with the responsibility to realize best scientific practice not only by the software developer but also by the users.

References

Audigier, V., & Resche-Rigon, M. (2018). `micemd`: Multiple imputation by chained equations with multilevel data [Computer software manual]. https://CRAN.R-project.org/package=micemd (R Package Version 1.2.0).

Audigier, V., White, I. R., Jolani, S., Debray, T. P. A., Quartagno, M., Carpenter, J., et al. (2017). *Multiple imputation for multilevel data with continuous and binary variables*. https://ui.adsabs.harvard.edu/abs/2017arXiv170200971A/abstract

Bartlett, J. W., Seaman, S. R., White, I. R., & Carpenter, J. R. (2015). Multiple imputation of covariates by fully conditional specification: Accommodating the substantive model. *Statistical Methods in Medical Research, 24*(4), 462–487.

Bolker, B. M., Brooks, M. E., Clark, C. J., Geange, S. W., Poulsen, J. R., Stevens, M. H. H., et al. (2009). Generalized linear mixed models: A practical guide for ecology and evolution. *Trends in Ecology & Evolution, 24*(3), 127–135.

Bottai, M. and Zhen, H. (2013). Multiple imputation based on conditional quantile estimation. *Epidemiology, Biostatistics and Public Health, 10*(1), 1–18.

Dahl, F. A. (2007). Convergence of random k-nearest-neighbour imputation. *Computational Statistics & Data Analysis, 51*(12), 5913–5917.

de Jong, R. (2012). Robust multiple imputation (Doctoral dissertation, University of Hamburg, Germany, 2012). https://ediss.sub.uni-hamburg.de/volltexte/2012/5971/

de Jong, R., van Buuren, S., & Spiess, M. (2016). Multiple imputation of predictor variables using generalized additive models. *Communications in Statistics – Simulation and Computation, 45*(3), 968–985.

Eilers, P. H. C., & Marx, B. D. (1996). Flexible smoothing with B-splines and penalties. *Statistical Science, 11*(2), 89–121.

Epskamp, S., Borsboom, D., & Fried, E. I. (2018). Estimating psychological networks and their accuracy: A tutorial paper. *Behavior Research Methods, 50*(1), 195–212.

Erdman, D., Jackson, L., & Sinko, A. (2008). Zero-inflated poisson and zero-inflated negative binomial models using the COUNTREG procedure. In SAS Institute (Ed.), *Proceedings of the SAS ® Global Forum 2008 Conference*. Cary, NC: SAS Institute. https://support.sas.com/resources/papers/proceedings/pdfs/sgf2008/322-2008.pdf

Geraci, M. (2014). Linear quantile mixed models: The `lqmm` package for Laplace quantile regression. *Journal of Statistical Software, 57*(13), 1–29.

Geraci, M. (2016a). Estimation of regression quantiles in complex surveys with data missing at random: An application to birthweight determinants. *Statistical Methods in Medical Research, 25*(4), 1393–1421.

Geraci, M. (2016b). `Qtools`: A collection of models and tools for quantile inference. *R Journal, 8*(2), 117–138.

Geraci, M., & McLain, A. (2018). Multiple imputation for bounded variables. *Psychometrika, 83*(4), 919–940.

Goldstein, H., Carpenter, J. R., & Browne, W. J. (2014). Fitting multilevel multivariate models with missing data in responses and covariates that may include interactions and non-linear terms. *Journal of the Royal Statistical Society: Series A (Statistics in Society), 177*(2), 553–564.

Hallquist, M. N., & Wiley, J. F. (2019). `MplusAutomation`: An R Package for facilitating large-scale latent variable analyses in Mplus. *Structural Equation Modeling, 25*(4), 621–638.

Harris, I. R. (1989). Predictive fit for natural exponential families. *Biometrika, 76*(4), 675–684.

He, Y., & Raghunathan, T. E. (2012). Multiple imputation using multivariate *gh* transformations. *Journal of Applied Statistics, 39*(10), 2177–2198.

Hilbe, J. M. (2011). *Negative binomial regression* (2nd ed.). Cambridge, UK: Cambridge University Press.

Horton, N. J., Lipsitz, S. R., & Parzen, M. (2003). A potential for bias when rounding in multiple imputation. *The American Statistician, 57*(4), 229–232.

Huisman, M. (2009). Imputation of missing network data: Some simple procedures. *Journal of Social Structure, 10*(1), 1–29.

Kleinke, K. (2016). *Multiple imputation of multilevel data by two-level predictive mean matching*. Paper presented at the 50th Congress of the German Psychological Society (DGPs), Leipzig, Germany.

Kleinke, K. (2017). Multiple imputation under violated distributional assumptions—a systematic evaluation of the assumed robustness of predictive mean matching. *Journal of Educational and Behavioral Statistics, 42*(4), 371–404.

Kleinke, K., & Reinecke, J. (2013a). *countimp 1.0—A multiple imputation package for incomplete count data* (Technical Report). Bielefeld: University of Bielefeld, Faculty of Sociology.

Kleinke, K., & Reinecke, J. (2013b). Multiple imputation of incomplete zero-inflated count data. *Statistica Neerlandica, 67*(3), 311–336.

Kleinke, K., & Reinecke, J. (2015a). Multiple imputation of multilevel count data. In U. Engel, B. Jann, P. Lynn, A. Scherpenzeel, & P. Sturgis (Eds.), *Improving survey methods: Lessons from recent research* (pp. 381–396). New York, NY: Routledge, Taylor & Francis.

Kleinke, K., & Reinecke, J. (2015b). Multiple imputation of overdispersed multilevel count data. In U. Engel (Ed.), *Survey measurements. Techniques, data quality and sources of error* (pp. 209–226). Frankfurt: Campus/The University of Chicago Press.

Kleinke, K., Stemmler, M., Reinecke, J., & Lösel, F. (2011). Efficient ways to impute incomplete panel data. *Advances in Statistical Analysis, 95*(4), 351–373.

Koenker, R. (2004). Quantile regression for longitudinal data. *Journal of Multivariate Analysis, 91*(1), 74–89.

Koenker, R. (2005). *Quantile regression*. New York, NY: Cambridge University Press.

Koenker, R., & Hallock, K. F. (2001). Quantile regression. *Journal of Economic Perspectives, 15*(4), 143–156.

Krause, R. W., Huisman, M., & Snijders, T. A. B. (2018). Multiple imputation for longitudinal network data. *Italian Journal of Applied Statistics, 30*(1), 33–58.

Lambert, D. (1992). Zero-inflated Poisson regression, with an application to defects in manufacturing. *Technometrics, 34*(1), 1–14.

Mullahy, J. (1986). Specification and testing of some modified count data models. *Journal of Econometrics, 33*(3), 341–365.

Reinecke, J., & Weins, C. (2013). The development of delinquency during adolescence: A comparison of missing data techniques. *Quality & Quantity, 47*(6), 3319–3334.

Resche-Rigon, M., & White, I. R. (2016). Multiple imputation by chained equations for systematically and sporadically missing multilevel data. *Statistical Methods in Medical Research, 27*(6), 1634–1649.

Rigby, R. A., & Stasinopoulos, M. D. (2005). Generalized additive models for location, scale and shape. *Journal of the Royal Statistical Society: Series C (Applied Statistics), 54*(3), 507–554.

Rigby, R. A., Stasinopoulos, M. D., & Voudouris, V. (2013). Discussion: A comparison of GAMLSS with quantile regression. *Statistical Modelling, 13*(4), 335–348.

Robitzsch, A., Grund, S., & Henke, T. (2017). `miceadds`: Some additional multiple imputation functions, especially for `mice` [Computer software manual]. https://CRAN.R-project.org/package=miceadds (R Package Version 2.8-24).
Rubin, D. B. (1987). *Multiple imputation for nonresponse in surveys*. New York, NY: Wiley.
Rubin, D. B. (1996). Multiple imputation after 18+ years. *Journal of the American Statistical Association, 91*(434), 473–489.
Salfrán, D. (2018). Multiple imputation for complex data sets (Doctoral dissertation, University of Hamburg, Germany). https://ediss.sub.uni-hamburg.de/volltexte/2018/9058/
Salfrán, D., & Spiess, M. (2017). `ImputeRobust`: Robust multiple imputation with generalized additive models for location scale and shape [Computer software manual]. https://CRAN.R-project.org/package=ImputeRobust (R Package Version 1.2).
Salfrán, D. & Spiess, M. (2018). Generalized additive model multiple imputation by chained equations with package `imputerobust`. *The R Journal, 10*(1), 61–72.
Schenker, N., & Taylor, J. M. G. (1996). Partially parametric techniques for multiple imputation. *Computational Statistics & Data Analysis, 22*(4), 425–446.
Seddig, D., & Reinecke, J. (2017). Exploration and explanation of adolescent self-reported delinquency trajectories in the Crimoc study. In A. Blokland & V. van der Geest (Eds.), *The Routledge international handbook of life-course criminology* (pp. 159–178). New York, NY: Routledge.
Siddique, J., & Belin, T. R. (2008). Multiple imputation using an iterative hot-deck with distance-based donor selection. *Statistics in Medicine, 27*(1), 83–102.
Stasinopoulos, M. D., & Rigby, R. A. (2007). Generalized additive models for location scale and shape (GAMLSS) in R. *Journal of Statistical Software, 23*(7), 1–46.
Stasinopoulos, M. D., Rigby, R. A., Heller, G. Z., Voudouris, V., & De Bastiani, F. (2017). *Flexible regression and smoothing*. Boca Raton, FL: CRC.
van Buuren, S. (2012). *Flexible imputation of missing data*. Boca Raton, FL: Chapmann & Hall/CRC.
van Buuren, S. (2013). Multiple imputation of multilevel data. Paper presented at the Conference on Recent Advances in Multiple Imputation, with Emphasis on Dealing with Deviations from MAR or Exchangeability, Utrecht, the Netherlands.
van Buuren, S., & Groothuis-Oudshoorn, K. (2011). `mice`: Multivariate imputation by chained equations in R. *Journal of Statistical Software, 45*(3), 1–67.
Vink, G., Lazendic, G., & van Buuren, S. (2015). Partitioned predictive mean matching as a large data multilevel imputation technique. *Psychological Test and Assessment Modeling, 57*(4), 577–594.
Yu, L. M., Burton, A., & Rivero-Arias, O. (2007). Evaluation of software for multiple imputation of semi-continuous data. *Statistical Methods in Medical Research, 16*(3), 243–258.
Zeileis, A., Kleiber, C., & Jackman, S. (2008). Regression models for count data in R. *Journal of Statistical Software, 27*(8), 1–25.

Appendix A
Matrix Algebra, Random Variables and Some Technical Results

A.1 Matrix Algebra

This section gives a short summary of the notation and states some basic results in matrix algebra used in this book but without proofs. More detailed presentations of matrix algebra from a statistical point of view can be found in most books on multivariate analysis. For an extensive treatment including proofs, see, e.g., Gentle (2017), Harville (1997).

A.1.1 Vectors and Matrices

A.1.1.1 Matrices

A matrix is a rectangular array of numbers $a_{11}, a_{12}, \ldots, a_{kl}, \ldots, a_{KL}$. Matrices are represented by boldface upper-case letters. If a matrix **A** has K rows and L columns, where K and L are also called the (row and column) dimensions of **A**, we denote this matrix as an $\mathbf{A}_{K \times L}$ or the $(K \times L)$ matrix **A**, or simply **A** if the dimensions follow from the context. A $(K \times L)$ matrix is also called a matrix of order $(K \times L)$. The elements of a matrix are denoted by small letters with subscripts indicating the row and column position of the element. The elements of the matrices considered here are all real, hence we only deal with real matrices.

K. Kleinke et al., *Applied Multiple Imputation*,
Statistics for Social and Behavioral Sciences,
https://doi.org/10.1007/978-3-030-38164-6

A $(K \times L)$ matrix $\mathbf{A}$ may be written as

$$\mathbf{A} = \begin{pmatrix} a_{11} & a_{12} & \cdots & a_{1L} \\ a_{21} & a_{22} & \cdots & a_{2L} \\ \vdots & \vdots & \ddots & \vdots \\ a_{K1} & a_{K2} & \cdots & a_{KL} \end{pmatrix} = (a_{kl}) \, ,$$

where a_{kl} is the element of the kth row and the lth column, $k = 1, \ldots, K, l = 1, \ldots, L$.

An example of a (2×3)-matrix is

$$\mathbf{A} = \begin{pmatrix} 2 & 0 & 5 \\ 1 & -3 & 2 \end{pmatrix} \, .$$

A.1.1.2 Transpose of a Matrix, Symmetric Matrix

The transpose of a matrix $\mathbf{A}$ is a matrix $\mathbf{A}^T$ which results from interchanging rows and columns:

$$\mathbf{A} = \begin{pmatrix} a_{11} & a_{12} & \cdots & a_{1L} \\ a_{21} & a_{22} & \cdots & a_{2L} \\ \vdots & \vdots & \ddots & \vdots \\ a_{K1} & a_{K2} & \cdots & a_{KL} \end{pmatrix} \qquad \mathbf{A}^T = \begin{pmatrix} a_{11} & a_{21} & \cdots & a_{K1} \\ a_{12} & a_{22} & \cdots & a_{K2} \\ \vdots & \vdots & \ddots & \vdots \\ a_{1L} & a_{2L} & \cdots & a_{KL} \end{pmatrix} \, .$$

The transpose satisfies the properties:

$$(\mathbf{A}^T)^T = \mathbf{A}, \quad (\mathbf{A} + \mathbf{B})^T = \mathbf{A}^T + \mathbf{B}^T \quad \text{and} \quad (\mathbf{AB})^T = \mathbf{B}^T \mathbf{A}^T \, .$$

A matrix $\mathbf{A}$ is called symmetric if $\mathbf{A}^T = \mathbf{A}$.

A.1.1.3 Vectors

Vectors are special matrices with one column ($L = 1$) or one row ($K = 1$), and are denoted by small boldface letters,

$$\mathbf{a} = \begin{pmatrix} a_1 \\ a_2 \\ \vdots \\ a_K \end{pmatrix} \quad \text{(column vector), and} \quad \mathbf{b}^T = \begin{pmatrix} b_1 & b_2 & \cdots & b_L \end{pmatrix} \quad \text{(row vector)} \, .$$

Examples are $\mathbf{a} = \begin{pmatrix} 2 \\ 0 \\ 5 \end{pmatrix}$ and $\mathbf{b}^T = \begin{pmatrix} 1 & -3 & 2 \end{pmatrix}$.

Note that a row vector is written as a transposed column vector.

A.1.1.4 Partitioned Matrices

If $\mathbf{a}_k^T$, $k = 1, \ldots, K$ denote the rows of the $(K \times L)$ matrix $\mathbf{A}$, then $\mathbf{A}$ may be written as

$$\mathbf{A} = \begin{pmatrix} \mathbf{a}_1^T \\ \mathbf{a}_2^T \\ \vdots \\ \mathbf{a}_K^T \end{pmatrix} .$$

If $\mathbf{a}_l$, $l = 1, \ldots, L$ denote the columns of the $(K \times L)$ matrix $\mathbf{A}$, then $\mathbf{A}$ may be written as

$$\mathbf{A} = \begin{pmatrix} \mathbf{a}_1 & \mathbf{a}_2 & \cdots & \mathbf{a}_L \end{pmatrix} .$$

The row vectors $\mathbf{a}_k^T$ and the column vectors $\mathbf{a}_l$ are sub-matrices of $\mathbf{A}$. A matrix $\mathbf{A}$ may be written in terms of more general sub-matrices $\mathbf{A}_{pq}$, $p = 1, \ldots, q = 1, \ldots$. For example,

$$\mathbf{A} = \begin{pmatrix} \mathbf{A}_{11} & \mathbf{A}_{12} & \mathbf{A}_{13} \\ \mathbf{A}_{21} & \mathbf{A}_{22} & \mathbf{A}_{23} \end{pmatrix} ,$$

where $\mathbf{A}_{p1}$, $\mathbf{A}_{p2}$ and $\mathbf{A}_{p3}$ are of the same row dimension, possibly different for each $p = 1, 2$, $\mathbf{A}_{1q}$ and $\mathbf{A}_{2q}$ are of the same column dimension, possibly different for each $q = 1, 2, 3$.

A.1.1.5 Square Matrices

A matrix $\mathbf{A}_{(K \times L)}$ is square if $K = L$. In this case we may also write $\mathbf{A}_K$. The elements a_{kl}, $k = l$, of a square matrix are called diagonal elements, elements a_{kl} for which $k \neq l$ are called off-diagonal elements.

A square matrix $\mathbf{A}$ is a diagonal matrix if $a_{kl} \neq 0$ for $k = l$ and $a_{kl} = 0$ for $k \neq l$. For diagonal matrix $\mathbf{A}$, we write $\mathbf{A} = \text{diag}(a_1, \ldots, a_K)$, omitting the second index.

A.1.1.6 Some Useful Specific Matrices

A particular diagonal matrix is the identity matrix $\mathbf{I}_K$, where all diagonal elements are equal to one and the off-diagonal elements are zero. For example,

$$\mathbf{I}_3 = \begin{pmatrix} 1 & 0 & 0 \\ 0 & 1 & 0 \\ 0 & 0 & 1 \end{pmatrix} .$$

$\mathbf{J}_{K \times L}$ denotes a $(K \times L)$ matrix of ones, $\mathbf{0}_{K \times L}$ denotes a $(K \times L)$ matrix of zeros.

A.1.2 Basic Operations

A.1.2.1 Equality

Two $(K \times L)$ matrices $\mathbf{A}$ and $\mathbf{B}$ are equal, $\mathbf{A} = \mathbf{B}$, if each element of $\mathbf{A}$ is equal to the corresponding element of $\mathbf{B}$.

A.1.2.2 Addition

The sum of two matrices $\mathbf{A}$ and $\mathbf{B}$ of the same dimensions is given by $\mathbf{A} + \mathbf{B} = (a_{kl} + b_{kl})$.

Summation satisfies:

$$(\mathbf{A} + \mathbf{B} + \mathbf{C}) = (\mathbf{A} + \mathbf{B}) + \mathbf{C} = \mathbf{A} + (\mathbf{B} + \mathbf{C}) = (\mathbf{A} + \mathbf{C}) + \mathbf{B} = \mathbf{A} + \mathbf{B} + \mathbf{C} .$$

A.1.2.3 Subtraction

The difference of two matrices $\mathbf{A}$ and $\mathbf{B}$ of the same dimensions is given by $\mathbf{A} - \mathbf{B} = (a_{kl} - b_{kl})$.

Subtraction satisfies:

$$(\mathbf{A} - \mathbf{B} - \mathbf{C}) = (\mathbf{A} - \mathbf{B}) - \mathbf{C} = \mathbf{A} - (\mathbf{B} + \mathbf{C}) = (\mathbf{A} - \mathbf{C}) - \mathbf{B} = \mathbf{A} - \mathbf{B} - \mathbf{C} .$$

A.1.2.4 Scalar Multiplication

The product of a scalar x and a matrix $\mathbf{A}$ is $x\mathbf{A} = (xa_{kl})$.

A.1.2.5 Inner Product, Orthogonal and Orthonormal Vectors

The inner product of two vectors **a** and **b** of the same dimension is given by

$$\mathbf{a}^T\mathbf{b} = \sum_{k=1}^{K} a_k b_k \,.$$

Two vectors **a** and **b** are said to be orthogonal if $\mathbf{a}^T\mathbf{b} = 0$. They are said to be orthonormal if $\mathbf{a}^T\mathbf{b} = 0$ and $\mathbf{a}^T\mathbf{a} = \mathbf{b}^T\mathbf{b} = 1$.

A.1.2.6 Outer Product

The outer product of two vectors $\mathbf{a}_K$ and $\mathbf{b}_K$ is given by

$$\mathbf{a}\mathbf{b}^T = \begin{pmatrix} a_1b_1 & a_1b_2 & \cdots & a_1b_L \\ a_2b_1 & a_2b_2 & \cdots & a_2b_L \\ \vdots & \vdots & \ddots & \vdots \\ a_Kb_1 & a_Kb_2 & \cdots & a_Kb_L \end{pmatrix} .$$

Note that there is no restriction with respect to the dimensions of the two vectors.

A.1.2.7 Multiplication

The product of two matrices $\mathbf{A}_{(K\times L)}$ and $\mathbf{B}_{(L\times M)}$, where $k = 1, \ldots, K$, $l = 1, \ldots, L$ and $m = 1, \ldots, M$, is

$$\mathbf{AB} = \begin{pmatrix} \sum_{l=1}^{L} a_{1l}b_{l1} & \sum_{l=1}^{L} a_{1l}b_{l2} & \cdots & \sum_{l=1}^{L} a_{1l}b_{lM} \\ \sum_{l=1}^{L} a_{2l}b_{l1} & \sum_{l=1}^{L} a_{2l}b_{l2} & \cdots & \sum_{l=1}^{L} a_{2l}b_{lM} \\ \vdots & \vdots & \ddots & \vdots \\ \sum_{l=1}^{L} a_{Kl}b_{l1} & \sum_{l=1}^{L} a_{Kl}b_{l2} & \cdots & \sum_{l=1}^{L} a_{Kl}b_{lM} \end{pmatrix} .$$

The k, mth element of this matrix is the inner product of the vector given by the kth row of **A** and the mth column of **B**.

Multiplication satisfies:

$$(\mathbf{AB})\mathbf{C} = \mathbf{A}(\mathbf{BC}) = \mathbf{ABC} \quad \text{and} \quad (\mathbf{A}+\mathbf{B})\mathbf{C} = \mathbf{AC} + \mathbf{BC} \,.$$

But $\mathbf{AB} \neq \mathbf{BA}$, in general.

A.1.2.8 Trace of a Symmetric Matrix

Let $\mathbf{A}$ be a $(K \times K)$ matrix with diagonal elements a_{kk}, $k = 1, \ldots, K$. Then the trace of $\mathbf{A}$ is $\mathrm{tr}(\mathbf{A}) = \sum_{k=1}^{K} a_{kk}$.

Let $\mathbf{A}$ and $\mathbf{B}$ be both $(K \times K)$ matrices, $\mathbf{C} = (d_{kl})$ be a $(K \times L)$, $\mathbf{D} = (d_{lk})$ be a $(L \times K)$ matrix, and x be a scalar. Properties of the trace function are:

$\mathrm{tr}(x\,\mathbf{A}) = x\,\mathrm{tr}(\mathbf{A})$,
$\mathrm{tr}(\mathbf{A} \pm \mathbf{B}) = \mathrm{tr}(\mathbf{A}) \pm \mathrm{tr}(\mathbf{B})$,
$\mathrm{tr}(\mathbf{CD}) = \mathrm{tr}(\mathbf{DC}) = \sum_{k=1}^{K} \sum_{l=1}^{L} c_{kl} d_{lk}$.

A.1.3 Properties of Matrices

A.1.3.1 Determinant

Instead of a definition, we introduce the determinant of a square matrix $\mathbf{A}$ by a computational approach (see, e.g., Harville 1997 for a more detailed treatment). The determinant of a $(K \times K)$ matrix $\mathbf{A}_K = (a_{kl})$ is denoted as $|\mathbf{A}|$ or $\det(\mathbf{A})$. Let $\mathbf{A}_{(kl)}$ be the submatrix $\mathbf{A}_{K-1}$ obtained by deleting the kth row and the lth column. The determinant $|\mathbf{A}_{(kl)}|$ of this submatrix is called the minor and $(-1)^{k+l}|\mathbf{A}_{(kl)}|$ is called the cofactor of element a_{kl}. The determinant of $\mathbf{A}_K$ can be calculated as follows:

$$\text{if} \quad K = 1: \quad |\mathbf{A}| = a \quad \text{for} \quad A_1 = (a)$$

and, for $k = 1, \ldots, K$,

$$\text{if} \quad K \geq 2: \quad |\mathbf{A}| = \sum_{l=1}^{K} (-1)^{k+l} a_{kl} |\mathbf{A}_{(kl)}|$$

or, correspondingly for $l = 1, \ldots, K$,

$$\text{if} \quad K \geq 2: \quad |\mathbf{A}| = \sum_{k=1}^{K} (-1)^{k+l} a_{kl} |\mathbf{A}_{(kl)}| \,.$$

For example, let

$$\mathbf{A} = \begin{pmatrix} 3 & 1 & 2 \\ 1 & 4 & 3 \\ 2 & 3 & 5 \end{pmatrix} .$$

The determinant can be calculated by fixing, e.g., $k = 1$,

$$|\mathbf{A}| = (-1)^2 a_{11} |\mathbf{A}_{(11)}| + (-1)^3 a_{12} |\mathbf{A}_{(12)}| + (-1)^4 a_{13} |\mathbf{A}_{(13)}|$$

and noting that

$$|\mathbf{A}_{(11)}| = (-1)^2 \cdot 4 \cdot 5 + (-1)^3 \cdot 3 \cdot 3 = 11$$
$$|\mathbf{A}_{(12)}| = (-1)^2 \cdot 1 \cdot 5 + (-1)^3 \cdot 3 \cdot 2 = -1$$
$$|\mathbf{A}_{(13)}| = (-1)^2 \cdot 1 \cdot 3 + (-1)^3 \cdot 4 \cdot 2 = -5$$

and therefore

$$|\mathbf{A}| = (-1)^2 \cdot 3 \cdot 11 + (-1)^3 \cdot 1 \cdot (-1) + (-1)^4 \cdot 2 \cdot (-5) = 24 .$$

A.1.3.2 (Non-)singular Matrix

A square matrix $\mathbf{A}$ is denoted as nonsingular if $|\mathbf{A}| \neq 0$. Otherwise it is denoted as singular.

A.1.3.3 Linear Combinations and Linear Dependence

Consider $(K \times 1)$ vectors $\mathbf{a}_1, \ldots, \mathbf{a}_L$ as columns in a $(K \times L)$ matrix $\mathbf{A}$. Vector $\mathbf{b}$ is called a linear combination of $\mathbf{a}_1, \ldots, \mathbf{a}_L$ if $\mathbf{b} = \mathbf{Ax}$ for some (real) vector $\mathbf{x} = (x_1, \ldots, x_L)^T$. A trivial solution if $\mathbf{b} = \mathbf{0}$ would be $\mathbf{x} = \mathbf{0}$.

The set of vectors $\mathbf{a}_1, \ldots, \mathbf{a}_L$ and thus the columns of $\mathbf{A}$ are said to be linearly dependent if there exists a vector $\mathbf{x} \neq \mathbf{0}$ such that $\mathbf{Ab} = \mathbf{0}$. Otherwise the set of vectors is said to be linearly independent.

As an example

$$\mathbf{A}_1 = \begin{pmatrix} 2 & 1 \\ 4 & 2 \end{pmatrix} \quad \text{and} \quad \mathbf{x} = \begin{pmatrix} 1 \\ -2 \end{pmatrix} \quad \text{gives} \quad \begin{pmatrix} 2 \\ 4 \end{pmatrix} \cdot 1 + \begin{pmatrix} 1 \\ 2 \end{pmatrix} \cdot (-2) = \begin{pmatrix} 0 \\ 0 \end{pmatrix} .$$

Thus, the columns of $\mathbf{A}_1$ are linearly dependent. On the other hand, the columns of

$$\mathbf{A}_2 = \begin{pmatrix} 2 & 0 \\ 4 & 2 \end{pmatrix}$$

are linearly independent, because $\mathbf{A}_2\mathbf{b}$ is a $\mathbf{0}_{2\times 1}$-vector only if $\mathbf{x} = \mathbf{0}$.

A.1.3.4 Rank of a Matrix

The row rank of a matrix $\mathbf{A}$ is equal to the maximum number of linearly independent rows of $\mathbf{A}$. The column rank of a matrix $\mathbf{A}$ is equal to the maximum number of linearly independent columns of $\mathbf{A}$. The row rank of a matrix is equal to its column rank. This number is called the rank of $\mathbf{A}$, or rank($\mathbf{A}$).

Some properties:

A $(K \times K)$ matrix $\mathbf{A}$ is nonsingular if rank($\mathbf{A}$) $= K$ and is singular if rank($\mathbf{A}$) $< K$.

For any $(K \times L)$-matrix it holds that the rank of $\mathbf{A}^T\mathbf{A}$ is equal to the rank of $\mathbf{A}\mathbf{A}^T$ which is equal to the rank of $\mathbf{A}$. If $K > L$ and $\mathbf{A}$ has full column rank, the rank of $\mathbf{A}^T\mathbf{A}$ is thus L and $\mathbf{A}^T\mathbf{A}$ is nonsingular.

A.1.3.5 Eigenvalues and Eigenvectors

Consider a square matrix $\mathbf{A}_K$. If there exist a $(K \times 1)$ vector $\mathbf{x}$, $\mathbf{x} \neq \mathbf{0}_{K\times 1}$ and a scalar λ such that

$$\mathbf{A}\mathbf{x} = \lambda\mathbf{x} \qquad \text{or, equivalently,} \qquad (\mathbf{A} - \lambda\mathbf{I})\mathbf{x} = \mathbf{0}$$

then λ is called an eigenvalue of $\mathbf{A}$ and $\mathbf{x}$ an eigenvector corresponding to λ.

If $\mathbf{x}$, $\mathbf{x} \neq \mathbf{0}_{K\times 1}$, is an eigenvector of $\mathbf{A}$, then $c\mathbf{x}$, $c \neq 0$, is also an eigenvector of $\mathbf{A}$ and belongs to the same eigenvalue λ as $\mathbf{x}$. However, for any eigenvector $\mathbf{x}$ there is only one eigenvalue λ such that $(\mathbf{A} - \lambda\mathbf{I})\mathbf{x} = \mathbf{0}$ holds.

The linear system $\mathbf{B}\mathbf{x} = \mathbf{0}$, where $\mathbf{B} = \mathbf{A} - \lambda\mathbf{I}$, is solved either for $\mathbf{x} = \mathbf{0}$ or if not all rows (columns) of $\mathbf{B}$ are linearly independent, i.e. if rank($\mathbf{B}$) $< K$. In the latter case $|\mathbf{B}| = 0$ (otherwise $|\mathbf{B}| \neq 0$) and the system $\mathbf{B}\mathbf{x} = \mathbf{0}$ has an infinite number of solutions in $\mathbf{x}$. Therefore, a non-trivial solution ($\mathbf{x} \neq \mathbf{0}$) of

$$(\mathbf{A} - \lambda\mathbf{I})\mathbf{x} = \mathbf{0}$$

exists if and only if

$$|\mathbf{A} - \lambda\mathbf{I}| = 0\,.$$

The latter is a polynomial in λ of degree K. The K roots, $\lambda_1, \ldots, \lambda_K$, are the—not necessarily all distinct—eigenvalues of $\mathbf{A}$.

Some properties:

All eigenvalues of a symmetric matrix are real.

The trace of a $(K \times K)$ matrix $\mathbf{A}$ is equal to the sum of its eigenvalues.

The determinant of a $(K \times K)$ matrix $\mathbf{A}$ is the product of its eigenvalues.

A.1.3.6 Non-negative and Positive (semi-)definite Matrices

A $(K \times K)$ matrix $\mathbf{A}$ is non-negative definite if $\mathbf{x}^T\mathbf{A}\mathbf{x} \geq 0$ for any real $\mathbf{x}$. The matrix $\mathbf{A}$ is positive definite if $\mathbf{x}^T\mathbf{A}\mathbf{x} > 0$ for every $\mathbf{x}$ and $\mathbf{x}^T\mathbf{A}\mathbf{x} = 0$ only for the null vector $\mathbf{x} = \mathbf{0}$. $\mathbf{A}$ is positive semidefinite if $\mathbf{x}^T\mathbf{A}\mathbf{x} \geq 0$ for every $\mathbf{x}$ and $\mathbf{x}^T\mathbf{A}\mathbf{x} = 0$ only for some $\mathbf{x} \neq \mathbf{0}$. Thus, a non-negative matrix $\mathbf{A}$ is said to be positive semidefinite if it is not positive definite.

Any positive definite matrix is nonsingular.

A square matrix is positive definite if its eigenvalues are $\lambda_k > 0$ for all $k = 1, \ldots, K$. A square matrix is positive semidefinite if $\lambda_k \geq 0$ for all $k = 1, \ldots, K$ and $\lambda_k = 0$ for at least one k.

$\mathbf{A}^T\mathbf{A}$ is positive semidefinite. To see this, let $\mathbf{x}$ be an $(L \times 1)$ vector, $\mathbf{A}$ a $(K \times L)$ matrix and $\mathbf{b} = \mathbf{A}\mathbf{x}$, then

$$\mathbf{x}^T\mathbf{A}^T\mathbf{A}\mathbf{x} = (\mathbf{A}\mathbf{x})^T\mathbf{A}\mathbf{x} = \mathbf{b}^T\mathbf{b} = \sum_{k=1}^{K} b_k^2 \geq 0 \,.$$

A $(K \times K)$ matrix $\mathbf{A}$ is negative definite if $-\mathbf{A}$ is positive definite.

A.1.3.7 Inverse of a Matrix

The inverse of a (square) matrix $\mathbf{A}$ is the unique matrix $\mathbf{A}^{-1}$ that satisfies $\mathbf{A}\mathbf{A}^{-1} = \mathbf{A}^{-1}\mathbf{A} = \mathbf{I}$. The inverse exists if and only if $\mathbf{A}$ is nonsingular or, equivalently, if and only if $|\mathbf{A}| \neq 0$.

A.1.3.8 Spectral Decomposition of a Symmetric Matrix

Any symmetric matrix $\mathbf{A}_K$ can be written as $\mathbf{A} = \boldsymbol{\Gamma}\boldsymbol{\Lambda}\boldsymbol{\Gamma}^T$, where $\boldsymbol{\Lambda}$ is a diagonal matrix with eigenvalues $\lambda_1, \ldots, \lambda_K$ of $\mathbf{A}$ on the diagonal and $\boldsymbol{\Gamma}$ a matrix whose columns are the corresponding orthonormal eigenvectors. Note that $\boldsymbol{\Gamma}^T\boldsymbol{\Gamma} = \mathbf{I}_K$. Expression $\mathbf{A} = \boldsymbol{\Gamma}\boldsymbol{\Lambda}\boldsymbol{\Gamma}^T$ is also denoted as the spectral decomposition of the $(K \times K)$ symmetric matrix $\mathbf{A}$.

A.1.3.9 Symmetric Square Root of a Matrix

Consider a $(K \times K)$ symmetric non-negative definite matrix $\mathbf{A}$. There exists a $(K \times K)$ symmetric non-negative definite matrix $\mathbf{B}$ such that $\mathbf{A} = \mathbf{B}\mathbf{B}$, where $\mathbf{B} = \boldsymbol{\Gamma}\text{diag}(\lambda_1^{1/2}, \ldots, \lambda_K^{1/2})\boldsymbol{\Gamma}^T$ is unique, $\boldsymbol{\Gamma}$ is the matrix of orthonormal eigenvectors of $\mathbf{A}$ and $\lambda_1, \ldots, \lambda_K$ are the corresponding eigenvalues of $\mathbf{A}$.

A.2 Random Variables and Statistics

In this book we do not differentiate notationally between random variables and their realization, if this is unambiguously clear from the context. For the ease of presentation we also use a simplified notation. For example, we ignore dependence of density or probability functions on parameters if convenient. In addition, we will often not distinguish between (absolutely) continuous and discrete random variables. Thus, we often use integrals in formulas to represent probabilities of events, expectations or marginal distributions even if discrete variables may be involved. If discrete variables are involved, integration would have to be replaced by summation. In addition, throughout we assume that each random variable considered follows a cumulative distribution function, ignore any reference to the underlying probability space and assume that all necessary moments exist and are finite. More extensive treatments of measure and probability theory can be found in most books on advanced statistics, e.g. Mardia, Kent, and Bibby (1979). A more detailed and basic treatment may be found, e.g., in Ash and Doléans-Dade (2000).

A.2.1 Sample Moments

For a scalar variable u, the sample mean $\bar{u}$ and variance s_u^2 are, respectively,

$$\bar{u} = \frac{1}{n}\sum_{i=1}^{n} u_i \quad \text{and} \quad s_u^2 = \frac{1}{n-1}\sum_{i=1}^{n}(u_i - \bar{u})^2 \,. \tag{A.1}$$

The sample covariance of two scalar variables v and u is

$$s_{vu} = \frac{1}{n-1}\sum_{i=1}^{n}(v_i - \bar{v})(u_i - \bar{u}) \,. \tag{A.2}$$

Let $\mathbf{u}_i = (u_{i1}, \ldots, u_{ip}, \ldots, u_{iP})^T$ and $\mathbf{U} = \left(\mathbf{u}_1 \cdots \mathbf{u}_n\right)^T$, then the sample mean is

$$\bar{\mathbf{u}} = \frac{1}{n}\left(\sum_{i=1}^{n}\mathbf{u}_i\right) = n^{-1}\mathbf{U}^T\mathbf{1} \,. \tag{A.3}$$

The sample covariance matrix with $i = 1, \ldots, n$ units can be calculated by

$$\mathbf{S} = \frac{n}{n-1}\left[\left(\sum_{i=1}^{n}\mathbf{u}_i\mathbf{u}_i^T/n\right) - \bar{\mathbf{u}}\bar{\mathbf{u}}^T\right] = \frac{1}{n-1}\left[\sum_{i=1}^{n}(\mathbf{u}_i - \bar{\mathbf{u}})(\mathbf{u}_i - \bar{\mathbf{u}})^T\right]$$
$$= (n-1)^{-1}\left[\left(\mathbf{U} - n^{-1}\mathbf{J}\mathbf{U}\right)^T\left(\mathbf{U} - n^{-1}\mathbf{J}\mathbf{U}\right)\right] = (n-1)^{-1}\left[\mathbf{U}^T\mathbf{U} - n\bar{\mathbf{u}}\bar{\mathbf{u}}^T\right] .$$

A.2.2 Random Variables

A.2.2.1 Basics

Let $\mathbf{u} = (u_1, \ldots, u_p, \ldots, u_P)^T$ be a $(P \times 1)$-dimensional random vector (or variable), where the components u_p are unidimensional random variables. Two important types of variables are discrete and (absolutely) continuous variables (we will in general omit the adverb 'absolutely').

Let $\mathbf{u}$ be a continuous random variable. We assume that a joint (probability) density function $f(\mathbf{u})$ exists such that

$$F(\mathbf{u}) = \int_{-\infty}^{\mathbf{u}} f(\mathbf{x})\, d\mathbf{x}\,, \tag{A.4}$$

where $F(\mathbf{u})$ is the cumulative distribution function, the value of which at the point $\mathbf{u}$ can be interpreted as the probability that each variable in $\mathbf{u}$ takes on values of at most the values $u_1, \ldots, u_p, \ldots, u_P$. In case of a P-dimensional variable $\mathbf{u}$, the integral sign in (A.4) is short for P-fold integration and $d\mathbf{x}$ denotes the product of P differential elements.

If all the elements in $\mathbf{u}$ are discrete, then the density function $f(\mathbf{u})$ has to be replaced by the probability function which gives the probability of observing specific values $\mathbf{u}$ and is often denoted by $\Pr(\cdot)$. In addition, integration in (A.4) is replaced by P-fold summation. Note that the probability functions of the binary response indicators are denoted by $g(\cdot)$ in this book.

A repeatedly used concept is that of a marginal distribution. Write $\mathbf{u} = (\mathbf{u}_1^T \;\; \mathbf{u}_2^T)^T$, where $\mathbf{u}_1$ is a P_1- and $\mathbf{u}_2$ is a $P_2 = (P - P_1)$-dimensional vector, respectively. Then the marginal function of $\mathbf{u}_1$ is

$$f(\mathbf{u}_1) = \int f(\mathbf{u}_1, \mathbf{u}_2)\, d\mathbf{u}_2$$

and, correspondingly, the marginal function of $\mathbf{u}_2$ is

$$f(\mathbf{u}_2) = \int f(\mathbf{u}_1, \mathbf{u}_2)\, d\mathbf{u}_1\,.$$

Note that $f(\mathbf{u}_1)$, $f(\mathbf{u}_2)$ and $f(\mathbf{u})$ may be very different density functions.

In the case of a two-dimensional variable, $(x \;\; y)^T$, the distribution of x would be denoted as the marginal distribution of x and the distribution of y would be called the marginal distribution of y.

For a given value $\mathbf{u}_2$ the density of $\mathbf{u}_1$ conditional on $\mathbf{u}_2$ is

$$f(\mathbf{u}_1 \mid \mathbf{u}_2) = \frac{f(\mathbf{u}_1, \mathbf{u}_2)}{f(\mathbf{u}_2)}\,, \qquad f(\mathbf{u}_2) > 0$$

and correspondingly the density of $\mathbf{u}_2$ conditional on $\mathbf{u}_1$ is

$$f(\mathbf{u}_2 \mid \mathbf{u}_1) = \frac{f(\mathbf{u}_2, \mathbf{u}_1)}{f(\mathbf{u}_1)}, \qquad f(\mathbf{u}_1) > 0 .$$

The variables $\mathbf{u}_1$ and $\mathbf{u}_2$ are independent if $f(\mathbf{u}_1, \mathbf{u}_2) = f(\mathbf{u}_1) f(\mathbf{u}_2)$ for all possible $\mathbf{u}_1$ and $\mathbf{u}_2$, in which case $f(\mathbf{u}_1 \mid \mathbf{u}_2) = f(\mathbf{u}_1)$ and $f(\mathbf{u}_2 \mid \mathbf{u}_1) = f(\mathbf{u}_2)$.

A.2.2.2 Population Moments

The expectation or mean of variable u with density function $f(u)$ is

$$E(u) = \mu_u = \int_{-\infty}^{\infty} u f(u)\, du ,$$

and its variance is

$$\mathrm{var}(u) = \sigma_u^2 = \int_{-\infty}^{\infty} (u - \mu_u)^2 f(u)\, du .$$

The covariance of two continuous random variables u and v with common density function $f(u, v)$ is given by

$$\mathrm{cov}(u, v) = \sigma_{u,v} = \int_{-\infty}^{\infty} \int_{-\infty}^{\infty} (u - \mu_u)(v - \mu_v) f(u, v)\, du\, dv ,$$

where $\mu_v = E(v)$.

If u or v is discrete, then the corresponding integrals has to be replaced by a sum.

Let $\mathbf{u} = (u_1 \cdots u_p \cdots u_P)^T$ be a continuous random vector with density function $f(\mathbf{u})$. Then its expectation or mean is

$$E(\mathbf{u}) = \boldsymbol{\mu} = (E(u_1), \ldots, E(u_P))^T = (\mu_1, \ldots, \mu_P)^T .$$

Its covariance matrix is

$$\mathrm{Var}(\mathbf{u}) = E\left\{[\mathbf{u} - E(\mathbf{u})][\mathbf{u} - E(\mathbf{u})]^T\right\} = E(\mathbf{u}\mathbf{u}^T) - E(\mathbf{u})E(\mathbf{u})^T ,$$

with elements $\sigma_{u_p}^2 = E(u_p^2) - E(u_p)^2$ on the diagonal and $\sigma_{u_p,u_q} = E(u_p u_q) - E(u_p)E(u_q)$, $p, q = 1, \ldots, P$ and $p \neq q$, the covariances of u_p and u_q as off-diagonal elements.

Any covariance matrix Var(**u**) is positive semidefinite (cf. Sect. A.1.3), because for any real vector **b** of suitable dimension

$$\mathbf{b}^T \text{Var}(\mathbf{u})\mathbf{b} = \mathbf{b}^T E(\mathbf{v}\mathbf{v}^T)\mathbf{b} = E(\mathbf{b}^T \mathbf{v}\mathbf{v}^T \mathbf{b}) = E[(\mathbf{b}^T \mathbf{v})^2] \geq 0 ,$$

where $\mathbf{v} = (\mathbf{u} - E(\mathbf{u}))$.

A.2.3 Some Results on Expectations, Variances and Covariances

Let u and v be random variables and assume that all necessary moments exist, then

$$\begin{aligned} E(u) &= E[E(u \mid v)] \qquad \text{(also known as `law of iterated expectations')} \\ \text{var}(u) &= E[\text{var}(u \mid v)] + \text{var}[E(u \mid v)] \,. \end{aligned} \tag{A.5}$$

Let r be a binary random variable and $\pi = \Pr(r = 1)$, then

$$\begin{aligned} E(u) =& \pi E(u \mid r = 1) + (1 - \pi)E(u \mid r = 0) \\ E[\text{var}(u \mid r)] =& \pi[E(u^2 \mid r = 1) - E(u \mid r = 1)^2] \\ &+ (1 - \pi)[E(u^2 \mid r = 0) - E(u \mid r = 0)^2] \end{aligned} \tag{A.6}$$

and

$$\begin{aligned} \text{var}[E(u \mid r)] =& E[E(u \mid r)^2] - E[E(u \mid r)]^2 \\ =& \pi E(u \mid r = 1)^2 + (1 - \pi)E(u \mid r = 0) \\ &- [\pi E(u \mid r = 1) + (1 - \pi)E(u \mid r = 0)]^2 \\ =& \pi(1 - \pi)[E(u \mid r = 1) - E(u \mid r = 0)]^2 \,. \end{aligned} \tag{A.7}$$

Replacing v in (A.5) with r, inserting (A.6) and (A.7), simplifying and rearranging terms leads to

$$\begin{aligned} \text{var}(u) =& \pi(1 - \pi)[E(u \mid r = 1) - E(u \mid r = 0)]^2 \\ &+ \pi \,\text{var}(u \mid r = 1) + (1 - \pi) \,\text{var}(u \mid r = 0) \,. \end{aligned}$$

The variance of a sum of two random variables, $u + v$, is

$$\text{var}(u + v) = \text{var}(u) + \text{var}(v) + 2\text{cov}(u, v) \,,$$

and therefore

$$\text{cov}(u, v) = \frac{1}{2}[\text{var}(u+v) - \text{var}(u) - \text{var}(v)] \; .$$

The variance of $u + v$ can be written as

$$\text{var}(u+v) = E[\text{var}(u+v \mid r)] + \text{var}[E(u+v \mid r)] \; ,$$

where

$$\begin{aligned} E[\text{var}(u+r \mid r)] =& \text{var}(u) - \pi(1-\pi)[E(u \mid r=1) - E(u \mid r=0)]^2 \\ &+ \text{var}(v) - \pi(1-\pi)[E(v \mid r=1) - E(v \mid r=0)]^2 \\ &+ 2\pi \,\text{cov}(u, v \mid r=1) + 2(1-\pi)\,\text{cov}(u, v \mid r=0) \end{aligned}$$

and

$$\begin{aligned} \text{var}[E(u+v \mid r)] =& \pi(1-\pi)[E(u \mid r=1) - E(u \mid r=0)]^2 \\ &+ \pi(1-\pi)[E(v \mid r=1) - E(v \mid r=0)]^2 \\ &+ 2\pi(1-\pi)\{[E(u \mid r=1) - E(u \mid r=0)] \\ &\times [E(v \mid r=1) - E(v \mid r=0)]\} \; . \end{aligned}$$

Therefore

$$\begin{aligned} \text{cov}(u, v) =& \pi(1-\pi)\{[E(u \mid r=1) - E(u \mid r=0)][E(v \mid r=1) - E(v \mid r=0)]\} \\ &+ \pi \,\text{cov}(u, v \mid r=1) + (1-\pi)\,\text{cov}(u, v \mid r=0) \; . \end{aligned} \tag{A.8}$$

A.2.4 Normal Distribution

The density function of a unidimensional normally distributed variable u is

$$f(u) = \frac{1}{\sigma_u \sqrt{2\pi}} \exp\left[-\frac{1}{2}\frac{(u-\mu_u)^2}{\sigma_u^2}\right] \qquad -\infty < u < \infty \; ,$$

with variance $\sigma_u^2 > 0$ and $\mu_u = E(u)$, $-\infty < \mu_u < \infty$, the population mean or expectation. Let $z = (u-\mu_u)/\sigma_u$, then z follows a standard normal distribution with $E(z) = 0$ and $\sigma_z^2 = 1$. The density of the standard normal distribution is denoted as $\phi(z)$.

The two-dimensional or bivariate normal density is

$$f(u, v) = \frac{\exp\left[-\frac{1}{2(1-\rho^2)}\left(\frac{(u-\mu_u)^2}{\sigma_u^2} - \frac{2\rho(u-\mu_u)(v-\mu_v)}{\sigma_u\sigma_v} + \frac{(v-\mu_v)^2}{\sigma_v^2}\right)\right]}{2\sigma_u\sigma_v\pi\sqrt{1-\rho^2}}$$

$$-\infty < u, v < \infty ,$$

with variances $\sigma_u^2, \sigma_v^2 > 0$, means $-\infty < \mu_u, \mu_v < \infty$ and correlation $-1 < \rho < 1$. Let $z_1 = (u - \mu_u)/\sigma_u$ and $z_2 = (v - \mu_v)/\sigma_v$, then $\mathbf{z} = (z_1 \quad z_2)^T$ follows a bivariate standard normal distribution with $E(z_1) = E(z_2) = 0$ and $\sigma_{z_1}^2 = \sigma_{z_2}^2 = 1$. The density of the bivariate standard normal distribution is denoted as $\phi(z_1, z_2)$.

Let $\mathbf{u}$ be multivariate or, more precisely, P-variate normally distributed with expectation $\boldsymbol{\mu}$ and covariance matrix $\boldsymbol{\Sigma}$, i.e.

$$\mathbf{u} \sim N(\boldsymbol{\mu}, \boldsymbol{\Sigma}) .$$

Then any linear combination $\mathbf{Au} + \mathbf{b}$, where $\mathbf{A}$ is a fixed matrix and $\mathbf{b}$ is a fixed vector, is normally distributed with expectation $\mathbf{A}\boldsymbol{\mu} + \mathbf{b}$ and covariance matrix $\mathbf{A}\boldsymbol{\Sigma}\mathbf{A}^T$. This implies that any subset of $\mathbf{u}$ is multivariate normally distributed (e.g., Mardia et al., 1979). The converse, however, is not true: Non-normal multivariate distributions may have normal marginal distributions (e.g., Kotz, Balakrishnan, & Johnson, 2000, pp. 112–113).

A.2.5 *Conditional Normal Distribution*

Consider the partition

$$\mathbf{u} = \begin{pmatrix} \mathbf{u}_1 \\ \mathbf{u}_2 \end{pmatrix} ,$$

and, correspondingly,

$$\boldsymbol{\mu} = \begin{pmatrix} \boldsymbol{\mu}_1 \\ \boldsymbol{\mu}_2 \end{pmatrix} \quad \text{and} \quad \boldsymbol{\Sigma} = \begin{pmatrix} \boldsymbol{\Sigma}_{11} & \boldsymbol{\Sigma}_{12} \\ \boldsymbol{\Sigma}_{21} & \boldsymbol{\Sigma}_{22} \end{pmatrix} .$$

Then the conditional distribution of $\mathbf{u}_1$ given $\mathbf{u}_2$ is

$$\mathbf{u}_1 \mid \mathbf{u}_2 \sim N(\boldsymbol{\mu}_1 + \boldsymbol{\Sigma}_{12}\boldsymbol{\Sigma}_{22}^{-1}(\mathbf{u}_2 - \boldsymbol{\mu}_2), \boldsymbol{\Sigma}_{11} - \boldsymbol{\Sigma}_{12}\boldsymbol{\Sigma}_{22}^{-1}\boldsymbol{\Sigma}_{21}) .$$

Let $\boldsymbol{\theta}_0 = \boldsymbol{\mu}_1 - \boldsymbol{\Sigma}_{12}\boldsymbol{\Sigma}_{22}^{-1}\boldsymbol{\mu}_2$ and $\boldsymbol{\theta}_1 = \boldsymbol{\Sigma}_{12}\boldsymbol{\Sigma}_{22}^{-1}$, then we can write

$$\mathbf{u}_1 = \boldsymbol{\theta}_0 + \mathbf{u}_2^T\boldsymbol{\theta}_1 + \mathbf{v}, \qquad \mathbf{v} \sim N(\mathbf{0}, \boldsymbol{\Sigma}_{11} - \boldsymbol{\Sigma}_{12}\boldsymbol{\Sigma}_{22}^{-1}\boldsymbol{\Sigma}_{21}) \text{ independent from } \mathbf{u}_2$$

(e.g., Mardia et al., 1979).

In particular, if $\mathbf{u} = \begin{pmatrix} y & x & z \end{pmatrix}^T$,

$$\boldsymbol{\mu} = \begin{pmatrix} \mu_y \\ \mu_x \\ \mu_z \end{pmatrix} \quad \text{and} \quad \boldsymbol{\Sigma} = \begin{pmatrix} \sigma_y^2 & \sigma_{yx} & \sigma_{yz} \\ \sigma_{xy} & \sigma_x^2 & \sigma_{xz} \\ \sigma_{zy} & \sigma_{zx} & \sigma_z^2 \end{pmatrix}$$

then

$$y = \beta_0 + x\beta_1 + z\beta_2 + v, \qquad v \sim N(\mathbf{0}, \sigma_v^2) \text{ independent from } x \text{ and } z ,$$

where

$$\beta_0 = \mu_y - \mu_x\beta_1 - \mu_z\beta_2 , \qquad \beta_1 = \frac{\sigma_{yx}\sigma_z^2 - \sigma_{yz}\sigma_{xz}}{\sigma_x^2\sigma_z^2 - \sigma_{xz}^2} ,$$

$$\beta_2 = \frac{\sigma_{yz}\sigma_x^2 - \sigma_{yx}\sigma_{xz}}{\sigma_x^2\sigma_z^2 - \sigma_{xz}^2} \quad \text{and} \quad \sigma_v^2 = \sigma_y^2 - \frac{\sigma_x^2\sigma_{yz}^2 - 2\sigma_{yx}\sigma_{yz}\sigma_{xz} + \sigma_z^2\sigma_{yx}^2}{\sigma_x^2\sigma_z^2 - \sigma_{xz}^2} .$$

If $\mathbf{u} = (u_1 \quad u_2)^T$ and both, u_1 and u_2, are scalar

$$u_1 = \theta_0 + u_2\theta_1 + v, \qquad v \sim N(0, \sigma_{u_1}^2 - \sigma_{u_1u_2}^2\sigma_{u_2}^{-2}) \text{ independent from } u_2 , \tag{A.9}$$

where $\theta_0 = \mu_{u_1} - \mu_{u_2}\theta_1$ and $\theta_1 = \sigma_{u_1u_2}/\sigma_{u_2}^2$.

A.2.6 *Truncated Normal Distribution and Normal Sample Selection Model*

A.2.6.1 Truncated Normal Distribution

Suppose r^* is normally distributed with expectation μ_{r^*} and variance $\sigma_{r^*}^2$, and

$$r = \begin{cases} 1 \text{ if } r^* > c \\ 0 \text{ else} \end{cases} .$$

Then the (marginal) probability for $r = 1$ is equal to the probability that $r^* > c$, i.e.

$$\Pr(r = 1) = \Pr(r^* > c) = 1 - \Phi(\tilde{c}) ,$$

where $\Phi(\cdot)$ is the standard normal distribution function and $\tilde{c} = (c - \mu_{r^*})/\sigma_{r^*}$. The conditional distribution of $r^* \mid r^* > c$, which is equivalent to $r^* \mid r = 1$, is called a one-sided truncated normal distribution, with density

$$f(r^* \mid r = 1) = f(r^* \mid r^* > c) = \begin{cases} \dfrac{\dfrac{1}{\sigma_{r^*}} \phi\left(\dfrac{r^* - \mu_{r^*}}{\sigma_{r^*}}\right)}{1 - \Phi(\tilde{c})} & \text{if} \quad r^* > c \\ 0 & \text{otherwise} \end{cases}$$

and

$$\mu_{r^*,(1)} = E(r^* \mid r = 1) = E(r^* \mid r^* > c) = \mu_{r^*} + \sigma_{r^*} \frac{\phi(\tilde{c})}{1 - \Phi(\tilde{c})}$$

$$\sigma^2_{r^*,(1)} = \mathrm{var}(r^* \mid r = 1) = \mathrm{var}(r^* \mid r^* > c) = \sigma^2_{r^*} \left[1 + \frac{\tilde{c}\,\phi(\tilde{c})}{1 - \Phi(\tilde{c})} - \left(\frac{\phi(\tilde{c})}{1 - \Phi(\tilde{c})}\right)^2\right]$$

(cf. Kotz et al., 2000, pp. 311–312). Correspondingly, $r^* \mid r^* \leq c$, which is equivalent to $r^* \mid r = 0$, follows a one-sided truncated normal distribution with density function

$$f(r^* \mid r = 0) = f(r^* \mid r^* \leq c) = \begin{cases} \dfrac{\dfrac{1}{\sigma_{r^*}} \phi\left(\dfrac{r^* - \mu_{r^*}}{\sigma_{r^*}}\right)}{\Phi(\tilde{c})} & \text{if} \quad r^* \leq c \\ 0 & \text{otherwise} \end{cases}$$

with

$$\mu_{r^*,(0)} = E(r^* \mid r = 0) = E(r^* \mid r^* \leq c) = \mu_{r^*} - \sigma_{r^*} \frac{\phi(\tilde{c})}{\Phi(\tilde{c})}$$

and

$$\sigma^2_{r^*,(0)} = \mathrm{var}(r^* \mid r = 0) = \mathrm{var}(r^* \mid r^* \leq c) = \sigma^2_{r^*} \left[1 - \frac{\tilde{c}\,\phi(\tilde{c})}{\Phi(\tilde{c})} - \left(\frac{\phi(\tilde{c})}{\Phi(\tilde{c})}\right)^2\right].$$

A.2.6.2 Normal Sample Selection Model

Suppose $\mathbf{u} = \left(y\ x\ r^*\right)^T$ is normally distributed with

$$\boldsymbol{\mu} = \begin{pmatrix} \mu_y \\ \mu_x \\ \mu_{r^*} \end{pmatrix}, \qquad \boldsymbol{\Sigma} = \begin{pmatrix} \sigma_y^2 & \sigma_{yx} & \sigma_{yr^*} \\ \sigma_{yx} & \sigma_x^2 & \sigma_{xr^*} \\ \sigma_{yr^*} & \sigma_{xr^*} & \sigma_{r^*}^2 \end{pmatrix} \tag{A.10}$$

and

$$r = \begin{cases} 1 \text{ if } r^* > c \\ 0 \text{ else} \end{cases} .$$

Then (cf. (A.9))

$$y = \theta_0 + r^*\theta_1 + v, \qquad v \sim N(0, \sigma_v^2) \text{ independent from } r^* , \tag{A.11}$$

where $\theta_0 = \mu_y - \mu_{r^*}\theta_1$, $\theta_1 = \sigma_{yr^*}/\sigma_{r^*}^2$ and $\sigma_v^2 = \sigma_y^2 - \sigma_{yr^*}^2\sigma_{r^*}^{-2}$, conditional mean $\mu_{y,(1)} = E(y \mid r = 1) = E(y \mid r^* > c)$,

$$\begin{aligned} \mu_{y,(1)} &= \theta_0 + E(r^* \mid r^* > c)\theta_1 + E(v \mid r^* > c) = \theta_0 + E(r^* \mid r^* > c)\theta_1 \\ &= \mu_y + \frac{\sigma_{yr^*}}{\sigma_{r^*}} \frac{\phi(\tilde{c})}{1 - \Phi(\tilde{c})}, \qquad \sigma_{r^*} > 0 , \end{aligned}$$

where $E(v \mid r^* > c) = E(v) = 0$, $\tilde{c} = (c - \mu_{r^*})/\sigma_{r^*}$ and conditional variance

$$\begin{aligned} \sigma_{y,(1)}^2 &= \theta_1^2 \text{var}(r^* \mid r^* > c) + \text{var}(v \mid r^* > c) \\ &= \sigma_y^2 + \frac{\sigma_{yr^*}^2}{\sigma_{r^*}^2} \left(\frac{1}{\sigma_{r^*}^2} \text{var}(r^* \mid r^* > c) - 1\right) \\ &= \sigma_y^2 + \frac{\sigma_{yr^*}^2}{\sigma_{r^*}^2} \left[\frac{\tilde{c}\,\phi(\tilde{c})}{1 - \Phi(\tilde{c})} - \left(\frac{\phi(\tilde{c})}{1 - \Phi(\tilde{c})}\right)^2 \right] \end{aligned}$$

because v is independent from r^*. Correspondingly,

$$\begin{aligned} \mu_{y,(0)} &= \theta_0 + E(r^* \mid r^* \le c)\theta_1 + E(v \mid r^* \le c) = \theta_0 + E(r^* \mid r^* \le c)\theta_1 \\ &= \mu_y - \frac{\sigma_{yr^*}}{\sigma_{r^*}} \frac{\phi(\tilde{c})}{\Phi(\tilde{c})} \end{aligned}$$

and

$$\begin{aligned}\sigma^2_{y,(0)} &= \theta_1^2 \mathrm{var}(r^* \mid r^* \leq c) + \mathrm{var}(v \mid r^* \leq c) \\ &= \sigma_y^2 - \frac{\sigma^2_{yr^*}}{\sigma^2_{r^*}} \left[\frac{\tilde{c}\,\phi(\tilde{c})}{\Phi(\tilde{c})} + \left(\frac{\phi(\tilde{c})}{\Phi(\tilde{c})} \right)^2 \right] .\end{aligned}$$

With

$$\mathrm{cov}(y, x \mid r = 1) = \frac{1}{2}[\mathrm{var}(y + x \mid r = 1) - \mathrm{var}(y \mid r = 1) - \mathrm{var}(x \mid r = 1)]$$

and

$$\mathrm{var}(y + x \mid r = 1) = \sigma_y^2 + \sigma_x^2 + 2\sigma_{yx} + (\sigma_{yr^*} + \sigma_{xr^*})^2/\sigma^2_{r^*} \left[\frac{\tilde{c}\,\phi(\tilde{c})}{1 - \Phi(\tilde{c})} - \left(\frac{\phi(\tilde{c})}{1 - \Phi(\tilde{c})} \right)^2 \right]$$

the conditional covariance of $y, x \mid r = 1$ is

$$\sigma_{yx,(1)} = \sigma_{yx} + \frac{\sigma_{yr^*}\sigma_{xr^*}}{\sigma^4_{r^*}} \left(\mathrm{var}(r^* \mid r^* > c) - \sigma^2_{r^*}\right)$$

and, if $\sigma_{xr^*} \neq 0$, may be written as

$$\sigma_{yx,(1)} = \sigma_{yx} + \frac{\sigma_{yr^*}}{\sigma_{xr^*}} \left(\sigma^2_{x|r=1} - \sigma_x^2\right) ,$$

or, if $\sigma_{yr^*} \neq 0$, as

$$\sigma_{yx,(1)} = \sigma_{yx} + \frac{\sigma_{xr^*}}{\sigma_{yr^*}} \left(\sigma^2_{y|r=1} - \sigma_y^2\right) .$$

Correspondingly, the conditional covariance of $y, x \mid r = 0$ is

$$\sigma_{yx,(0)} = \sigma_{yx} + \frac{\sigma_{yr^*}\sigma_{xr^*}}{\sigma^4_{r^*}} \left(\mathrm{var}(r^* \mid r^* \leq c) - \sigma^2_{r^*}\right)$$

and, if $\sigma_{xr^*} \neq 0$,

$$\sigma_{yx,(0)} = \sigma_{yx} + \frac{\sigma_{yr^*}}{\sigma_{xr^*}} \left(\sigma^2_{x|r=0} - \sigma_x^2\right)$$

or, if $\sigma_{yr^*} \neq 0$,

$$\sigma_{yx,(0)} = \sigma_{yx} + \frac{\sigma_{xr^*}}{\sigma_{yr^*}} \left(\sigma^2_{y|r=0} - \sigma_y^2\right) .$$

A.3 Estimation

Several approaches have been developed to generate estimators for unknown parameters in statistical models. Two well-known approaches are least squares estimation and the maximum-likelihood (ML) method. Both will be introduced in the following two sections. At the end of the second section we give some intermediate results for Examples 2.6 and 2.7 in Chap. 2.

Advantageous properties of an estimator $\hat{\boldsymbol{\theta}}$ for an unknown parameter in finite samples in a model-based frequentist approach are (at least approximate) unbiasedness of the estimator itself ($E(\hat{\boldsymbol{\theta}}) = \boldsymbol{\theta}_0$), where $\boldsymbol{\theta}_0$ is the unknown true parameter value, but also of its variance and a known (at least approximative) distribution of $\hat{\boldsymbol{\theta}}$. Given these properties, it is often desirable for the variance of $\hat{\boldsymbol{\theta}}$ to be small as the inferences are more precise as compared to estimators with larger variance.

On the other hand, in many cases finite properties cannot be derived. Then asymptotic ($n \rightarrow \infty$) properties are of interest, like asymptotic unbiasedness, consistency and an approximation to the variance and distribution of $\hat{\boldsymbol{\theta}}$ in large samples. Roughly speaking, an estimator is consistent if the probability that it deviates from the true value by more than an arbitrary small value goes to zero as $n \rightarrow \infty$.

A.3.1 Least Squares

A.3.1.1 Ordinary Least Squares

The least squares principle allows estimation in a large class of statistical models. In this section we consider ordinary least squares (OLS) and generalized least squares (GLS) estimation in linear regression models.

Assume a linear regression model with dependent variables collected in an $(n \times 1)$-dimensional vector $\mathbf{y} = (y_1 \cdots y_n)^T$, an $(n \times (P+1))$-matrix $\mathbf{X} = (\mathbf{x}_1 \cdots \mathbf{x}_n)^T$ of covariates or predictor variables including a column of ones, $\mathbf{x}_i = (1 \;\; x_{i,1} \cdots x_{i,P})^T$, $i = 1, \ldots, n$, and an n-dimensional vector of random errors $\boldsymbol{\epsilon} = (\epsilon_1 \cdots \epsilon_n)^T$. Assume further

$$\mathbf{y} = \mathbf{X}\boldsymbol{\beta}_0 + \boldsymbol{\epsilon} \; , \tag{A.12}$$

where $\boldsymbol{\beta}_0 = (\beta_{0,c} \;\; \beta_{0,1} \cdots \beta_{0,P})^T$ is the unknown parameter of interest.

To estimate $\boldsymbol{\beta}_0$ we may adopt the least squares principle and minimize the function

$$q(\mathbf{e}) = \sum_{i=1}^{n} e_i^2 = \mathbf{e}^T\mathbf{e} = (\mathbf{y} - \mathbf{X}\boldsymbol{\beta})^T(\mathbf{y} - \mathbf{X}\boldsymbol{\beta})$$

with respect to $\boldsymbol{\beta}$, where $\mathbf{e} = \mathbf{y} - \mathbf{X}\boldsymbol{\beta}$ and $e_i = y_i - \mathbf{x}_i^T\boldsymbol{\beta}$. The solution to this minimization problem is found by taking the first derivative of $q(\mathbf{e})$ with respect to $\boldsymbol{\beta}$, set the $P + 1$ derivatives equal to zero (the corresponding equations are called 'estimating equations') and solve this system of equations for $\boldsymbol{\beta}$. The estimating equations are

$$\mathbf{0} = \mathbf{X}^T(\mathbf{y} - \mathbf{X}\boldsymbol{\beta})$$

and are solved by

$$\hat{\boldsymbol{\beta}}_{\text{OLS}} = (\mathbf{X}^T\mathbf{X})^{-1}\mathbf{X}^T\mathbf{y}$$

if $(\mathbf{X}^T\mathbf{X})$ is nonsingular which is the case if the columns in $\mathbf{X}$ are linearly independent (see Sect. A.1.3).

If we assume $E(\boldsymbol{\epsilon} \mid \mathbf{x}) = E(\boldsymbol{\epsilon}) = \mathbf{0}$, $\text{var}(\boldsymbol{\epsilon}) = \sigma_0^2\mathbf{I}$, fix $\mathbf{X}$ at its observed values and estimate σ_0^2 which is needed, e.g., to calculate confidence intervals, by $\hat{\sigma}^2 = (\mathbf{y} - \mathbf{X}\hat{\boldsymbol{\beta}}_{\text{OLS}})^T(\mathbf{y} - \mathbf{X}\hat{\boldsymbol{\beta}}_{\text{OLS}})/(n - P - 1)$, then it can be shown that

1. $E(\hat{\boldsymbol{\beta}}_{\text{OLS}}) = \boldsymbol{\beta}_0$, i.e. $\hat{\boldsymbol{\beta}}_{\text{OLS}}$ is unbiased,
2. $\text{var}(\hat{\boldsymbol{\beta}}_{\text{OLS}}) = \sigma_0^2(\mathbf{X}^T\mathbf{X})^{-1}$,
3. the variances of the elements of $\hat{\boldsymbol{\beta}}_{\text{OLS}}$, i.e. estimators $\hat{\beta}_{\text{OLS},p}$, are minimal among unbiased estimators which are linear in $\mathbf{y}$ and
4. $E(\hat{\sigma}^2) = \sigma_0^2$, i.e. the estimator of the error variance is also unbiased.

Thus, the variance of $\hat{\boldsymbol{\beta}}_{\text{OLS}}$ can be estimated by $\widehat{\text{var}}(\hat{\boldsymbol{\beta}}_{\text{OLS}}) = \hat{\sigma}^2(\mathbf{X}^T\mathbf{X})^{-1}$. The assumption that all errors have the same variance σ^2 is also known as the assumption of homoscedasticity.

If the above assumptions hold, then $\hat{\boldsymbol{\beta}}_{\text{OLS}}$ is said to be BLUE, which is short for 'best linear unbiased estimator'. If in addition to the above assumptions we assume ϵ_i, $i = 1, \ldots, n$, follow the same normal distribution, then it can be shown that $\hat{\boldsymbol{\beta}}_{\text{OLS}}$ is normally distributed even in small samples. If the normality assumption cannot be justified then, in large samples, one might resort to asymptotic properties.

The above results hold even if n is finite. If $n \to \infty$, it can be shown that $\hat{\boldsymbol{\beta}}_{\text{OLS}}$ and $\hat{\sigma}^2$ are both consistent and $\hat{\boldsymbol{\beta}}_{\text{OLS}}$ is asymptotically normally distributed under weak conditions without assuming normality of ϵ_i, $i = 1, \ldots, n$. Its variance can again be estimated by $\widehat{\text{var}}(\hat{\boldsymbol{\beta}}_{\text{OLS}}) = \hat{\sigma}^2(\mathbf{X}^T\mathbf{X})^{-1}$.

In addition, under small modifications similar results can be shown if the predictors are treated as random (e.g., Cameron & Trivedi, 2005).

A.3.1.2 Generalized Least Squares

The assumption $\text{var}(\boldsymbol{\epsilon}) = \sigma^2\mathbf{I}$ for some $\sigma^2 > 0$ might be violated. For example, the error variances might differ over units i and/or the errors may be correlated, for example, if observations are clustered. Then assumption $\mathrm{var}(\boldsymbol{\epsilon}) = \sigma^2\mathbf{I}$ is replaced by $\mathrm{var}(\boldsymbol{\epsilon}) = \sigma^2\boldsymbol{\Sigma}$ where $\boldsymbol{\Sigma}$ is a positive definite matrix.

Since $\boldsymbol{\Sigma}$ is positive definite, we can define new variables $\tilde{\mathbf{y}} = \boldsymbol{\Sigma}^{-1/2}\mathbf{y}$, $\widetilde{\mathbf{X}} = \boldsymbol{\Sigma}^{-1/2}\mathbf{X}$, $\tilde{\boldsymbol{\epsilon}} = \boldsymbol{\Sigma}^{-1/2}\boldsymbol{\epsilon}$, where $\boldsymbol{\Sigma}^{-1/2}$ is the inverse of the positive square root of $\boldsymbol{\Sigma}$, and rewrite model (A.12) correspondingly. The covariance matrix of the error term in the transformed model is then

$$\boldsymbol{\Sigma}^{-1/2}\mathrm{var}(\boldsymbol{\epsilon})\boldsymbol{\Sigma}^{-1/2} = \boldsymbol{\Sigma}^{-1/2}(\sigma^2\boldsymbol{\Sigma})\boldsymbol{\Sigma}^{-1/2} = \sigma^2\mathbf{I}\,.$$

Thus, the transformed model coincides with model (A.12). Applying the OLS-estimator to the transformed model gives the generalized least squares (GLS) estimator in the untransformed model

$$\hat{\boldsymbol{\beta}}_{\mathrm{GLS}} = (\mathbf{X}^T\boldsymbol{\Sigma}^{-1}\mathbf{X})^{-1}\mathbf{X}^T\boldsymbol{\Sigma}^{-1}\mathbf{y}$$

and

$$\mathrm{var}(\hat{\boldsymbol{\beta}}_{\mathrm{GLS}}) = \sigma^2(\mathbf{X}^T\boldsymbol{\Sigma}^{-1}\mathbf{X})^{-1}\,.$$

It can again be shown that $\hat{\boldsymbol{\beta}}_{\mathrm{GLS}}$ is a best linear estimator (BLUE). It should be noted that $\hat{\boldsymbol{\beta}}_{\mathrm{OLS}}$ is also unbiased even if $\mathrm{var}(\boldsymbol{\epsilon}) = \sigma^2\boldsymbol{\Sigma}$, but it is not BLUE anymore. Hence, $\hat{\boldsymbol{\beta}}_{\mathrm{GLS}}$ allows more precise inferences in that case if all necessary assumptions are met.

If the errors ϵ_i and $\epsilon_{i'}$, $i \neq i'$ are uncorrelated, then $\boldsymbol{\Sigma}$ reduces to a diagonal matrix. If in addition the diagonal elements are not all equal to one, then the model allows for different variances, i.e. heteroscedasticity of the errors.

Note that σ^2 and $\boldsymbol{\Sigma}$ are usually unknown and need to be estimated. In that case it can be shown that, given all assumptions are met, $\hat{\boldsymbol{\beta}}_{\mathrm{GLS}}$ is consistent and approximately normally distributed with a covariance matrix that can consistently be estimated.

A.3.2 *Maximum Likelihood*

According to the maximum likelihood principle parameter estimators are created as functions of variables $\mathbf{u}_i$, $i = 1, \ldots, n$, such that the density or probability function of the variables treated as random in $\mathbf{u}_i$, $i = 1, \ldots, n$, conditional on those that are held fixed is maximized. Let $\mathbf{u}$ be a vector collecting all $\mathbf{u}_i$, $i = 1, \ldots, n$. We call an estimator $\hat{\boldsymbol{\theta}}(\mathbf{u})$, or $\hat{\boldsymbol{\theta}}$ for short, ML estimator if it maximizes the likelihood function

$$L(\boldsymbol{\theta}; \mathbf{u}) = f(\mathbf{u} \mid \boldsymbol{\theta})$$

i.e.,

$$L(\hat{\boldsymbol{\theta}}; \mathbf{u}) \geq L(\boldsymbol{\theta}; \mathbf{u}) \quad \text{for all possible } \boldsymbol{\theta} \in \boldsymbol{\Theta}$$

where $f(\mathbf{u} \mid \boldsymbol{\theta})$ is the density or probability function of $\mathbf{u}$, depending on whether the variables in $\mathbf{u}$ treated as random are continuous or discrete and $\boldsymbol{\Theta}$ is the set of possible parameter values, the parameter space. The above likelihood function simplifies to

$$L(\boldsymbol{\theta}; \mathbf{u}) = \prod_{i=1}^{n} f(\mathbf{u}_i \mid \boldsymbol{\theta})$$

if units $i = 1, \ldots, n$ are independent.

Instead of the likelihood function itself, it is usually more convenient to work with the log-likelihood function, a monotone function of the likelihood that does not affect the resulting estimator,

$$l(\boldsymbol{\theta}; \mathbf{u}) = \sum_{i=1}^{n} \log f(\mathbf{u}_i \mid \boldsymbol{\theta}) \; .$$

The ML estimator $\hat{\boldsymbol{\theta}}$ can then be found by setting the vector of partial derivatives of the log-likelihood function to zero and solving for $\boldsymbol{\theta}$,

$$\mathbf{s}(\hat{\boldsymbol{\theta}}; \mathbf{u}) = \left. \frac{\partial\, l(\boldsymbol{\theta}; \mathbf{u})}{\partial\, \boldsymbol{\theta}} \right|_{\boldsymbol{\theta}=\hat{\boldsymbol{\theta}}} = \mathbf{0}$$

where $\mathbf{s}(\hat{\boldsymbol{\theta}}; \mathbf{u})$ are also called maximum likelihood equations or vector of score functions. Assuming a solution exists, this strategy gives a (local) maximum if the matrix of second partial derivatives, the Hessian matrix, $\mathbf{H}(\hat{\boldsymbol{\theta}}; \mathbf{u})$, is negative definite. If a solution has to be found iteratively and if there may be more than one solution to the score functions, a global maximum may be found by using different starting values and comparing the log-likelihood functions at these points.

An important result in the ML context is that if the distribution of $\mathbf{u}$ at the true parameter value differs from the distribution at every other possible value—this is called identification—then, the 'true' log-likelihood function, the limit distribution $E[\log f(\mathbf{u} \mid \boldsymbol{\theta})]$, has a unique maximum at the true value $\boldsymbol{\theta}_0$. Under some technical conditions the log-likelihood function converges for $n \to \infty$ to this limit distribution and the ML estimator converges to the true parameter value. As a general result it can be shown that, given all necessary assumptions are met, the distribution of $\sqrt{n}(\hat{\boldsymbol{\theta}} - \boldsymbol{\theta}_0)$ converges, under some technical conditions, to a (multivariate) normal distribution with mean zero and covariance matrix $\mathbf{I}^{-1}(\boldsymbol{\theta}_0)$, where $\mathbf{I}(\boldsymbol{\theta}_0)$ is the Fisher information matrix or information for short

$$\mathbf{I}(\boldsymbol{\theta}_0) = \int_{-\infty}^{\infty} \left[\frac{\partial \log f(\mathbf{u} \mid \boldsymbol{\theta})}{\partial \boldsymbol{\theta}} \right]_{\boldsymbol{\theta}=\boldsymbol{\theta}_0} \left[\frac{\partial \log f(\mathbf{u} \mid \boldsymbol{\theta}_0)}{\partial \boldsymbol{\theta}} \right]_{\boldsymbol{\theta}=\boldsymbol{\theta}_0}^T f(\mathbf{u} \mid \boldsymbol{\theta}_0)\, d\mathbf{u} \,,$$

i.e. the expectation of the outer product of the score function at $\boldsymbol{\theta} = \boldsymbol{\theta}_0$, or equivalently if all assumptions are met, by the information matrix equality,

$$\mathbf{I}(\boldsymbol{\theta}_0) = -E[\mathbf{H}(\boldsymbol{\theta}_0; \mathbf{u})] = -\int_{-\infty}^{\infty} \left. \frac{\partial^2 \log f(\mathbf{u} \mid \boldsymbol{\theta})}{\partial \boldsymbol{\theta}\, \partial \boldsymbol{\theta}} \right|_{\boldsymbol{\theta}=\boldsymbol{\theta}_0} f(\mathbf{u} \mid \boldsymbol{\theta}_0)\, d\mathbf{u}$$

at $\boldsymbol{\theta} = \boldsymbol{\theta}_0$. A further advantageous property of ML estimators is that they are asymptotically efficient within a large class of estimators. This means that inferences are (asymptotically) at least as precise as inferences based on many other estimators. For a detailed discussion, see Newey and McFadden (1994).

With these results, the distribution of $\hat{\boldsymbol{\theta}}$ can be approximated by a normal distribution with mean $\boldsymbol{\theta}_0$ and covariance matrix $n^{-1}\mathbf{I}^{-1}(\boldsymbol{\theta}_0)$ in large samples. To estimate the Fisher information and thus the covariance matrix of $\hat{\boldsymbol{\theta}}$, one may use minus the mean of individual contributions to the Hessian matrix with $\boldsymbol{\theta}_0$ replaced by $\hat{\boldsymbol{\theta}}$, the observed (Fisher) information,

$$\mathbf{I}_1(\hat{\boldsymbol{\theta}}) = -n^{-1} \sum_{i=1}^{n} \left. \frac{\partial^2 \log f(\mathbf{u}_i \mid \boldsymbol{\theta})}{\partial \boldsymbol{\theta}\, \partial \boldsymbol{\theta}} \right|_{\boldsymbol{\theta}=\hat{\boldsymbol{\theta}}}$$

or

$$\mathbf{I}_2(\hat{\boldsymbol{\theta}}) = n^{-1} \sum_{i=1}^{n} \left[\frac{\partial \log f(\mathbf{u}_i \mid \boldsymbol{\theta})}{\partial \boldsymbol{\theta}} \right]_{\boldsymbol{\theta}=\hat{\boldsymbol{\theta}}} \left[\frac{\partial \log f(\mathbf{u}_i \mid \boldsymbol{\theta})}{\partial \boldsymbol{\theta}} \right]_{\boldsymbol{\theta}=\hat{\boldsymbol{\theta}}}^T .$$

For completely observed data sets or if missing values are MCAR, the expected value of $\mathbf{I}_1(\hat{\boldsymbol{\theta}})$, the expected Fisher information at $\hat{\boldsymbol{\theta}}$,

$$E(\mathbf{I}_1(\hat{\boldsymbol{\theta}})) = -\, E \left. \left(\frac{\partial^2 \log f(\mathbf{u} \mid \boldsymbol{\theta})}{\partial \boldsymbol{\theta}\, \partial \boldsymbol{\theta}} \right) \right|_{\boldsymbol{\theta}=\hat{\boldsymbol{\theta}}} .$$

may be used (cf. Welsh 1996, p. 73, sec. 4.2.9; Lehmann 1998, sec. 7.2). Note that the expectation of $\mathbf{I}_1(\hat{\boldsymbol{\theta}})$ is taken with respect to $f(\mathbf{u} \mid \boldsymbol{\theta})$, no other process like a selection or missing data mechanism is considered.

A.3.2.1 Some Results for Example 2.6

In Example 2.6 (see p. 37) we estimate μ_2, the mean of a variable $u_{i,2}$, which is surveyed together with another variable $u_{i,1}$. We assume that $\mathbf{u}_i = (u_{i,1}\ u_{i,2})^T$,

$i = 1, \ldots, n$ are independent bivariate normally distributed and that with the exception of μ_2 all other parameters of a bivariate normal distribution are known. The density function of the observed variables ignoring the missing data mechanism can be written as

$$f(\mathbf{u} \mid \boldsymbol{\theta}) = \prod_{i=1}^{n} f(u_{i,1}, u_{i,2} \mid \boldsymbol{\theta})^{r_i} f(u_{i,1} \mid \mu_1, \sigma_1^2)^{1-r_i}$$

where $\mathbf{u} = (\mathbf{u}_1^T \ \cdots \ \mathbf{u}_n^T)^T$, $\boldsymbol{\theta} = (\mu_1 \ \mu_2 \ \sigma_1^2 \ \sigma_2^2 \ \rho_{1,2})^T$ with $\mu_1 = E(u_{i,1})$, $\mu_2 = E(u_{i,2})$, $\sigma_1^2 = \text{var}(u_{i,1})$, $\sigma_2^2 = \text{var}(u_{i,2})$ and $\rho_{1,2}$ is the correlation of $u_{i,1}$ and $u_{i,2}$. Further, r_i is a binary variable indicating whether $u_{i,2}$ is observed ($r_i = 1$) or not ($r_i = 0$).

With known $\rho_{1,2}$, $\mu_1 = 0$, $\sigma_1^2 = 1$, $\sigma_2^2 = 1$ and ignoring the missing data mechanism, the log-likelihood function can be written as

$$l(\mu_2) = \text{const} - \frac{1}{2(1-\rho_{1,2}^2)} \sum_{i=1}^{n} r_i \left[u_{i,1}^2 - 2\rho_{1,2} u_{i,1}(u_{i,2} - \mu_2) + (u_{i,2} - \mu_2)^2 \right] ,$$

where const is a term not depending on μ_2. Let $n_{(1)}$ be the number of observed values $u_{i,2}$. Setting the first derivative with respect to μ_2 equal to zero and solving for μ_2 leads to

$$\hat{\mu}_2 = n_{(1)}^{-1} \sum_{i=1}^{n} r_i (u_{i,2} - \rho_{1,2} u_{i,1}) .$$

As an estimator of its covariance matrix we use minus the inverse of the second derivative of the log-likelihood with respect to μ_2 so that

$$\text{var}(\hat{\mu}_2) = (1 - \rho_{1,2}^2)/n_{(1)} .$$

Note that $\hat{\mu}_2$ is unbiased and normally distributed even in small data sets if there are no missing values. It is still unbiased if the missing values are MCAR or MAR because

$$\begin{aligned}
E(\hat{\mu}_2) &= E\{E[E(\hat{\mu}_2 \mid \mathbf{u}_1, \mathbf{r}) \mid \mathbf{r}]\} \\
&= E\{E[n_{(1)}^{-1} \sum_{i=1}^{n} r_i (E(u_{i,2} \mid u_{i,1}, r_i) - \rho_{1,2} u_{i,1}) \mid \mathbf{r}]\} \\
&= E\{E[n_{(1)}^{-1} \sum_{i=1}^{n} r_i ((\mu_2 + \rho_{1,2} u_{i,1}) - \rho_{1,2} u_{i,1}) \mid \mathbf{r}]\} \\
&= E\Big[\Big(\sum_{i=1}^{n} r_i\Big)^{-1} \sum_{i=1}^{n} r_i \mu_2\Big] = \mu_2 .
\end{aligned}$$

A.3.2.2 Some Results for Example 2.7

In Example 2.7 (see p. 39) we estimate μ_2 and $\rho_{1,2}$ assuming all other parameters of a bivariate normal distribution to be known. Let r_i be the response indicator with $r_i = 1$ if $u_{i,2}$ is observed and $r_i = 0$ otherwise, and $n_{(1)}$ be the number of observed values $u_{i,2}$. With known $\mu_1 = 0$, $\sigma_1^2 = 1$, $\sigma_2^2 = 1$ and ignoring the missing data mechanism, the log-likelihood function is (cf. Sect. A.3.2.1)

$$\begin{aligned} l(\mu_2, \rho_{1,2}) = \text{const} &- \frac{n_{(1)}}{2} \log(1 - \rho_{1,2}^2) \\ &- \frac{1}{2(1 - \rho_{1,2}^2)} \sum_{i=1}^{n} r_i \left[u_{i,1}^2 - 2\rho_{1,2} u_{i,1}(u_{i,2} - \mu_2) + (u_{i,2} - \mu_2)^2 \right] , \end{aligned}$$

where const is a term not depending on μ_2 or $\rho_{1,2}$. Taking the first derivatives leads to the estimating equations

$$0 = \sum_{i=1}^{n} r_i [(u_{i,2} - \mu_2) - \rho_{1,2} u_{i,1}]$$

for μ_2 and

$$0 = n_{(1)} \rho_{1,2}(1 - \rho_{1,2}^2) - \sum_{i=1}^{n} r_i (u_{i,1} - \rho_{1,2}(u_{i,2} - \mu_2))(\rho_{1,2} u_{i,1} - (u_{i,2} - \mu_2))$$

for $\rho_{1,2}$, which have to be solved iteratively. The matrix of second derivatives can be used to calculate the observed information,

$$\mathbf{I}_1(\hat{\mu}_2, \hat{\rho}_{1,2}) = \begin{pmatrix} \hat{\imath}_{11} & \hat{\imath}_{12} \\ \hat{\imath}_{12} & \hat{\imath}_{22} \end{pmatrix} ,$$

where

$$\hat{\imath}_{11} = -\frac{n_{(1)}}{1 - \hat{\rho}_{1,2}^2} , \quad \hat{\imath}_{12} = -\frac{1}{(1 - \hat{\rho}_{1,2}^2)^2} \sum_{i=1}^{n} r_i [u_{i,1}(1 + \hat{\rho}_{1,2}^2) - 2\hat{\rho}_{1,2}(u_{i,2} - \hat{\mu}_2))]$$

and

$$\begin{aligned} \hat{\imath}_{22} =& \frac{n_{(1)}(1 + \hat{\rho}_{1,2}^2)}{(1 - \hat{\rho}_{1,2}^2)^2} - \frac{1}{(1 - \hat{\rho}_{1,2}^2)^3} \\ &\times \sum_{i=1}^{n} r_i [(1 + 3\hat{\rho}_{1,2}^2)(u_{i,1}^2 + (u_{i,2} - \hat{\mu}_2)^2) - 3\hat{\rho}_{1,2}(2 + \hat{\rho}_{1,2}^2) u_{i,1}(u_{i,2} - \hat{\mu}_2)] . \end{aligned}$$

The diagonal elements of the inverse of minus $\mathbf{I}_1(\hat{\mu}_2, \hat{\rho}_{1,2})$ can then be used as estimators for the variances of $\hat{\mu}_2$ and $\hat{\rho}_{1,2}$. Ignoring the missing data mechanism while taking the expectation of the Hessian matrix gives the Fisher information under ignorability conditional on $\mathbf{r}$ at the points $\hat{\mu}_2$ and $\hat{\rho}_{1,2}$

$$E(\hat{\imath}_{11}) = -\frac{n_{(1)}}{1-\hat{\rho}_{1,2}^2}, \quad E(\hat{\imath}_{12}) = 0 \quad \text{and} \quad E(\hat{\imath}_{22}) = -\frac{n_{(1)}(1-2\hat{\rho}_{1,2}^4)}{(1-\hat{\rho}_{1,2}^2)^3}.$$

A.3.3 Information Criteria

Akaike's Information Criterion (AIC; Akaike, 1998) is defined as follows:

$$\text{AIC} = -2LL + 2p \tag{A.13}$$

with LL as the logarithm of the Likelihood value obtained from the model estimation and p as the number of model parameters. The Bayesian Information Criterion (BIC; Schwarz, 1978) extends the AIC via the sample size n to:

$$\text{BIC} = -2LL + p\ln(n). \tag{A.14}$$

The sample-size adjusted BIC (aBIC) which is provided by the program M*plus* replaces n with $(n+2)/24$ and was found to give superior performance for model selection (Yang, 2006). The information criteria can be used for descriptive model comparisons. The lower the value, the better is the correspondence between empirical data structure (observed mean vector and covariance matrix of the variables in the model) and the model-implied estimates, i. e., the model estimated mean vector and covariance matrix. In case of different model specifications model comparisons based on the LL value are limited because with each additional (also redundant) parameter the value of the LL would always decrease. The number of parameters (and in case of BIC and aBIC the sample size) serve as so-called penalty terms preventing the information criteria to decrease when adding redundant parameters to the model.

A.4 Multiple Imputation: Some Technical Results

In this section we present a derivation and a simplification used in Chap. 4.

A.4.1 Derivation of (4.6), (4.8) and (4.9)

Under ignorability of the missing data mechanism, the numerator of (4.5) simplifies further to

$$\int\int f(\mathbf{u} \mid \boldsymbol{\theta}) g(\mathbf{r} \mid \mathbf{u}, \boldsymbol{\gamma}) p(\boldsymbol{\theta}, \boldsymbol{\gamma})\, d\boldsymbol{\theta}\, d\boldsymbol{\gamma}$$
$$= \Big[\int g(\mathbf{r} \mid \mathbf{u}_{(1)}, \boldsymbol{\gamma}) p(\boldsymbol{\gamma})\, d\boldsymbol{\gamma}\Big]\Big[\int f(\mathbf{u} \mid \boldsymbol{\theta}) p(\boldsymbol{\theta})\, d\boldsymbol{\theta}\Big]$$

and correspondingly the denominator to

$$\int\int\int f(\mathbf{u} \mid \boldsymbol{\theta}) g(\mathbf{r} \mid \mathbf{u}, \boldsymbol{\gamma}) p(\boldsymbol{\theta}, \boldsymbol{\gamma})\, d\boldsymbol{\theta}\, d\boldsymbol{\gamma}\, d\mathbf{u}_{(0)}$$
$$= \int \Big[\int g(\mathbf{r} \mid \mathbf{u}, \boldsymbol{\gamma}) p(\boldsymbol{\gamma})\, d\boldsymbol{\gamma}\Big]\Big[\int f(\mathbf{u} \mid \boldsymbol{\theta}) p(\boldsymbol{\theta})\, d\boldsymbol{\theta}\Big] d\mathbf{u}_{(0)}$$
$$= \Big[\int g(\mathbf{r} \mid \mathbf{u}_{(1)}, \boldsymbol{\gamma}) p(\boldsymbol{\gamma})\, d\boldsymbol{\gamma}\Big]\Big[\int\int f(\mathbf{u} \mid \boldsymbol{\theta}) p(\boldsymbol{\theta})\, d\boldsymbol{\theta}\, d\mathbf{u}_{(0)}\Big].$$

Hence, if the missing data mechanism is ignorable, we can write (4.5) as

$$f(\mathbf{u}_{(0)} \mid \mathbf{u}_{(1)}, \mathbf{r}) = \int \frac{\int f(\mathbf{u} \mid \boldsymbol{\theta}) p(\boldsymbol{\theta})}{\int\int f(\mathbf{u} \mid \boldsymbol{\theta}) p(\boldsymbol{\theta})\, d\mathbf{u}_{(0)}}\, d\boldsymbol{\theta}$$
$$= \int f(\mathbf{u}_{(0)}, \boldsymbol{\theta} \mid \mathbf{u}_{(1)})\, d\boldsymbol{\theta}$$
$$= \int f(\mathbf{u}_{(0)} \mid \mathbf{u}_{(1)}, \boldsymbol{\theta}) p(\boldsymbol{\theta} \mid \mathbf{u}_{(1)})\, d\boldsymbol{\theta}\ ,$$

(cf. (4.6)).

A.4.2 Simplification of $f(\mathbf{u}_{(0)} \mid \mathbf{u}_{(1)}, \boldsymbol{\theta})$ and $p(\boldsymbol{\theta} \mid \mathbf{u}_{(1)})$

Let cob be short for the set of units for which all values in u are observed and $\overline{\text{cob}}$ denote the set of units for which at least one u is not observed. Then

$$f(\mathbf{u}_{(0)}, \mathbf{u}_{(1)} \mid \boldsymbol{\theta}) = \prod_i f(\mathbf{u}_{i,(0)}, \mathbf{u}_{i,(1)} \mid \boldsymbol{\theta})$$
$$= \prod_i f(\mathbf{u}_{i,(0)} \mid \mathbf{u}_{i,(1)}, \boldsymbol{\theta}) f(\mathbf{u}_{i,(1)} \mid \boldsymbol{\theta})$$
$$= \Big[\prod_{i \in \overline{\text{cob}}} f(\mathbf{u}_{i,(0)} \mid \mathbf{u}_{i,(1)}, \boldsymbol{\theta})\Big]\Big[\prod_{i \in \text{cob}} f(\mathbf{u}_{i,(1)} \mid \boldsymbol{\theta})\Big]$$

$$
\begin{aligned}
f(\mathbf{u}_{(1)} \mid \boldsymbol{\theta}) &= \int f(\mathbf{u}_{(0)}, \mathbf{u}_{(1)} \mid \boldsymbol{\theta})\, d\mathbf{u}_{(0)} \\
&= \prod_i \int f(\mathbf{u}_{i,(0)}, \mathbf{u}_{i,(1)} \mid \boldsymbol{\theta})\, d\mathbf{u}_{i,(0)} \\
&= \Big[\prod_{i \in \overline{\text{cob}}} \int f(\mathbf{u}_{i,(0)} \mid \mathbf{u}_{i,(1)}, \boldsymbol{\theta})\, d\mathbf{u}_{i,(0)} \Big] \Big[\prod_{i \in \text{cob}} f(\mathbf{u}_{i,(1)} \mid \boldsymbol{\theta}) \Big] \\
&= \prod_{i \in \text{cob}} f(\mathbf{u}_{i,(1)} \mid \boldsymbol{\theta})
\end{aligned}
$$

and therefore

$$
\begin{aligned}
f(\mathbf{u}_{(0)} \mid \mathbf{u}_{(1)}, \boldsymbol{\theta}) &= \Big[\prod_i f(\mathbf{u}_{i,(0)}, \mathbf{u}_{i,(1)} \mid \boldsymbol{\theta}) \Big] \Big/ \Big[\prod_{i \in \text{cob}} f(\mathbf{u}_{i,(1)} \mid \boldsymbol{\theta}) \Big] \\
&= \prod_{i \in \overline{\text{cob}}} f(\mathbf{u}_{i,(0)} \mid \mathbf{u}_{i,(1)}, \boldsymbol{\theta})
\end{aligned}
$$

(cf. (4.8)).

Similarly, let pob be short for the set of units with at least one u observed. Then

$$
\begin{aligned}
p(\boldsymbol{\theta} \mid \mathbf{u}_{(1)}) &= \frac{\int \big[\prod_i f(\mathbf{u}_{i,(0)}, \mathbf{u}_{i,(1)} \mid \boldsymbol{\theta}) \big]\, p(\boldsymbol{\theta})\, d\mathbf{u}_{(0)}}{\int \int \big[\prod_i f(\mathbf{u}_{i,(0)}, \mathbf{u}_{i,(1)} \mid \boldsymbol{\theta}) \big]\, p(\boldsymbol{\theta})\, d\mathbf{u}_{(0)}\, d\boldsymbol{\theta}} \\
&= \frac{\prod_i \int f(\mathbf{u}_{i,(0)}, \mathbf{u}_{i,(1)} \mid \boldsymbol{\theta})\, p(\boldsymbol{\theta})\, d\mathbf{u}_{i,(0)}}{\int \big[\prod_i \int f(\mathbf{u}_{i,(0)}, \mathbf{u}_{i,(1)} \mid \boldsymbol{\theta})\, p(\boldsymbol{\theta})\, d\mathbf{u}_{i,(0)} \big]\, d\boldsymbol{\theta}} \\
&= \frac{\prod_{i \in \text{pob}} f(\mathbf{u}_{i,(1)} \mid \boldsymbol{\theta})\, p(\boldsymbol{\theta})}{\int \prod_{i \in \text{pob}} f(\mathbf{u}_{i,(1)} \mid \boldsymbol{\theta})\, p(\boldsymbol{\theta})\, d\boldsymbol{\theta}}
\end{aligned}
$$

leading to (4.9).

References

Akaike, H. (1998). Information theory and an extension of the maximum likelihood principle. In E. Parzen, K. Tanabe, & G. Kitagawa (Eds.), *Selected papers of Hirotugu Akaike* (pp. 199–213). New York, NY: Springer.

Ash, R. B., & Doléans-Dade, C. A. (2000). *Probability and measure theory* (2nd ed.). San Diego, CA: Academic Press.

Cameron, A. C., & Trivedi, P. K. (2005). *Microeconometrics: Methods and applications*. Cambridge, UK: University Press.

Gentle, J. E. (2017). *Matrix algebra* (2nd ed.). Cham: Springer.

Harville, D. A. (1997). *Matrix algebra from a statistician's perspective*. New York, NY: Springer.

Kotz, S., Balakrishnan, N., & Johnson, N. L. (2000). *Continuous multivariate distributions. Volume 1: Models and applications* (2nd ed.). New York, NY: Wiley.

Lehmann, E. L. (1998). *Elements of large-sample theory*. New York, NY: Springer.

Mardia, K. V., Kent, J. T., & Bibby, J. M. (1979). *Multivariate analysis*. London, UK: Academic Press.

Newey, W. K., & McFadden, D. L. (1994). Large sample estimation and hypothesis testing. In R. F. Engle & D. L. McFadden (Eds.), *Handbook of econometrics* (Vol. IV, pp. 2111–2245). Amsterdam: Elsevier.

Schwarz, G. (1978). Estimating the dimension of a model. *The Annals of Statistics, 6*(2), 461–464.

Welsh, A. H. (1996). *Aspects of statistical inference*. New York, NY: Wiley.

Yang, C.-C. (2006). Evaluating latent class analysis models in qualitative phenotype identification. *Computational Statistics & Data Analysis, 50*(4), 1090–1104.

Glossary

ACA	Available case analysis
CCA	Complete case analysis
GAMLSS	Generalized additive models for location, scale and shape
iid	Independent and identically distributed
MAR	Missing at random
MCAR	Missing completely at random
MI	Multiple imputation
ML	Maximum likelihood
MNAR	Missing not at random
OLS	Ordinary least squares

K. Kleinke et al., *Applied Multiple Imputation*,
Statistics for Social and Behavioral Sciences,
https://doi.org/10.1007/978-3-030-38164-6

Index

K. Kleinke et al., *Applied Multiple Imputation*, Statistics for Social and Behavioral Sciences,
https://doi.org/10.1007/978-3-030-38164-6

The manufacturer's authorised representative in the EU is Springer Nature Customer Service Centre GmbH, Europaplatz 3, 69115 Heidelberg, Germany. If you have any concerns regarding our products, please contact ProductSafety@springernature.com

Printed and bound by CPI Group (UK) Ltd, Croydon, CR0 4YY
22/09/2026
02221057-0012